Law in Public Health Practice

LAW IN PUBLIC HEALTH PRACTICE

Edited by

Richard A. Goodman
Public Health Law Program
Centers for Disease Control
 and Prevention
Atlanta, Georgia

Mark A. Rothstein
Institute for Bioethics, Health Policy,
 & Law
University of Louisville School of
 Medicine
Louisville, Kentucky

Richard E. Hoffman
Department of Preventive Medicine
 and Biometrics
University of Colorado
 Health Sciences Center
Denver, Colorado

With the assistance of:
Karen L. Foster
National Center for
 Environmental Health
Centers for Disease Control
 and Prevention
Atlanta, Georgia

Wilfredo Lopez
Office of General Counsel
New York City Department of Health
New York, New York

Gene W. Matthews
Office of the General Counsel
Centers for Disease Control
 and Prevention
Atlanta, Georgia

OXFORD
UNIVERSITY PRESS
2003

OXFORD

Oxford University Press

Oxford   New York
Auckland   Bangkok   Buenos Aires   Cape Town   Chennai
Dar es Salaam   Delhi   Hong Kong   Istanbul   Karachi   Kolkata
Kuala Lumpur   Madrid   Melbourne   Mexico City   Mumbai   Nairobi
São Paulo   Singapore   Taipei   Tokyo   Toronto

Copyright © 2003 by Oxford University Press, Inc.

Published by Oxford University Press, Inc.
198 Madison Avenue, New York, New York 10016
http://www.oup-usa.org

Oxford is a registered trademark of Oxford University Press

Library of Congress Cataloging-in-Publication Data
Law in public health preactice / edited by Richard A. Goodman . . . [et al.] ; with the
assistance of Karen Foster.
p.cm.   Includes bibliographical references and indes.
ISBN 0-19-514871-1
1. Public health laws—United States.   2. Public health personnel—Legal status, laws,
etc.—United States.   3. Public health administration—United States.   I. Goodman, Richard
A. (Richard Alan), 1949–

KF3775.L384 2003
344.73'04—cd21   2002022044

9 8 7 6 5 4 3 2

Printed in the United States of America
on acid-free paper

Preface

> While the modern health officer must be an educator and a states-
> man, rather than merely a police officer, many of his duties are
> still necessarily concerned with law enforcement. . . . Health offi-
> cers must be familiar not only with the extent of their powers and
> duties, but also with the limitations imposed upon them by law.
> With such knowledge available and widely applied by health au-
> thorities, public health will not remain static, but will progress.
>
> James A. Tobey (*Public Health Law*. New York:
> The Commonwealth Fund, 1947)

In his classic text on public health law in 1947, James Tobey offered the above perspective on the relevance of law to public health practice. Tobey's notion of more than 50 years ago may be even more pertinent now as public health enters the twenty-first century. Even before the events of September 11, 2001, forced an intensified review of legal authorities for ensuring public health preparedness for emergencies, health departments and public health practitioners had begun increasing their efforts to use law more effectively as a tool for improving the public's health. Examples of such efforts include litigation and other approaches to curbing the effects of the epidemic of tobacco use; the role of environmental law to address myriad environmental hazards; and the complementary roles of science, regulatory authorities, and laws in improving food safety and preventing food-borne infectious diseases, as well as addressing newly emergent infectious disease threats such as the West Nile virus.

The legal basis of public health practice in the United States substantially antedates key public health developments during the last century and even the landmark 1905 U.S. Supreme Court case of *Jacobson v. Massachusetts*. For example, one of the amazing ironies in U.S. public health history is the past and continuing influence of smallpox on law in relation to public health. As public health scholar Dr. Donald Hopkins made clear in *Princes & Peasants*, his treatise on smallpox in history, the legal and epidemiologic strategy of local quarantine to prevent the spread of smallpox was employed on Long Island as early as 1662. In 1731, the Massachusetts Bay Colony passed "An Act to Prevent Persons from Concealing the Small Pox." Moreover, smallpox was at the root of the *Jacobson* case itself—a decision in which the Supreme Court upheld Massachusetts' statutory requirement for smallpox vaccination as a valid application of the state's police power. Now, more than two decades after the eradication of smallpox from natural circulation on the planet, we are confronted with the need to examine legal authorities necessary for countering the potential deliberate use of smallpox and other infectious disease pathogens as weapons of mass destruction.

But infectious diseases are not the sole focus of law in public health practice. The law also has evolved in response to and frames virtually every other problem on the continuum of public health. For example, the law has provided mandates and served as a pivotal public health tool for addressing myriad environmental problems, including lead contamination in paint and the resulting hazards for children; the use of lead as a gasoline additive and its consequent potentiation of air pollution; and the invidious scourge of toxic waste sites. The increasing importance of law as a tool for addressing other noninfectious concerns—such as lung disease, certain cancers, and cardiovascular conditions—is suggested by the roles law and litigation have played in combating the impact of tobacco use on U.S. and global public health.

During workshops on public health law sponsored by the Centers for Disease Control and Prevention (CDC) in 1999 and 2000, major public health stakeholders—groups including health officers, epidemiologists, public health lawyers, educators, and legislators—recognized the need to strengthen the legal foundation for public health practice. The set of tools available to public health practitioners has grown steadily during the past decade and now reflects an expanding array of disciplines, including, economics and prevention effectiveness, health communications, and informatics. Public health stakeholders recognized that the field can benefit from adding legal skills, knowledge, and resources to practitioners' tool kits.

Responding to the call of public health stakeholders and others, this book aims to emphasize the law in relation to the practice of public health at local, state, and federal levels. The book is intended especially for practitioners and students of public health practice. Public health practitioners are those whose work is directed toward improvement of the public's health. Among their ranks are public health nurses, sanitarians, health educators, industrial hygienists, epidemiologists, physicians, veterinarians, dentists, administrators, managers, and, lawyers.

This book has twin aims. First, because law is a primary determinant for public health and public health practice in the United States, we have tried to identify, define, and clarify the complex principles of law as they bear on the practice of public health. Second, by enhancing the understanding of the legal principles underlying U.S. public health practice, we hope to show how the law may be applied with greater effectiveness and prudence as a tool to improve the public's health.

A word about the development of this book. For obvious reasons multiple authorship poses challenges to the task of organizing and completing any volume, but the nature of our aims demanded a multiauthored approach. Perhaps because of the challenges it posed, the book does not have a true precedent in the field of public health. We have attempted to produce an interdisciplinary volume that bridges two disparate worlds: the realm of law and lawyers, and the realm of public health practice and technicians. The co-editors themselves are a reflection of these different perspectives and disciplines. Two are physicians whose professional experiences have encompassed work at the state and federal levels and involvement with local health departments, community organizations, the legislature, and public health and medical academia. Three are lawyers whose experiences run the gamut from providing legal counsel to health agencies at the federal and municipal levels, to applied legal and policy research, training of students of health and public health practice, and interacting with legislators and public health policy makers. And Karen Foster, the managing editor, has over two-decades' experience in editing and producing public health publications, including the CDC's *Morbidity and Mortality Weekly Report.*

This book is divided into three sections that progress from fundamental principles to specific areas of public health practice. The first section provides a foundation in the basic principles and concepts underlying the relation between law and public health practice. It covers such topics as constitutional and statutory bases for public health practice, administrative and regulatory law, and criminal law—as well as the overarching areas of bioethics and international law. The second section covers the law in relation to core functions of public health practice that are multidisciplinary. It deals with the interaction between practitioners and legal counsel, law underlying public health surveillance, outbreak investigations, public health research, confidentiality and privacy, managed care in public health, interventions in emergency response, and special populations. The third section offers a detailed examination of the law in nine prominent areas of public health: genetics, vaccinations, food-borne diseases, blood-borne and sexually transmitted infections, tobacco use, reproductive health, environmental hazards, injuries, and the workplace. To ensure a consistent approach to the law in relation to each of these practice areas, each chapter in this section has a uniform format that includes background to the subject, key legal authorities, legal issues and controversies, practice considerations, and emerging issues.

The contributing authors represent the ranks of the legal and public health practitioners for whom this book is intended and the editors want to thank them sincerely for their efforts. They worked under a tight time line, which, for many, was complicated by the events of September 2001. People within the CDC who have been key in their support of this project, include Martha Katz, Kathy Cahill, Bill Gimson, Howard Green, Dr. Ed Baker, Debbie Jones, Patti Seikus, and Dr. Tony Moulton. Drs. Michelle Leverett and Tony Moulton also reviewed material at the editors' request. We appreciate the extremely useful suggestions of Dr. Barry Levy, which helped give early shape to the book. Finally, we are especially grateful to Jeff House of Oxford University Press for his sustained encouragement, ideas, and numerous constructive suggestions at all stages of the book's development.

Atlanta, Georgia	R.A.G.
Louisville, Kentucky	M.A.R.
Denver, Colorado	R.E.H.
New York, New York	W.L.
Atlanta, Georgia	G.W.M.
Atlanta, Georgia	K.L.F.

Contents

PART II   THE LAW AND CORE PUBLIC HEALTH FUNCTIONS

PART III   THE LAW IN CONTROLLING AND PREVENTING DISEASES, INJURIES, AND DISABILITIES

Contributors

BEBE J. ANDERSON, J.D.
Staff Attorney
The Center for Reproductive Law and
  Policy
New York, New York

RUTH GAARE BERNHEIM, J.D.,
  M.P.H.
Executive Director
Institute for Practical Ethics
Assistant Professor of Medical Education
University of Virginia
Charlottesville, Virginia

LAURA M. BESKOW, M.P.H.
Career Development Award Recipient—
  Association of Teachers of Preventive
  Medicine
Office of Genomics and Disease
  Prevention
Centers for Disease Control and
  Prevention
Atlanta, Georgia

GUTHRIE S. BIRKHEAD, M.D.,
  M.P.H.
Director
AIDS Institute
Director
Center for Community Health
New York State Department of Health
Associate Professor of Epidemiology
School of Public Health, University at
  Albany
Albany, New York

RICHARD J. BONNIE, L.L.B.
Director
Institute of Law, Psychiatry, and Public
  Policy
John S. Battle Professor of Law
School of Law
University of Virginia
Charlottesville, Virginia

JAMES W. BUEHLER, M.D.
Associate Director for Science
National Center for HIV, STD, and TB
   Prevention
Centers for Disease Control and
   Prevention
Atlanta, Georgia

CHRISTINE P. BUMP
J.D./M.P.H. candidate
Emory University School of Law
Atlanta, Georgia

MARTIN S. CETRON, M.D.
Deputy Director
Division of Global Migration and
   Quarantine
National Center for Infectious Diseases
Centers for Disease Control and
   Prevention
Atlanta, Georgia

TOM CHRISTOFFEL, J.D.
Boulder, Colorado
Professor (Retired)
School of Public Health
University of Illinois at Chicago
Chicago, Illinois

RONALD M. DAVIS, M.D., M.A.
Director
Center for Health Promotion and Disease
   Prevention
Henry Ford Health System
Detroit, Michigan

RICHARD A. DAYNARD, J.D., PH.D.
Professor of Law
Northeastern University School of Law
Boston, Massachusetts

NANETTE R. ELSTER, J.D., M.P.H.
Assistant Professor
Institute for Bioethics, Health Policy, and
   Law
University of Louisville School of
   Medicine
Louisville, Kentucky

KEVIN FAIN, J.D.
Associate Chief Counsel
Office of the Chief Counsel
Food and Drug Administration
Rockville, Maryland

HENRY FALK, M.D., M.P.H.
Assistant Administrator
Agency for Toxic Substances and Disease
   Registry
Atlanta, Georgia

DAVID P. FIDLER, J.D., M.PHIL.,
   B.C.L.
Professor of Law
Indiana University School of Law
Bloomington, Indiana

DAVID W. FLEMING, M.D.
Deputy Director for Science and Public
   Health
Centers for Disease Control and
   Prevention
Atlanta, Georgia

KAREN L. FOSTER, M.A.
Technical Writer-Editor
Office of Communication
National Center for Environmental
   Health
Centers for Disease Control and
   Prevention
Atlanta, Georgia

RICHARD A. GOODMAN, M.D.,
   J.D., M.P.H.
Public Health Law Program
Public Health Practice Program Office
Senior Advisor for Science and Policy
Financial Management Office
Centers for Disease Control and
   Prevention
Atlanta, Georgia

LAWRENCE O. GOSTIN, J.D.,
L.L.D. (HON.)
Professor of Law, Georgetown
  University
Professor of Public Health, The Johns
  Hopkins University
Director, Center for Law and the
  Public's Health
Washington, D.C.

MARK A. GOTTLIEB, J.D.
Staff Attorney
Tobacco Control Resource Center
Northeastern University School of Law
Boston, Massachusetts

FRANK P. GRAD, J.D.
Professor Emeritus
Columbia University School of Law
New York, New York

MARTA GWINN, M.D., M.P.H.
Senior Medical Epidemiologist
Office of Genomics and Disease
  Prevention
Centers for Disease Control and
  Prevention
Atlanta, Georgia

ALAN R. HINMAN, M.D., M.P.H.
Principal Investigator
All Kids Count
Center for Innovation in Health
  Information Systems
Task Force for Child Survival and
  Development
Atlanta, Georgia

RICHARD E. HOFFMAN, M.D.,
M.P.H.
Associate Professor Adjoint
Department of Preventive Medicine and
  Biometrics
University of Colorado Health Sciences
  Center
Denver, Colorado
Former Chief Medical Officer and State
  Epidemiologist
Colorado Department of Public Health
  and Environment
Denver, Colorado

HEATHER H. HORTON, J.D.,
M.H.A.
Attorney Advisor
Office of the General Counsel
Centers for Disease Control and
  Prevention
Atlanta, Georgia

PETER D. JACOBSON, J.D., M.P.H.
Associate Professor
University of Michigan School of Public
  Health
Ann Arbor, Michigan

BRIAN KAMOIE, J.D.
Assistant Research Professor
Hirsh Health Law and Policy Program
The George Washington University
School of Public Health and Health
  Services
Washington, D.C.

ROBERT L. KLINE, J.D.
Staff Attorney
Tobacco Control Resource Center
Northeastern University School of Law
Boston, Massachusetts

CHRIS S. KOCHTITZKY, M.S.P.
Associate Director for Policy
Division of Emergency and
* Environmental Health Service*
National Center for Environmental
* Health*
Centers for Disease Control and
* Prevention*
Atlanta, Georgia

JEFFREY P. KOPLAN, M.D.,
M.P.H.
Director
Centers for Disease Control and
* Prevention*
Atlanta, Georgia

ZITA LAZZARINI, J.D., M.P.H.
Director
Division of Medical Humanities, Health
* Law, and Ethics*
University of Connecticut Health Center
Farmington, Connecticut

JOHN R. LIVENGOOD, M.D.,
M.PHIL.
Deputy Associate Director for Science
Centers for Disease Control and
* Prevention*
Atlanta, Georgia

PAUL A. LOCKE, J.D., DR.P.H.,
M.P.H.
Deputy Director and General Counsel
Trust for America's Health
Washington, D.C.

WILFREDO LOPEZ, J.D.
General Counsel
New York City Department of Health
New York, New York

KEVIN M. MALONE, J.D.,
M.H.S.A.
Senior Attorney
Office of the General Counsel
Centers for Disease Control and
* Prevention*
Atlanta, Georgia

GENE W. MATTHEWS, J.D.
Legal Advisor to CDC
Office of the General Counsel
Centers for Disease Control and
* Prevention*
Atlanta, Georgia

JAMES J. MISRAHI, J.D.
Attorney Advisor
Office of the General Counsel
Centers for Disease Control and
* Prevention*
Atlanta, Georgia

BENJAMIN MOJICA, M.D., M.P.H.
Deputy Commissioner
Division of Health
New York City Department of Health
New York, New York

VERLA S. NESLUND, J.D.
Director
Office of the Executive Secretariat
Centers for Disease Control and
* Prevention*
Atlanta, Georgia

PHILLIP NIEBURG, M.D., M.P.H.
Visiting Scholar
Center for Biomedical Ethics
University of Virginia
Charlottesville, Virginia

WENDY E. PARMET, J.D.
Professor of Law
Northeastern University School of Law
Boston, Massachusetts

TONY D. PEREZ
Director
Division of Global Migration and
* Quarantine*
National Center for Infectious Diseases
Centers for Disease Control and
* Prevention*
Atlanta, Georgia

ROBERT M. PESTRONK, M.P.H.
Health Officer Director
Genesee County Health Department
Flint, Michigan

EDWARD P. RICHARDS, J.D., M.P.H.
Professor of Law
Louisiana State University
Baton Rouge, Louisiana

GARY RISCHITELLI, M.D., J.D., M.P.H.
Assistant Scientist
The Center for Research in Occupational and Environmental Toxicology
Oregon Health and Science University
Portland, Oregon

SARA ROSENBAUM, J.D.
Hirsh Professor of Health Law and Policy
School of Public Health and Health Services
The George Washington University
Washington, D.C.

MARK A. ROTHSTEIN, J.D.
Director
Institute for Bioethics, Health Policy, and Law
University of Louisville School of Medicine
Louisville, Kentucky

SARAH SCOTT, J.D.
General Counsel
Office of Chief Medical Examiner
New York, New York

JEREMY SOBEL, M.D., M.P.H.
Medical Epidemiologist
Division of Bacterial and Mycotic Diseases
National Center for Infectious Diseases
Centers for Disease Control and Prevention
Atlanta, Georgia

PAUL V. STANGE, M.P.H.
Policy Advisor
Office of HealthCare Partnerships
Division of Prevention Research and Analytic Methods
Epidemiology Program Office
Centers for Disease Control and Prevention
Atlanta, Georgia

T. HOWARD STONE, J.D., LL.M.
Associate Professor
Institute for Bioethics, Health Policy, and Law
University of Louisville School of Medicine
Louisville, Kentucky

EDWARD L. SWEDA, JR., J.D.
Senior Attorney
Tobacco Control Resource Center
Northeastern University School of Law
Boston, Massachusetts

STEPHEN P. TERET, J.D., M.P.H.
Professor and Director
Center for Law and the Public's Health
Johns Hopkins Bloomberg School of Public Health
Baltimore, Maryland

LYNNE S. WILCOX, M.D., M.P.H.
Director,
Division of Reproductive Health
National Center for Chronic Disease Prevention and Health Promotion
Centers for Disease Control and Prevention
Atlanta, Georgia

Glossary of Selected Legal Terms Used in This Book

administrative law: the body of law created by administrative agencies through rules, regulations, orders, and procedures designed to further legislatively enacted policy goals.

administrative orders (also known as **health hold orders**): orders issued by a health department to a third party to remedy a condition that threatens public health. Depending on state law, the orders can be issued under the health department's police power without specific legislation, under a specific law granting the power to issue general orders, or under specific administrative regulations.

burden of proof: the allocation of responsibility to demonstrate that a matter alleged in a court is factually true and to the level of confidence in the allegation required in that particular setting. The level of confidence may be called the *standard of proof* (includes *preponderance of evidence*, *clear and convincing evidence*, and *beyond a reasonable doubt*).

*Reprinted from *Black's Law Dictionary*, Pocket Edition (BA Garner, Editor-in-Chief), ©1996, with permission of The West Group.

case law: court-produced bodies of legal opinions that guide the application of the law.

chain of custody of evidence: a legal requirement to ensure the identity and integrity of evidence obtained during an investigation to be admissible in court.

civil commitment: a statutorily structured process by which persons with qualifying conditions are legally confined within a designated facility either because they pose a danger to themselves or to protect the safety of others.

Code of Federal Regulations (C.F.R.): official source for federal regulations implementing U.S. congressional statutes.

common law: judge-made law that is modified case by case over generations.

contract:* an agreement between two or more parties creating obligations that are enforceable or otherwise recognizable at law.

crime: an act performed in violation of a specific law passed by the legislature that provides for punishment for violating a duty that an individual owes a community.

customary international law: unwritten rules of international law that develop through general and consistent state practice supported by the sense that following the practice is legally required.

defendant:* a person sued in a civil proceeding or accused in a criminal proceeding.

dicta: discussion in a court decision that addresses an issue outside the direct facts presented by the case and therefore outside the court's holding, and thus is of no precedential value in directing future court decisions.

due process, procedural: fundamental protection provided by the Due Process Clause of the U.S. Constitution, or comparable clause in a state constitution, that requires government officials and their agents to follow fair and even-handed procedures when enforcing laws. Basic elements of due process are determined by the nature of the rights and can include notice to the person involved, opportunity for a hearing or similar proceeding, and the right to representation by counsel.

due process, substantive: fundamental protection provided by the Due Process Clause of the U.S. Constitution that ensures that a law's overall effect on an individual's fundamental rights, such as the right to procreate and the right to marry, is justified or justifiable.

federalism: the system of government in the United States that is based on the concept of dual sovereignty between the states and the federal government.

felony: a crime punishable by a prison term of 1 year or longer and high fines

habeas corpus:* a writ employed to bring a person before a court, most frequently to ensure that the party's imprisonment is not illegal.

home rule:* a state legislative provision or action allocating a measure of autonomy to a local government, conditional on its acceptance of terms.

immunity, qualified: doctrine that provides that government officials who are performing discretionary functions are immune from civil liability if their actions do not violate clearly established statutory or constitutional rights of which a reasonable person would be aware.

immunity, sovereign:* a government's immunity from being sued in its own courts without its consent.

injunction: a court order requiring an actor to stop a defined activity that may be prohibited by law or to follow certain prescribed actions to comply with applicable law.

international law: the rules that regulate the relationships among sovereign states and other actors, such as international organizations and individuals, in the international system.

inter alia: among other things.

law: rules that are subject to the enforcement power of a government entity. Law includes the structures, norms, and rules that a society uses to resolve disputes, govern itself, and order relations between members of the society.

litigation:* the process of carrying on a lawsuit or the lawsuit itself.

least restrictive alternative: a view that an intrusion by a regulatory authority into an individual liberty should be limited and reasonable.

memorandum of understanding: an agreement or consensus among parties that does not create an enforceable promise nor specify legal remedies if one party violates the requirements of the agreement.

misdemeanor: a crime punishable by a fine of up to $500, imprisonment for up to 1 year in the county jail, or both

negligence: the failure to do something that a reasonable person, guided by the considerations that normally regulate human affairs, would do or the doing of something that a reasonable person would not do.

nuisance, public: an activity that unreasonably interferes with the public's use and enjoyment of a public place or that harms the health, safety, and welfare of the community.

parens patriae: doctrine under which the state asserts authority over a child's welfare.

police power: the residual power held by the states to enact legislation and regulations to protect the public health, welfare, and morals and to promote the common good

preemption: the legal effect that results when a superior governmental unit blocks an inferior governmental unit from regulating a particular area. The rationale of preemption is to provide national uniformity in certain areas.

prima facie case:* the plaintiff's production of enough evidence to allow the fact-trier to infer the fact at issue and rule in the plaintiff's favor.

prosecutor: public official who represents the government in a criminal case.

strict liability: legal doctrine under which parties are responsible, without proof or fault on their part, for injuries caused by abnormally dangerous activities under their control or products they have manufactured, distributed, or sold.

strict scrutiny: in constitutional law, the standard applied to fundamental rights (such as voting rights) in due process analysis and to suspect classifications (such as race) and classifications based on exercise of a fundamental right in equal protection analysis. Under strict scrutiny, the state must establish that it has a compelling interest that justifies and necessitates the law in question.

subpoena:* a court order commanding the appearance of a witness, subject to penalty for noncompliance.

taking:* in constitutional law, the government's actual or effective acquisition of private property either by ousting the owner and claiming title or by destroying the property or severely impairing its utility.

tort: a civil wrong in which the victim suffers injury to his or her person or damage to his or her property as a result of intentional, negligent, or abnormally dangerous conduct of the injuring party.

treaty: a written agreement between countries, the obligations of which are binding under international law.

United States Code (U.S.C.): official source for statutory law passed by the U.S. Congress.

warrant requirement: the necessity, based on the Fourth Amendment of the U.S. Constitution, for law enforcement officials to obtain a warrant to search private property.

Introduction: The Interdependency of Law and Public Health

WENDY E. PARMET

For many public health practitioners, law is an alien discipline, a separate field with its own language and its own values. Likewise, lawyers—to the extent they think about public health (and few do)—share this sense of separation. Few lawyers know anything about the history, perspectives, goals, or skills of the public health professional.

This mutual ignorance is unfortunate because law and public health are interdependent fields. They share a history that is far richer and more intimate than many appreciate. Even today, when the fields appear remote, their fates remain intertwined.

The chapters that follow document the intimacy of the relation between law and public health and demonstrate the many ways in which law is relevant to specific public health concerns. In this brief introduction, I paint with a broader brush, forsaking an in-depth analysis of the laws relating to a particular public health field for a more general examination of the ways in which public health depends on law and, less obviously, the ways in which public health has contributed to the field of law. I then consider some impediments to the successful exploitation of the relation, as well as some things we can do to make the inevitable collaboration between law and public health as successful as possible.

DEFINING LAW AND PUBLIC HEALTH

Understanding the meanings of *law* and *public health* is essential to exploring their relation to each other. Both law and public health are complex terms, with myriad and contested meanings. Even though in this Introduction I cannot fully explore these meanings, I can make some tentative observations.

Law and public health are both professional disciplines as well as complex social phenomena. We can speak of "a law" as a rule enforceable by the positive power of the state.[1] Such rules may be formulated by judges, legislatures, or even administrative officials. However, the term *law* certainly implies more than that; it includes the structures, norms, and rules that a society uses to govern itself, resolve disputes, and construct the relationships between members of that society.[2] A law, therefore, can be a specific regulation that pertains to health (e.g., a law banning use of lead paint), or it can be a more diffuse norm (e.g., the idea of property), which sets the stage on which people lead their lives, conduct their work, and become ill or remain healthy.

Likewise, public health is an enormously complex phenomenon. A common definition provided by the Institute of Medicine begins, "Public health is what we, as a society, do collectively to assure the conditions for people to be healthy."[3] This definition emphasizes the active nature of public health. However, the term *public health* also can denote the health status of a population. For example, when we say that tobacco is a threat to the public health, we mean, of course, that tobacco use jeopardizes the health of a particular population. Many commentators agree that public health is distinguished from medicine by its focus on the health status of a population or a community rather than on a particular individual.[4]

Both law and public health are also disciplines and professions with their own skills and their own ways of seeing and describing the world. When we say that someone has "entered the law" or can "think like a lawyer" (the goal of most first-year law school programs), we suggest not only that he or she has particularized skills relating to the structures, norms, and rules by which society orders itself but also that he or she has acquired and internalized norms and perspectives common to the profession.[5] Likewise, public health professionals not only possess specialized skills, such as their abilities to use biostatistics and epidemiology, they also share a language and values regarding the importance and nature of health. Thus, when members of the two professions try to work together, they come with different skills and with significantly different world views.

IMPACT OF LAW ON PUBLIC HEALTH

In this age of scientific wonders, it is easy to assume that a community's health depends on scientific knowledge and technologic prowess. However, studies suggest that, until recently, medical technology and health care have played a relatively small role in determining the health of a population.[6] Indeed, if we look either historically or globally, we are apt to recognize that social and economic factors have usually played a far more robust role than health technology.

Pointing to individual behavioral and genetic factors as key determinants of health has become common.[7] However, as Geoffrey Rose has indicated, although the examination of individual health risks may be useful for learning who in a given society is likely to become ill, it is far less helpful in shedding light on why a particular society has a particular rate of illness.[8] Nor does protecting the health of the population at large often help.

Modern epidemiology, therefore, recognizes the importance of social structures in public health.[9] The construction and revision of those structures, of course, lies within the domain of law. To take an obvious example, smoking rates undisputably affect population health profoundly. Epidemiology, a core science of public health, teaches us that valuable lesson. Public health also teaches us how to educate people about smoking and how to help them choose to quit. However, the underlying social conditions that help determine how widely available cigarettes will be and how popular they will become, the way in which they are marketed, to whom they can be sold, and the degree to which they are taxed all lie outside the exclusive domain of public health and implicate issues of social policy and law. These are the issues that the lawyer is trained to assess, affect, and alter.

The recognition that public health protection often requires the positive intervention of law is not new. The earliest known civilizations engaged in public health activities—enforcing sanitation codes, regulating the food supply, and caring for the sick.[10] These activities, many of which affected the well-being of the communities themselves, were more likely to be founded on religious beliefs than on scientific understanding (although a rough empiricism undoubtedly informed many practices). For these early public health practitioners, the chief tool of public health was law. In the ancient world, the practice of public health depended first and foremost on the establishment of a legal system that could ensure the organization and use of civil authority to proscribe practices thought to threaten health and prescribe practices thought to complement it.[10] Then, as now, knowledge of what harms public health was helpful only when it was joined with the mechanisms, provided by law, for reducing those threats.

Public health's dependence on law was especially apparent in times of crisis. When plague threatened, law was the chief mechanism to support public health. Whether they relied on the enforcement of maritime quarantines or on the establishment of pest-houses, people have invariably depended on law's ability to structure responses and to enforce norms in response to public health threats.[11] Indeed, in times of crisis, the most potent variable distinguishing the community that survives a plague from that which does not is not the degree of scientific knowledge possessed by the community but rather the responsiveness and stability of its legal system. Thus, in the late nineteenth century, cities in the United States that had established well-organized boards of health and had granted them the requisite legal authority were far better able to endure the threats of cholera and other epidemics than were communities that lacked the legal structure to respond.[12]

The success of public health boards and practitioners has long depended on the laws that establish their offices, grant their authority, and appropriate their funds. As mechanisms of the state, public health offices depend absolutely on state laws for their existence, financial support, and authority. Law determines whether they can inspect restaurants, kill mosquitoes, or quarantine people with communicable diseases.

Laws also help provide the information that boards and researchers need to determine their public health policies. For many years, our epidemiologic understanding depended absolutely on laws mandating the keeping of vital statistics and the reporting of diseases. Even today, when researchers frequently rely on other sources of information, public health professionals depend on public health reporting laws, as well as on vital statistics laws, to provide the sentinel of new and emerging health threats.

However, believing that law's role in facilitating public health is limited to the enactment of so-called public health laws—those that relate to the creation and authorization of health offices, tracking of health information, and direct regulation of dangerous activities—is too easy. Although laws that relate to public health's so-called core functions (i.e., assessment, policy development, and assurance) are critically important, they just touch the legal foundations for public health.

As noted above, law most fundamentally consists of the publicly sanctioned norms and structures that organize human interactions. Thus, law derives from and helps constitute societies, providing them with the tools to order relationships, respond to events, and resolve disputes. In this most fundamental way, law is absolutely essential to public health. Without law, in some form, social chaos ensues. When social chaos exists, public health is imperiled, not only because violence erupts but also because there is no clean water, no wholesome food, and no social security necessary for the healthy rearing of children. Instead, stress, uncertainty, and environmental degradation threaten the well-being of individuals and their communities. Thus, we should not be surprised that, as law breaks down—as it did in the former republics of the Soviet Union in the early 1990s—public health declines.[13]

Even closer to home, in less extreme ways, law as a tool of social ordering is a sine qua non of public health. Consider, for example, the *Healthy People 2010* goal of eliminating disparities in health.[14] Is this a challenge for science or for law? Although scientific research might be useful, or even essential, in pinpointing specific factors responsible for disparities, science alone cannot resolve them. No magic pill can be administered to end racial discrepancies in health. Nor can public health officials, acting alone, using their public health skills, solve the problem. Instead, if any meaningful approach is devised to eliminate racial disparities, it will necessarily emerge from an assortment of social responses that will be informed by public health but prompted or thwarted by law. Thus, although public health studies and professionals will teach us what needs to be done and where some of the problems lie, we will need to turn to laws to address some of those problems. Perhaps some of those laws may involve core public health laws (such as laws providing for public health clinics in certain neighborhoods), but other laws relevant to the issue may appear to be remote from public health laws. Perhaps laws relating to affordable housing, zoning, workplace discrimination, or drug possession will play a role in abetting or retarding racial disparities. These and many other issues and responses in the domain of law may have to be addressed if the goals of *Healthy People 2010* are to be even partially realized.

Major public health initiatives, therefore, invariably implicate law. Law, understood both as a discipline and as a set of social tools, frequently can provide a powerful mechanism for dramatically changing the course of public health. The impact of litigation on the way cigarettes are marketed, regulated, and understood in the United States demonstrates the potential potency of one legal tool for addressing public health problems.[15]

On the other hand, law has not always been a friend to public health. Law can create barriers to public health. It can defend the interests of industries that threaten the public health, preserve the status quo, and place economic interests above public health. For example, early in the twentieth century, U.S. constitutional law was interpreted and applied to impose major restrictions on the abilities of states to regulate conditions in the workplace.[16] Today, the First Amendment may present a formidable obstacle to the strict (and perhaps effective) regulation of tobacco advertising. Thus, law always influences public health but not necessarily as an ally.

The barriers that law can create for public health result from more than happenstance. They emerge, in part, from the different world views cherished by each discipline. Although public health focuses primarily on the well-being of populations, U.S. law focuses on individuals and procedures. Thus, lawyers generally focus on protecting individual rights, including rights of property, provision of fair procedures, and imposition of limitations on governmental overreaching. As a result, law, particularly law as litigation, has often imposed limitations on public health initiatives—whether they are founded on sound science or mistaken prejudice. Public health officials, therefore, might be forgiven for assuming that law simply imposes a hurdle that stands in their way.

That law can also be used positively to enhance a community's well-being— and how that can be done—has less often been appreciated by either lawyers or public health practitioners. Recent developments, such as the use of litigation to challenge the tobacco industry and the work of lawyers to challenge bans against needle-exchange programs, should remind us that law not only can create the background environment necessary for public health but also can affirmatively support public health.

IMPACT OF PUBLIC HEALTH ON THE LAW

How does public health affect law? Law's dependence on public health, I suspect, is far less salient than public health's dependence on law, but it is nonetheless critical.

Without question, a minimal degree of public health is necessary for law to function well. Just as public health is imperiled when lawlessness exists, so too is law threatened when public health is jeopardized. During the yellow fever epidemic of 1793, for example, civil authority broke down in Philadelphia, threatening not only local law but also the fledgling constitution because Philadelphia was then the U.S. capitol.[11] In a true sense, law is a luxury that is made possible only when a modest degree of public health is achieved—and so the establishment and maintenance of public health may well be the first essential and necessary undertaking for law.

Law's dependence on public health, however, is not limited to preventing the anarchy that can accompany epidemics. Public health has served law and relates to law in many more subtle ways. For example, one of the continuing challenges in U.S. constitutional law has been to find widely agreed-on arbiters or principles that can help demarcate the boundaries between federal authority and state authority, and between the public sphere and the realm of individual autonomy. Throughout the nineteenth and early twentieth centuries, courts frequently used the idea of the health of the public as a defining component of the police power and to help distinguish federal from state powers and public from individual rights.[17] In a world of contested values and conflicting moral judgments, public health proved to be one of the most widely accepted rationales for communal action. In that role, public health played a critical, although often unrecognized, role in the development of U.S. constitutional law. Thus, doctrines as diverse as those relating to the Commerce Clause,[18] the right to privacy,[19] and the Fourth Amendment[20] have all been built on and enriched by considerations of public health. Constitutional law, therefore, owes a debt to public health that has yet to be acknowledged.

The discipline and expertise of public health have also proved critical to the development of bureaucratic organization and administrative law. Indeed, public health boards and agencies are among the most ancient of all administrative agencies. In fact, in many places medical police long predated and formed the model for what we have come to know as the police.[10] Thus, the tools government uses to enforce law and the tools courts use to review and limit that enforcement developed in the nursery of public health and have been founded in untold ways on understandings gleaned from the struggle to improve communal health.

DEVELOPMENTS IN THE EVOLVING RELATION BETWEEN LAW AND PUBLIC HEALTH

What do we take from this tale of interdependency? First, that law and public health have developed together and are interconnected in ways that are seldom appreciated. Unfortunately, neither the inevitability nor the depth of the relation can ensure its success. Although neither law nor public health can function without the other, they need not serve each other well. Indeed, history is rife with examples of legal rules and doctrines—from the enforcement of Jim Crow to the doctrine of substantive due process—that have undermined health.

In our own time, the question of whether law will help or hinder the reduction in racial health disparities, the struggle to reduce tobacco-related illnesses, or the challenge of emerging infections remains unclear. If law is to facilitate public health in each of these areas and in many others, the connections between law and public health need to be more transparent and better understood. One hundred years ago the relation between the two fields was readily apparent. Legal opinions were filled with discussion of public health, and public health officials clearly understood that the law was one of their chief tools.

Today, even though the relation is no less critical, it is far less salient. The field of public health has grown far from its roots in social organization. Increasingly connected to the sciences, both medical and social, public health as a field is in danger of overlooking the critical legal tools necessary to actually implement and achieve the lessons learned in the laboratory. Indeed, as public health scholars and practitioners increasingly rely on the tools of quantification and empirical analysis, the risk arises that legal insights, not easily subject to empirical verification, will become lost. Yet, public health policy often will succeed only if legal obstacles are overcome and legal tools used.

The field of law, however, has been even more neglectful than public health has been in recognizing the partnership. In the last half-century, the law has forsaken its traditional appreciation of public health. Where judges once wrote eloquently about public health, it seldom appears in opinions today. When courts do use the phrase, they give it little weight. That public health is both a discipline and a human good is rarely noted by our jurists and often forgotten by our legislators.

Law's neglect of public health is also evident in the academy. Few lawyers ever take a course in public health law or even in the law's impact on public health. The law school course that generally comes closest is the course on health law; but that, not surprisingly, has followed the market and focuses generally on the regulation and provision of medical services. Few text books in the field devote any attention to public health; and in those that do, public health is clearly a minor theme in the major tale of the medical marketplace. Moreover, the vast majority of lawyers do not take even that course. Instead, in their courses on torts and constitutional and administrative law, they learn the values of individual rights and the perspective that economic analysis bears on decision making. That those decisions may affect dramatically the health of a population and that a discipline exists that sheds light on the nature and degree of those effects are barely ever noted.

CONCLUSION

Given the interdependence of law and public health, the question is not whether the fields will affect one another but whether their relation will be positive and whether it will advance or retard public health law while fulfilling other goals, such as respect for individual liberty. Will lawyers draft regulations, decide cases, and enter into settlements that advance or threaten the public's health? Will public health officials use the law to achieve their goals, or will their ignorance of the law lead to policies that are either thrown out in the courts or ineffectively implemented?

Although no simple formula for success exists, the positive collaboration between law and public health surely requires that law and public health become reacquainted—in other words, public health officials and others who work to advance public health must have more than a passing knowledge of law. They must understand that law plays a key role in what they do; they must be sensitive to its inclusion; and they must know how to seek out and work with lawyers and others who work in and speak the language of law.

Ideally, lawyers too must become reacquainted with public health. In a more perfect world, all lawyers would know at least as much about public health as they know about the laws of the market. Today we expect law students and lawyers to possess a basic competency in economics. Perhaps some day we can make the same expectation with respect to public health. Even though few lawyers will become public health professionals, all lawyers should understand basic teachings of public health, recognize its relevance, and know when to seek the advice and expertise of public health professionals.

In addition, both lawyers and public health workers need to recognize the breadth and depth of their relationship. The convergence between law and public health cannot be viewed as limited to the powers of public health officials or to those laws that West Publishing (which publishes most case reports) designates as public health laws. We must instead cast our nets wide and explore the multiple ways in which structuring government, determining safety standards, allocating liability, envisioning equality, and resolving disputes influence a people's health. Likewise, lawyers must understand how private actions, contractual agreements, economic incentives, and claims of right all affect communal well-being.

To do all this, we need not only to talk more across disciplinary boundaries and rediscover our collective roots but also to develop new ways to explore and assess our interactions. We need to think creatively about developing new methodologies that borrow the best from both public health's association with the sciences and law's relation with the humanities.

Most importantly, each profession must endeavor to understand the values of the other. If law imposes limits on the policies of public health authorities, these limitations are not always deleterious to public health for they may help to preserve the individual rights and civic stability that are ultimately crucial to public health.[4] Likewise, public health challenges to legal norms may often be less threatening than lawyers may initially suppose. For as public health is improved and our understanding of it is enriched, so too are our human rights as well as legal discourse.

These are ambitious goals. They will not be achieved effortlessly. There is no magic pill. But this book and the concerted efforts that many organizations are undertaking can lead us toward a reinvigorated partnership between law and public health—a partnership that will be not only inevitable but also enviable.

References

1. Hart HLA. *The Concept of Law*. Oxford: Clarendon Press, 1961.
2. Sarat A, Kearns TR, eds. *Beyond the Great Divide: Forms of Legal Scholarship and Everyday Life*. Ann Arbor: University of Michigan Press, 1993.
3. Institute of Medicine, Committee for the Study of Future Health. *The Future of Public Health*. Washington, DC: National Academy Press, 1988.
4. Mann J. Medicine and public health. *Hastings Center Rep* 1996;3:6–13.
5. Terrell TP, Wildman JH. Rethinking professionalism. *Emory Law Journal* 1992;41: 403–32.
6. McMichael AJ, Beaglehole R. The changing global context of public health. *Lancet* 2000;356:495–9.
7. Marmot MG. Improvement of social environment to improve health. *Lancet* 1998; 351:57–60.
8. Rose G. *The Strategy of Preventive Medicine*. Oxford: Oxford University Press, 1992.
9. Koopman JS. Emerging objectives and methods in epidemiology. *Am J Public Health* 1996;86:630–2.
10. Porter D. *Health Civilization and the State: A History of Public Health from Ancient to Modern Times*. London: Routledge, 1999.
11. Parmet WE. Health care and the constitution: public health and the role of the state in the framing era. *Hastings Constitution Law Quarterly* 1993;20:267–335.
12. Leavitt JW. *The Healthiest City: Milwaukee and the Politics of Health Reform*. Princeton, NJ: Princeton University Press, 1982.

13. Garrett L. *Betrayal of Trust: The Collapse of Global Public Health.* New York: Hyperion, 2000.
14. U.S. Department of Health and Human Services. *Healthy people. What are its goals?* Available at www.health.gov/healthypeople/about/goals.htm. Accessed April 26, 2001.
15. Parmet WE, Daynard RA. The new public health litigation. *Annu Rev Public Health* 2000;21:437–54.
16. *Lochner v. New York*, 198 U.S. 45 (1905).
17. Parmet WE. From slaughter-house to Lochner: the rise and fall of the constitutionalization of public health. *Am J Legal History* 1996;40:476–505.
18. *Gibbons v. Ogden*, 22 U.S. (9 Wheat.) 1, 303 (1824).
19. *Roe v. Wade*, 410 U.S. 113 (1973).
20. *Camara v. Municipal Court*, 387 U.S. 583 (1967).

I

LEGAL BASIS FOR PUBLIC HEALTH PRACTICE

1

The Law and the Public's Health: The Foundations

LAWRENCE O. GOSTIN, JEFFREY P. KOPLAN, AND FRANK P. GRAD

The law has played a vital role in public health since the founding of the Republic when the principal threats to health and safety were epidemic diseases. Law creates public health agencies, designates their mission, provides their authority, and limits their actions to protect a sphere of freedom outlined by the Constitution. The law, therefore, has always been vital to public health. The field of public health law, however, has never been more important than after the catastrophic threats to health that occurred after the events of September 11, 2001, particularly the dangers from anthrax. Just as these threats, old and new, teach us about the importance of a strong public health infrastructure, they also remind us of the need for appropriate public health powers. Public health law, of course, is about not only power, but also restraint. Public health officials, to be effective, need to act with strong scientific evidence and with fairness and tolerance.

In this chapter, we present the foundations of public health law—its definition, infrastructure, constitutional underpinnings, and powers. For more in-depth examinations of selected foundational topics, we refer readers to additional texts and resources.[1-3] Before turning to a careful exploration of the legal basis of public health, we examine fundamental aspects of the field of public health.

3

THE POPULATION BASIS FOR PUBLIC HEALTH

Defining Public Health

The effort to capture the entire spectrum of public health activity in one definition is bound to be complex and challenging. The field of public health is
broad, and the mix of disciplines makes justice difficult to bestow on all of
them. The Institute of Medicine's 1988 report, *The Future of Public Health*
offers a good starting point by describing public health's mission as "fulfill[ing]
society's interest in assuring the conditions in which people can be healthy."[4]

Several important and distinctive concepts are packed into this phrase: public
health's collective action on society's behalf ("fulfill *society's interest*" and "*assuring* the conditions"), a broad view of the determinants of health ("the *conditions in which* people can be healthy"), and an emphasis on populations rather
than on individuals ("in which *people* can be healthy"). In addition to these
characteristics, public health is unique among health-related fields for the value
and emphasis it places on prevention, protection, community health, education,
and partnerships with varied organizations.

The mandate to "fulfill society's interests" and "assure" healthy conditions
and quality services puts public health in frequent and compelling contact with
the legal system. Likewise, "the conditions in which people can be healthy"
recognizes the salience of the root causes or determinants of health—particularly
those that may not be obvious, immediate, or perceived to be within the purview
of other parts of the health system. In practice, this requires attention to the
prevention of disease (not just to its detection and treatment) and to a view of
disease that acknowledges the health implications of income, education, employment, and community.

Although the public health system often works in close partnership with the
medical-care system to protect the public's health, many aspects of public health
are not only essential but also unique. Different approaches to tobacco are a
good example of these complementary approaches. Tobacco—the underlying
cause of one of every five deaths in the United States—is a serious public health
threat and causes a variety of diseases in smokers and others exposed to tobacco.
The medical-care system focuses on treating the emphysema, lung cancer, and
heart disease that result from tobacco use and provides individual counseling
and perhaps assistance with smoking cessation (e.g., prescribing a nicotine patch
for a smoker who wants to quit). The public health approach, on the other hand,
seeks to change social norms about smoking (e.g., through media campaigns
and by advocating smoke-free workplaces and public places) and has the goal
of preventing tobacco addiction in the first place, especially among children.

Both approaches are needed, but their emphasis is at different points on the
disease continuum (from prevention to treatment), and thus the two parts of the

system employ different tools. In the medical-care system, health-care providers focus on diagnosing and treating an individual patient. In the public health system, the "patient" is the community or an entire population. The diagnosis focuses on identifying risk factors and preventing disease or its consequences, and the treatment might involve policy changes, media campaigns, environmental changes, or enforcement of regulations. Medical care usually is offered according to a medical model in selected settings—such as physicians' offices, hospitals, and clinics—while public health involves numerous disciplines (medicine, epidemiology, economics, political science), settings (such as schools and workplaces), and tools (including the media, regulatory authority, and changes to policies, the environment, and individual behavior).

Public health also is unique in its status as a common good. National disease surveillance systems that track the health status of populations, laboratory tests and techniques that track strains of disease, and teams of epidemiologists and other scientists that can be deployed when outbreaks occur are all examples of functions that no single private or nonprofit entity could support and for which few, if any, market-based financial incentives exist. In this sense, the results of public health activities are truly common goods that benefit all of us, whether we are wealthy or poor, insured or uninsured, urban or rural, healthy or sick.

Public Health's Infrastructure

The 1988 Institute of Medicine report diagnosed a public health system in disarray and suggested three core functions for public health as a new framework to return public health to its roots: assessment, policy development, and assurance. The law is important in establishing each of these three vital roles within public health agencies. The three overlapping functions encompass the entire spectrum of public health activity, from surveillance functions that detect and monitor disease and injury patterns, to developing policies that promote health and prevent disease and disability, to ensuring that data-driven interventions address the health issues identified through assessment activities. The cycle is continuously renewed as assessment activities detect whether progress has been made, leading to a subsequent set of policy actions, interventions, and reassessment (Fig. 1–1). These core functions, in turn, were further delineated into more specific "essential services" of public health,[5] which have since formed the basis for planning documents (such as *Healthy People 2010*) and ongoing research on the status of public health practice.

Another way to describe public health is to consider its key components, or infrastructure. In a recent report to Congress,[6] The Centers for Disease Control and Prevention (CDC) identified three main components of the system's infrastructure, all of which work together to ensure that the public health system is fully prepared to carry out the core functions and essential services needed to

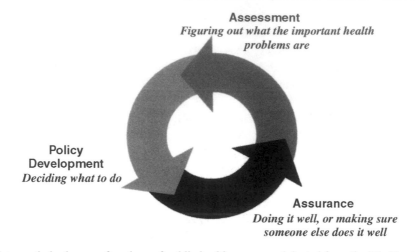

Assessment
Figuring out what the important health problems are

Policy Development
Deciding what to do

Assurance
Doing it well, or making sure someone else does it well

FIGURE 1–1. the core functions of public health. SOURCE: Adapted from the Washington State Public Health Improvement Plan

protect communities across the country from both routine and acute health events. These elements are (*1*) workforce capacity and competency, (*2*) information and data systems, and (*3*) organizational capacity.

Like the Institute of Medicine report that preceded it, the CDC status report on public health's infrastructure found many areas for concern. The report concluded that despite recent efforts and some improvements, the system's infrastructure "is still structurally weak in nearly every area." The Institute of Medicine's new report, *Assuring the Health of the Public in the 21st Century*, similarly draws attention to the inadequacy of the public health infrastructure to detect and respond effectively to disease threats.[7]

Although the public health system has indeed been underfunded for decades, its contributions have been impressive. As British physician Geoffrey Rose[8] has observed,

Measures to improve public health, relating as they do to such obvious and mundane matters as housing, smoking, and food, may lack the glamour of high-technology medicine, but what they lack in excitement they gain in their potential impact on health, precisely because they deal with the major causes of common disease and disabilities.

Public health's most dramatic accomplishment is the extension of the average life span, from 45 years at the turn of the twentieth century to nearly 80 years in 2002. Of these 35 years of "extra" longevity, only 5 or so can be attributed to advances in clinical medicine. Public health can take the credit for the other 30 years, thanks to improvements in sanitation, health education, the development of effective vaccines, and other advances (Table 1–1). U.S. census forms

TABLE 1–1. A Century of Public Health Accomplishment—United States, 1900–1999

30 years of increased longevity
Vaccinations
Healthier mothers and babies
Family planning
Safer and healthier foods
Fluoridation of drinking water
Control of infectious diseases
Decline in deaths from heart disease and stroke
Recognition of tobacco use as a health hazard
Motor vehicle safety
Safer workplaces

Source: Adapted from the CDC.[9]

now include three digits for recording a respondent's age—a tribute to the growing number of centenarians among us, now estimated to be approximately 70,000 Americans. Notice that for most of these achievements, law has played a vital role in relation to, for example, compulsory vaccinations, food and drug safety, regulation of the water supply, personal-control measures for contagious diseases, tobacco regulation (taxation, labeling and advertising, and tort actions), and regulation of car design and seatbelt use. Overall, these achievements highlight public health's protective role—the constant struggle to identify and minimize risk, whether it emanates from our own behaviors or those of others, the environments in which we live and work, our genetic legacy, or, as is often the case, some interplay among these.

Future Challenges

Of course, "fulfilling society's interest" is a task as immense as protecting the public's health (not only in the United States, but around the globe), and much remains undone. In the decades ahead, we are bound to face both known and unanticipated challenges. In the known category, challenges[10] include

- Achieving meaningful *changes in health-care systems*, including instituting a rational health-care system that balances equity, cost, and quality; and eliminating health disparities among racial and ethnic groups
- Focusing on the chronologic milestones of *childhood and old age* by investing in children's emotional and intellectual development and working to achieve not only a longer life span but also a longer "health span," one that offers a better quality of life, mobility, and independence for the growing population of seniors
- Addressing the *risks posed by our lifestyles and the environment*, such as

incorporating healthy eating and physical activity into daily life (to combat the twin epidemics of obesity and diabetes, among many other adverse health outcomes); responding to emerging infectious diseases (including new pathogens spread by travel, migration, and commerce, as well as microbial adaptation sped along by inappropriate use of antibiotics); and balancing economic growth with protection of our environment

• Applying what we already know and unlocking persistent mysteries about *the brain and human behavior* by recognizing and addressing the contributions of mental health to overall health and well-being and reducing the toll of violence (including homicide, suicide, and other types of violence) in society

• Exploring *new scientific frontiers* and applying *new scientific knowledge* (e.g., the mapping of the human genome) equitably, ethically, and responsibly

In many of these areas—including, for example, child development, mental health, obesity and physical activity, the environment, bioterrorism, and aging— promising science-based interventions are available and deserve support and broader implementation. In other areas, particularly the needs to delineate a rational health-care system, eliminate health disparities, curb violence, and manage new genetic knowledge, the course of action is less clear or even potentially divisive.

Like the public health achievements of the past, these future challenges will demand a blend of scientific innovation, technical and managerial expertise (especially regarding implementing health programs at the community level), persuasion, courage, and (last but not least) the skillful application of legal principles and tools. Public health's unique perspective can alter how these policy debates are framed and interpreted. By understanding and applying legal tools and principles that have already helped secure public health's achievements in the past century, the public health field can accelerate improvements in the public's health for decades to come.

CONCEPTUAL FOUNDATIONS OF PUBLIC HEALTH LAW

Public health law plays a unique role in ensuring the population's health. To demonstrate its importance, defining public health law and the public health law infrastructure are helpful.

Defining Public Health Law

A recent textbook defines public health law as "The study of the legal powers and duties of the state to assure the conditions for people to be healthy (e.g., to identify, prevent, and ameliorate risks to health in the population), and the limitations on the power of the state to constrain the autonomy, privacy, liberty, proprietary, or other legally protected interests of individuals for protection or promotion of community health."[1] This definition suggests five essential characteristics of public health law, which correspond with the characteristics of public health itself described in the previous section:

- *Government:* Public health activities are the primary (but not exclusive) responsibility of government. Government creates policy and enacts laws and regulations designed to safeguard community health.
- *Populations:* Public health focuses on the health of populations. Certainly, public health authorities are concerned with access and quality in medical care, but their principal concern is to create the conditions in which communities can be healthy.
- *Relationships:* Public health contemplates the relationship between the state and the population (or between the state and individuals who place themselves or the community at risk).
- *Services:* Public health deals with the provision of population-based services grounded on the scientific methodologies of public health (e.g., biostatistics and epidemiology).
- *Coercion:* Public health authorities possess the power to coerce individuals and businesses for the protection of the community rather than relying on a near universal ethic of voluntarism.

The Public Health Law Infrastructure

The public health law infrastructure includes public health laws (statutes principally at the state level that establish the mission, functions, powers, and structures of public health agencies) and laws about the public's health (laws and regulations that offer a variety of tools to prevent injury and disease and promote the public's health). The Institute of Medicine[2] and the Department of Health and Human Services[11] recommended reform of state public health laws. Public health laws are scattered across countless statutes and regulations at the state and local levels. Problems of antiquity, inconsistency, redundancy, and ambiguity render these laws ineffective, or even counterproductive, in advancing the population's health. In particular, health codes frequently are outdated, constructed in layers over different periods of time, and highly fragmented among the 50 states and the territories.[12]

Problem of antiquity

The most striking characteristic of state public health law—and the one that underlies many of its defects—is its overall antiquity. Certainly, some statutes are relatively recent in origin. However, much of public health law was framed in the late nineteenth and early to mid-twentieth centuries and contains elements that are 40 to 100 years old. Old public health statutes are often outmoded in ways that directly reduce their effectiveness and conformity with modern standards. These laws often do not reflect contemporary scientific understandings of injury and disease (e.g., surveillance, prevention, and response) or legal norms for protection of individual rights. Rather, public health laws use scientific and legal standards that prevailed when they were enacted. Society faces different sorts of risks today and deploys different methods of assessment and intervention. When many of these statutes were written, public health (e.g., epidemiology and biostatistics) and behavioral (e.g., client-centered counseling) sciences were in their infancy. Modern prevention and treatment methods did not exist.

Problem of multiple layers of law

Related to the problem of antiquity is the problem of multiple layers of law. The law in most states consists of successive layers of statutes and amendments, constructed in some cases over 100 years or more in response to existing or perceived health threats. This is particularly troublesome in the area of infectious diseases, which forms a substantial part of state health codes. Because communicable disease laws have been enacted piecemeal, in response to specific epidemics, (e.g., smallpox, yellow fever, cholera, tuberculosis, venereal diseases, polio, and acquired immunodeficiency syndrome [AIDS]), they tell the story of the history of disease control in the United States. The disparate legal structures of state public health laws can significantly undermine their effectiveness. Laws enacted piecemeal over time are inconsistent, redundant, and ambiguous.

Problem of inconsistency

Public health laws remain fragmented not only within states but also among them. Health codes within the states and territories have evolved independently, leading to profound variation in the structure, substance, and procedures for detecting, controlling, and preventing injury and disease. In fact, statutes and regulations among U.S. jurisdictions vary so significantly in definitions, methods, age, and scope that they defy orderly categorization. There is good reason for greater uniformity among the states in matters of public health. Health threats are rarely confined to single jurisdictions but pose risks within whole regions or the nation itself (e.g., air or water pollution, disposal of toxic waste, and the spread of infectious diseases, either naturally or through bioterrorist events).

One approach to rectifying inconsistencies in public health law is to reform laws so that they conform with modern scientific and legal standards, are more consistent within and among states, and more uniformly address different health threats. A single set of standards and procedures would add needed clarity and coherence to legal regulation and would reduce the opportunity for politically motivated disputes about how to classify newly emergent health threats.

Law as a Tool to Safeguard the Public's Health

Public health laws constitute the foundations for public health practice while providing tools for public health authorities. At least six models exist for legal intervention designed to prevent injury and disease and to promote the public's health. Although legal interventions can be effective, they often raise social, ethical, or constitutional concerns that warrant careful study.

Model 1 is the power to tax and spend. This power, given in federal and state constitutions, provides government with an important regulatory technique. The power to spend enables government to set conditions for the receipt of public funds. For example, the federal government grants highway funds to states on condition that they set the legal drinking age at 21 years.[13] The power to tax provides strong inducements to engage in beneficial behavior or refrain from risk behavior. For example, taxes on cigarettes significantly reduce smoking, particularly among young people.

Model 2 is the power to alter the informational environment. Government can add its voice to the marketplace of ideas through health promotion activities such as health communication campaigns; by providing relevant consumer information through labeling requirements; and by limiting harmful or misleading information through regulation of commercial advertising of unsafe products (e.g., cigarettes and alcoholic beverages).

Model 3 is direct regulation of individuals (e.g., seatbelt and motorcycle helmet laws), professionals (e.g., licenses), or businesses (e.g., inspections and occupational safety standards). Public health authorities regulate pervasively to reduce risks to the population.

Model 4 is indirect regulation through the tort system. Tort litigation can provide strong incentives for businesses to engage in less risky activities. Litigation has been used as a tool of public health to influence manufacturers of automobiles, cigarettes, and firearms. Litigation resulted in safer automobiles; reduced advertising and promotion of cigarettes to young people; and encouraged at least one manufacturer (Smith & Wesson) to develop safer firearms.

Model 5 is deregulation. The impact of laws may sometimes be detrimental to public health and may be an impediment to effective action. For example, criminal laws proscribe the possession and distribution of sterile syringes and needles. These laws, therefore, make engagement in human immunodeficiency virus (HIV) prevention activities more difficult for public health authorities.

The government, then, has many legal "levers" designed to prevent injury and disease and to promote the public's health. Legal interventions can be highly effective and need to be part of the public health officer's arsenal. At the same time, legal interventions can be controversial, raising important ethical, social, constitutional, and political issues. These conflicts are complex, important, and fascinating for students of public health law.

THE CONSTITUTIONAL UNDERPINNINGS OF
PUBLIC HEALTH LAW

No inquiry is more important to public health law than understanding the role of government in the constitutional design. If, as we have suggested, public health law principally addresses government's assurance of the conditions for the population's health, then what activities must government undertake? The question is complex, requiring an assessment of duty (what government must do), authority (what government is empowered, but not obligated, to do), and limits (what government is prohibited from doing). In addition, this query raises a corollary question: Which government is to act? Some of the most divisive disputes in public health are among the federal government, the states, and the localities about which government has the power to intervene.

Government Duties to Ensure the Public's Health

Given the importance of government in maintaining public health (and many other communal benefits), one might expect the U.S. Constitution to create affirmative obligations for government to act. Yet, by standard accounts, the Constitution is cast purely in negative terms. The Supreme Court remains faithful to this negative conception of the Constitution, even in the face of dire personal consequences. In *DeShaney v. Winnebago County Department of Social Services*,[14] the Supreme Court held that government has no affirmative duty to protect citizens. In that case, a 1-year-old child, Joshua DeShaney, was beaten so badly by his father that he was left profoundly retarded and institutionalized. The social services department was aware of the abuse but took no steps to prevent further injuries to Joshua.

The Supreme Court has applied this line of reasoning in cases that bitterly divided the Court. In *Webster v. Reproductive Health Services*,[15] the majority saw no government obligation to provide services—in this case, medical services—to the poor[16] when a Missouri statute barred state employees from performing abortions and banned the use of public facilities for such. Referring to *DeShaney*, the Court rejected a positive claim for basic government services: "[O]ur cases have recognized that the Due Process Clauses generally confer no affirmative right to governmental aid, even where such aid may be necessary to secure life, liberty, or property interests of which the government itself may not deprive the individual."[15] This negative theory of constitutional design, although well accepted, is highly simplified and, in the words of Justice Blackmun, represents "a sad commentary upon American life and constitutional principles."[14]

Federal Powers to Ensure the Conditions for Public Health

In theory, the United States is a government of limited powers, but the reality is quite different. The federal government possesses considerable authority to act and exerts extensive control in the realm of public health and safety. The Supreme Court, through an expansive interpretation of Congress's enumerated powers, has enabled the federal government to maintain a vast presence in public health—in matters ranging from biomedical research and the provision of health care to the control of infectious diseases, occupational health and safety, pure food and drugs, and environmental protection. The main constitutional powers for federal action in the realm of public health are the powers to tax and spend and to regulate interstate commerce.

At face value, the power to tax and spend has a single, overriding purpose: to raise revenue to provide for the good of the community. Without the ability to generate sufficient revenue, the legislature could not provide services such as transportation, education, medical services to the poor, sanitation, and environmental protection. The power to tax is also the power to regulate risk behavior and influence health-promoting activities. Broadly speaking, the tax code influences health-related behavior through tax relief and tax burdens. Tax relief encourages private health-promoting activity, and tax burdens discourage risk behavior.

Through various forms of tax relief, government provides incentives for private activities that it views as advantageous to community health. The tax code influences private health-related spending in many other ways: encouraging child care to enable parents to enter the work force; inducing investment in low-income housing; and stimulating charitable spending for research and care.

Taxation also regulates private behavior by economically penalizing risk-taking activities. Tax policy discourages a number of activities that government regards as unhealthy or dangerous. Consider excise or manufacturing taxes on tobacco, alcoholic beverages, or firearms. It is difficult to imagine a public health threat caused by human behavior or business activity that cannot be influenced by the taxing power. Similarly, the spending power does not simply grant Congress the authority to allocate resources; it is also an indirect regulatory device. Congress may prescribe the terms on which it disburses federal money to the states.

The Commerce Clause, more than any other enumerated power, affords Congress potent regulatory authority. The Commerce Clause gives Congress the power to regulate commerce "with foreign Nations, and among the several States, and with the Indian Tribes."[17] At face value, the Commerce Clause is limited to controlling the flow of goods and services across state lines. Yet, as interstate commerce has become ubiquitous; activities once considered purely local have come to have national effects and have accordingly come within Congress' commerce power. The Supreme Court's broad interpretation of the Commerce Clause has enabled national authorities to reach deeply into traditional realms of state public health power.

The Rehnquist Court, however, has begun to rethink the Commerce Clause as part of its agenda of gradually returning power from the federal government to the states. In the process, the Court has held that Congress lacks the power to engage in social and public health regulation primarily affecting intrastate activities. For example, the Court has held that Congress lacks the power to regulate firearms near schools[18] and to provide a remedy for victims of sexual violence.[19]

POLICE POWERS: STATE POWER TO REGULATE FOR THE PUBLIC'S HEALTH AND SAFETY

The "police power" is the most famous expression of the natural authority of sovereign governments to regulate private interests for the public good. One definition of the police power is

the inherent authority of the state (and, through delegation, local government) to enact laws and promulgate regulations to protect, preserve and promote the health, safety, morals, and general welfare of the people. To achieve these communal benefits, the state retains the power to restrict, within federal and state constitutional limits, private interests—personal interests in autonomy, privacy, association, and liberty as well as economic interests in freedom to contract and uses of property.[1]

The linguistic and historical origins of the concept of "police" demonstrate a close association between government and civilization: *politia* (the state), *polis* (city), and *politeia* (citizenship).[20] "Police" was meant to describe those powers that permitted sovereign government to control its citizens, particularly for promoting the general comfort, health, morals, safety, or prosperity of the public. The word had a secondary usage as well: "the cleansing or keeping clean." This use resonates with early twentieth century public health connotations of hygiene and sanitation.

States exercise police powers to ensure that communities live in safety and security, in conditions conducive to good health, with moral standards, and, generally speaking, without unreasonable interference with human well-being. Police powers legitimize state action to protect and promote broadly defined social goods.

Government, to achieve common goods, is empowered to enact legislation, regulate, and adjudicate in ways that necessarily limit, or even eliminate, private interests. Thus, government has inherent power to interfere with personal interests in autonomy, privacy, association, and liberty as well as economic interests in ownership, uses of private property, and freedom to contract. State power to restrict private rights is embodied in the common law maxim, *sic utere tuo ut alienum non laedas*, "use your own property in such a manner as not to injure that of another." The maxim supports the police power, giving government authority to determine safe uses of private property to diminish risks of injury and ill-health to others.[21] More generally, the police power affords government the authority to keep society free from noxious exercises of private rights. The state retains discretion to determine what is considered injurious or unhealthful and the manner in which to regulate, consistent with constitutional protections of personal interests.

The police powers have enabled states and their subsidiary municipal corporations to promote and preserve the public health in areas ranging from injury and disease prevention to sanitation, waste disposal, and water and air protections. Police powers exercised by the states include vaccination, isolation, and quarantine; inspection of commercial and residential premises; abatement of unsanitary conditions or other health nuisances; regulation of air and surface water contaminants; and restriction on the public's access to polluted areas, standards for pure food and drinking water, extermination of vermin, fluoridization of municipal water supplies, and licensure of physicians and other health-care professionals. These are the kinds of powers exercised daily by state and local public health agencies, as the following discussion demonstrates.

PUBLIC HEALTH POWERS: REGULATION OF PERSONS, PROFESSIONALS, AND BUSINESSES

The powers available to public health authorities in state statutes, as the previous discussion of police powers illustrates, are pervasive. Although systematically examining the full scope and complexity of the public health powers is not possible here, in this section we briefly outline selected principal authorities, many of which are detailed in subsequent chapters. These authorities group into the categories of the power to regulate persons, professionals, and businesses to safeguard the common good.

Regulation of Persons to Prevent Transmission of Communicable Disease: Autonomy, Privacy, and Liberty

Public health authorities have traditionally had a variety of powers to control personal behavior for preventing transmission of a communicable disease. These powers are essential to ensure effective surveillance and response to epidemics. The exercise of compulsory powers, however, also can interfere with autonomy, privacy, and liberty. As a society, we face hard trade-offs between the common good and the rights of individuals to a sphere of freedom. This section offers three illustrations of communicable disease powers: medical examination or testing, vaccination, and isolation or quarantine.

Medical examination and testing

State laws often provide public health authorities with the power to compel individuals to submit to testing or medical examination. Generally, testing and clinical examinations are not regarded as harsh legal requirements when the person may benefit. Some states require testing or examinations for sexually transmitted disease before marriage on the assumption that such testing can help prevent the spread of infection. Persons who engage in certain occupations, such as food handlers, nurses, and teachers, are required to submit to testing and examinations to be permitted to practice their occupation. Again, the rationale is that these examinations are useful in preventing disease (e.g., food handlers tested for typhoid or salmonellosis).

Compelling a person to undergo compulsory testing or examination is an invasion of autonomy and privacy and, therefore, requires a clear justification. Consider a recent Supreme Court decision that found compulsory drug testing of pregnant women to be a violation of the Fourth Amendment's proscription against unreasonable searches and seizures. Because the test information was shared with the police, the Court found that it lacked sufficient justification.[22] By analogy, a public health officer could not order a woman to undergo an examination for a sexually transmitted disease because there was no reason to believe she was infected.[23]

Compulsory vaccination

Compulsory vaccination has become a major tool of public health practice, even though its constitutionality was not upheld by the U.S. Supreme Court until the seminal case of *Jacobson v. Massachusetts* in 1905.[24] The principle established in upholding required smallpox vaccination has been applied in other compulsory vaccination requirements, with particular applicability to childhood diseases such as measles, rubella, and mumps.

Virtually all states permit religious exemptions from compulsory vaccination. State Supreme Courts (with the exception of Mississippi)[25] have permitted legislatures to create exemptions for religious beliefs.[26,27] Even so, courts sometimes strictly construe religious exemptions, insisting that the belief against compulsory vaccination must be "genuine," "sincere," and an integral part of the religious doctrine.[28] A minority of states also permit exemptions based on conscientious objections.

Isolation and quarantine

Public health authorities have the power to isolate or quarantine persons who are infected or exposed and who pose a danger to the public's health. It is a drastic remedy to prevent the spread of disease, and it is not used with any frequency today.

One tool for preventing the spread of infection is the exclusion of cases and contacts from populations that have not been exposed such as in schools or workplaces; sometimes isolation or quarantine requires a complete separation of the person from contact with others. As late as 1966, it was held that the health officer may make an isolation or quarantine order whenever he or she shall determine in a particular case that quarantine or isolation is necessary to protect the public health.[29] Still, the modern courts have required rigorous procedural due process before persons can be isolated or quarantined. In *Greene v. Edwards* (1980), the West Virginia Supreme Court reasoned that there is little difference between loss of liberty for mental health reasons and the loss of liberty for public health rationales.[30] Persons with an infectious disease, therefore, are entitled to similar procedural protections as persons with mental illness facing civil commitment. These procedural safeguards include the right to counsel, a hearing, and an appeal. Such rigorous procedural protections are justified by the fundamental invasion of liberty occasioned by long-term detention; the serious implications of erroneously finding a person dangerous; and the value of procedures in accurately determining the complex facts that are important to predicting future dangerous behavior.

Regulation of Professions and Businesses: Economic Liberty

Public health authorities have powers to regulate professions and businesses to safeguard the public's health and safety. These powers are important to ensure that professionals and businesses act in reasonably competent and safe ways. Professionals and businesses, however, also sometimes contest the validity of these powers because they interfere with economic freedoms to use property, enter into contracts, and pursue a profession. This section discusses several important regulatory powers: licensure, inspections, and nuisance abatement.

Licensure as a tool of public health

When a person is born, his or her birth certificate is likely to be signed by a licensed physician. When a person dies, he or she is buried by a mortician, also licensed by a state agency. Between birth and death, many other agencies with health responsibilities are regulated through the device of professional, occupational, or institutional licensure. A discussion of licensure therefore follows logically the subject of restrictions of the person because licensure is a restriction, an imposition of conditions limiting the person's freedom to carry on an activity, profession, occupation, or business of choice. The license requirement thus limits both the person's liberty and the use of the person's property. The imposition of such a restraint is justified because it protects the public health, safety, and welfare. Public health law, as an early field of administrative law, has used licensure effectively for many generations. The occupations and callings in the general area of public health are among the earliest of licensed occupations.

Licensure, like other police powers, is an authority afforded by the legislature. It authorizes a licensing agency, either a board of health, a board of regents, or a special professional or occupational board, to promulgate rules relating to license applications and to control the licensed activity. The licensing law that delegates powers to the licensing agency may prescribe narrow or broad powers, granting it limited ministerial scope, such as collection of fees, or it may delegate broad regulatory powers to set rules for the exercise of the activity and giving the agency broad regulatory powers. The task does not end with granting licenses. The licensing agency generally has the continuing obligation to supervise the particular licensed activity. The obligation includes both the formulation of policy and standard setting in the light of what may be rapidly changing technology in the field and what may be changing needs of the people for protection.

Three major uses of licensure exist in areas related to public health. The first two are primarily matters of public health control or regulation. The first involves the licensing of people engaged in public health professions or occupations, such as physicians, dentists, nurses, physiotherapists, occupational therapists, psychologists, X-ray technologists, nutritionists, and many other allied health professionals. The second category is institutional licensure, such as state licensure of hospitals, intermediate-care facilities, nursing homes, clinics and ambulatory-care centers, and other places where patient health services are delivered, such as clinical and X-ray laboratories, including pharmacies and other businesses directly involved in rendering services. The third category is business that is not directly involved in providing health care and goods related to health care. Many businesses affect public health, including milk pasteurizing, food, energy, and public waste treatment.

Because licenses involve limits on a person's freedom to engage in particular activities, and because licensure grants a particular group of persons and businesses something of a monopoly, broad licensing powers can be justified only to protect the public health, safety, and welfare. Thus, all of the constitutional limitations that apply to the police power generally clearly apply to the grant of licenses and to the scope and fairness of licensing regulations. Licensure, in particular, should not be used as a device for economic control. Occupational licensure that restricts access to the field may be used by the "ins" to entrench themselves and to keep out the "outs." Licensure is used by some occupational groups to restrict competition, and it ought not to be misused for this purpose.

Licenses are now generally regarded as protected property rights. A license to carry on a business or engage in an occupation or profession has great value to the person or business that holds it. The question whether the government can revoke a license at any time because it was considered a mere privilege is no longer valid. A license, particularly in the field of institutional and occupational license in public health, incorporates valuable rights. Such a license is protected by due process and cannot be revoked or suspended without proper notice and hearing.

Searches and inspections

Inspections are a common tool in public health designed to protect the population's health and safety. They are used to determine whether conditions exist that are deleterious to health and that violate public health standards or rules designed to bring about proper healthful performance of particular businesses, trades, and industries. Administrative inspections, unlike criminal law searches, are not primarily intended to uncover evidence to be used in the prosecution of a crime.

Although searches and inspections have a different emphasis, for constitutional purposes courts have generally regarded inspections as a lesser species of searches that must be conducted with constitutional safeguards. Inspections may uncover violations of health standards, for which violators may be prosecuted and penalties imposed. Inspections span the entire field of public health-related law. Inspections may be conducted to ensure health and safety in health care (e.g., hospitals and pharmacies), agriculture, nuclear power, food and drugs (Food and Drug Administration law), workplaces (Occupational Safety and Health Administration law), restaurants, housing, plumbing, and child care.

Sometimes inspections are referred to as administrative searches, but this term may sometimes be confusing in light of the use of the term *search*, which usually applies to criminal prosecutions. However, both searches and inspections are subject to review under the Fourth Amendment, which proscribes "unreasonable" searches and seizures. Before 1967, health and housing inspections were generally treated as reasonable searches, causing few constitutional problems. In *Camara v. Municipal Court of San Francisco* (1967), the U.S. Supreme Court held that the Fourth Amendment also applied to administrative searches and inspections.[31] Mr. Justice White, writing for the Court, held that a housing inspection was an intrusion on the privacy and security of individuals protected by the Fourth Amendment. Consequently, the public health authority must usually obtain a judicial warrant for an inspection. Inspection warrants, however, would normally be granted if the inspection is based on either the knowledge of an existing violation or a clear standard for routine inspections.

Although the Supreme Court has significantly changed the law of inspections, both before and after the decision in 1967 most inspections are carried out without a warrant because owners or occupants of premises generally will consent to inspections. Moreover, some exceptions exist to the inspection warrant requirement. For example, there is an exception for "pervasively regulated" businesses (e.g., firearms or alcoholic beverages). Pervasively regulated businesses are businesses so long and thoroughly regulated that persons who engage in the business have given up any "justifiable expectation of privacy."[32]

The control of nuisances and dangerous conditions

The vast field of tort law includes intentional or negligent injuries to persons and harm to property. It includes, for instance, medical malpractice and products liability affecting the manufacture of, *inter alia*, drugs and vaccines. The vastness and complexity of the broad area of torts prevents its general inclusion in this section, which focuses predominantly on public rather than private remedies.

The term *nuisance* covers both public and private nuisances. In the public health context, the primary concern is with public nuisances, a term that covers a variety of conditions that violate requirements of health and safety. A nuisance is a condition that constitutes an interference with the public right to pursue the normal conduct of life without the threat to health, comfort, and repose, ranging variously from matters of significant annoyance to conditions that impose significant risks to health and safety, for example, excessive noise, stenches, filth that attracts insects or rodents, and chemical wastes that contaminate the water supply. Facilities that generate smoke, soot, chemical odors, or other substances regarded as air pollutants may also be public nuisances. All these examples share interference with the rights of the public, and all are prohibited by law. Although any number of these examples would be treated in earlier days as common law nuisances, public nuisances are today defined by statute or ordinance[33,34] and are considered public offenses subject to criminal prosecution. Depending on the specific legislation, nuisances may also result in injunctive relief requiring "abatement."

The abatement of a public nuisance often involves the invasion of private property, so it must be clearly justified. If a health officer abates a nondangerous condition or acts excessively in light of the danger posed, then the purported abatement may constitute a "taking" or damaging of private property without due process of law, in violation of the Fourteenth Amendment. In such cases, the property owner may recover appropriate damages for the loss.[35]

The exercise of compulsory power clearly is a staple of public health law. Control over persons or property is necessary to promote the common good in a well-regulated society. At the same time, coercive measures infringe individual rights—autonomy, privacy, liberty, and property. Public health law, therefore, requires a careful examination of the tradeoffs between collective goods and personal freedoms.

THE FUTURE OF PUBLIC HEALTH LAW

Public health law is experiencing a renaissance in the United States. For example, the CDC has developed a public health law program (PHLP) designed to improve scientific understanding of the interaction between law and public health and to strengthen the legal foundation for public health practice. The

PHLP has established a CDC Collaborating Center for Law and the Public's Health at Georgetown and Johns Hopkins universities; awarded a series of grants to investigate the connections between law and the public's health; and hosted the first national conference on public health law. At the same time, scholarship in public health law is blossoming, and new links are being formed between public health practitioners and attorneys.

National and state authorities are awakening to the possibilities of law reform to improve the public's health. The Robert Wood Johnson "Turning Point" Program is supporting the "Public Health Statute Modernization National Collaborative," a consortium of states and national public health organizations.[36] The Collaborative is conducting a comprehensive analysis of the structure and appropriateness of state public health statutes and developing a model state public health statute.

The events of September 11, 2001, provoked a national debate about the adequacy of the public health law infrastructure, and both federal and state governments began to examine the need for emergency health powers legislation. The CDC asked the Center for Law and the Public's Health at Georgetown and Johns Hopkins Universities to draft the Model Emergency Health Powers Act, which has now been adopted in whole or in part by a number of states.[37] Policy makers are realizing that the law relating to public health must be clear and consistent and afford strong and effective powers to public health authorities. At the same time, the law must respect personal freedoms and treat groups with fairness and tolerance.

The law, of course, cannot guarantee better public health. However, by crafting a consistent and uniform approach, carefully delineating the mission and functions of public health agencies, designating a range of flexible powers, specifying the criteria and procedures for using those powers, and protecting against discrimination and invasion of privacy, the law can become a catalyst, rather than an impediment, to reinvigorating the public health system.

References

1. Gostin LO. *Public Health Law: Power, Duty, Restraint*. Berkeley: University of California Press, 2000.
2. Gostin LO. *Public Health Law and Ethics: A Reader*. Berkeley: University of California Press, 2002.
3. Grad F. *Public Health Law Manual*, 2nd ed. Washington, DC: American Public Health Association, 1990.
4. Institute of Medicine. *The Future of Public Health*. Washington, DC: National Academy Press, 1988.
5. Baker EL, Melton RJ, Stange PV, et al. Health reform and the health of the public. *JAMA* 1994;272:1276–82.
6. U.S. Department of Health and Human Services, Centers for Disease Control and

Prevention. *Public Health's Infrastructure: A Status Report.* Submitted to the Appropriations Committee of the U.S. Senate, 2001.

7. Institute of Medicine. *Assuring the Health of the Public in the 21st Century.* Washington, DC: National Academy Press, 2002.

8. Rose G. *The Strategy of Preventive Medicine.* Oxford: Oxford University Press, 1992: pp. 101.

9. CDC. Ten great public health achievements—United States, 1900–1999. *MMWR* 1999;48:241–3.

10. Koplan JP, Fleming DW. Current and future public health challenges. *JAMA* 2000; 284:1696–8.

11. U.S. Department of Health and Human Services. *Healthy People 2010.* Washington, DC: U.S. Department of Health and Human Services, 2000.

12. Gostin LO. Public health law reform. *Am J Public Health* 2001;91:1365–8.

13. *South Dakota v. Dole*, 483 U.S. 203 (1987).

14. *DeShaney v. Winnebago County Department of Social Services* 489 U.S. 189, 213 (1989).

15. *Webster v. Reproductive Health Services*, 492 U.S. 490, 507 (1989).

16. Tribe LH. The abortion funding conundrum: inalienable rights, affirmative duties, and the dilemma of dependence. Harvard Law Rev 1985;99:330–40.

17. U.S. Constitution, Article I, Section 8.

18. *United States v. Lopez*, 115 S. Ct. 1624 (1995).

19. *United States v. Morrison*, 120 S. Ct. 1740 (2000).

20. *Webster's Third New International Dictionary, Unabridged.* Springfield, MA: Merriam-Webster, 1986: pp. 1753.

21. *Commonwealth v. Alger, 7 Cush.* 53, 96 (Mass. 1851).

22. *Ferguson v. City of Charleston*, 121 S. Ct. 1281 (2001).

23. *Irwin v. Arrendale*, 17 Ga. App. 1, 5–6, 159 S.E.2d 719, 724 (1967).

24. *Jacobson v. Massachusetts*, 197 U.S. 11 (1905).

25. *Brown v. Stone*, 378 So.2d 218, 223 (Miss. 1979).

26. *Mason v. General Brown Cent. School Dist*, 851 F.2d 47 (2d Cir. 1988).

27. *Berg v. Glen Cove City Sch. Dist*, 853 F.Supp. 651 (E.D.N.Y. 1994).

28. *Brown v. City School Dist*, 429 N.Y.S.2d 355 (1980).

29. Application of Halko, 246 Cal. App.2d 553 (1966).

30. *Greene v. Edwards*, 263 S.E.2d 661, 663 (1980).

31. *Camara v. Municipal Court of San Francisco*, 381 U.S. 523 (1967).

32. *Colonnade Catering v. United States*, 397 U.S. 72 (1970).

33. *Lawton v. Steele*, 152 U.S. 133 (1894).

34. *State ex rel. Haas v. Dionne*, 42 Or. App. 851, 601 P.2d 894 (1979).

35. *Peters v. Township of Hopewell*, 534 F.Supp. 1324 (1982).

36. Turning Point. Available at http://www.turningpointprogram.org. Accessed December 18, 2001.

37. Model State Health Emergency Powers Act. Available at http://www.public healthlaw.net/MSEPHA/MSEPHA2.pdf. Accessed May 23, 2002.

2

Regulating Public Health: Principles and Applications of Administrative Law

PETER D. JACOBSON AND
RICHARD E. HOFFMAN

Public health practice frequently involves regulatory endeavors shaped by and grounded in administrative law. The core functions of public health practice are authorized, developed, and implemented through the regulatory process. Most public health actions, whether developing sanitation codes, responding to a disease outbreak, or enforcing environmental regulations, are subject to administrative law requirements. The foundation of public health practice is in the law, and public health's ability to regulate provides the key for understanding how to translate legal authority into practice.[1] Proper use of the regulatory process is therefore essential to successful public health practice and management.

In this chapter, we examine the key aspects and requirements of public health regulation. We focus on the administrative processes for state and local public health practitioners. Our goals are twofold: (1) to set forth the mechanics of the administrative process and (2) to provide a practical context for using the administrative process to the practitioner's advantage. Understanding and effectively using the administrative process will both facilitate public health practice and invite public support for public health policies.

BACKGROUND

Administrative law is the body of law created by administrative agencies through rules, regulations, orders, and procedures designed to further legislatively enacted policy goals.[2] All regulatory agencies, including public health departments, are responsible for implementing and enforcing legislation. By issuing and enforcing regulations, they create a body of administrative law. Administrative agencies must adhere to specific procedural requirements, set forth by the legislative branch, before taking any action. In conducting their business, administrative agencies operate on two levels. First, they issue rules. Second, they adjudicate challenges to how the rules are enforced.

Public health regulation dates back to the early days of the new American republic. The first federal health-related provision was passed on July 31, 1789, the first year Congress met under the new Constitution. It provided funding for quarantine inspections by charging all ships entering U.S. ports a 20¢ bill-of-health fee.[3] During the mid-nineteenth century, cities and then states established boards of health to oversee sanitation and quarantine requirements. In 1856, Louisiana created a statewide board of health. By 1873, Massachusetts, California, and Michigan had also formed state boards of health, and 19 states followed that model by 1879. States were primarily concerned with controlling infectious diseases, such as smallpox and yellow fever, and with improving sanitation. For example, early state regulations to combat smallpox and yellow fever involved the highly controversial actions of quarantines and smallpox inoculations (such as *Jacobson v. Massachusetts*, rejecting an individual's challenge to a law mandating smallpox inoculations).[4]

After the Civil War, the states became more active in regulating public health, especially in establishing a systematic public health infrastructure and creating mental health hospitals. The National Health Board was formed in 1879, and for 4 years it attempted to establish itself by aiding the states in their quarantine regulations. However, years of sparring with the state health departments and interdepartmental wars with the Marine Hospital Service were too much for this fledgling agency. By 1883, the National Health Board had disintegrated.[5]

National quarantine regulation was placed under the purview of the Marine Hospital Service in 1890. That agency oversaw marine quarantines, although it was limited to control of plague, cholera, typhus fever, yellow fever, smallpox, anthrax, and leprosy. In 1902, Congress passed an act reorganizing health care into the United States Public Health and Marine Hospital Service. The U.S. Public Health Service was adopted in 1912, but public health policy remained largely a state-based effort. Most public health activity in the twentieth century (and continuing into the twenty-first century) occurred at the state level. From designing and enforcing sanitation codes and maintaining responsibility for water and sewage inspections to designing disease-control strategies, state and local health departments have been the leading public health practitioners.

Until recently, public health has been exclusively the domain of governmental agencies. With the shift of health care to an increasingly market-based system and the rising distrust of government, the public health system has come under increasing pressure to involve the private sector (such as managed-care organizations) in providing public health services (see Chapter 9). Although the bulk of traditional public health services remains a government responsibility, many public health agencies are relying on partnerships with the private sector to achieve their public health goals. Public–private partnerships include programs such as Medicaid managed care and the formation of state public health institutes that are not attached to a government unit.[a]

REGULATING PUBLIC HEALTH

We use the term *regulation* to encompass both legislative and regulatory oversight of the public health system. As a government responsibility, the public health system depends on legislative authority for its practices and funding. Inherent in state sovereignty is the police power to protect the public's health and welfare. This has translated into a broad grant of authority from state legislatures to state and local health departments to prevent the spread of disease.

Regulatory agencies (both state and federal) are part of the executive branch, are created by legislatures, and exist largely to implement policy enacted by the legislative branch. Congress and state legislatures usually enact broad policy statements, delegating the details to the appropriate regulatory agency. Even though regulatory agencies are part of the executive branch, the nature and scope of specific legislation and the presence or absence of funding to implement legislative policies generally determine the agenda of a given regulatory agency. For instance, Congress used broad language to protect patient privacy under the Health Information and Privacy Act Amendments (HIPAA) but did not specify how the goals of the act should be accomplished. The details of developing regulatory guidance for and implementation of HIPAA were delegated to the U.S. Department of Health and Human Services.

At the federal level, many of the administrative agencies are independent of the executive branch, even though the executive branch exerts substantial control over regulatory policy through political appointments. Regulatory agencies at the state and local levels are usually not independent of the executive branch. In fact, the executive branch often sets state public health policy, although local agencies may have either congruent or independent authority subject only to local boards of health.

The justification for public health regulation has been the need for the state to exercise its police powers to act in the public's health to prevent the spread of infectious diseases; prevent injuries; protect against environmental harms; destroy contaminated products; and, in some instances, provide safety net services of last resort. The range of public health responsibilities at the beginning of the twenty-first century is remarkably expansive. Government has always assumed responsibility for protecting the public's health. Because no market has developed to provide these services, government agencies retain the authority to issue and enforce appropriate regulations.

In contrast, the general justification for regulating private health care is to redress market failure,[6] that is, where market competition is not working or where barriers exist to competition that can be eliminated only by government or other non-market institutions.[7] In the private sector, self-regulatory entities have emerged to oversee how health care is delivered. In the 1950s, the Joint Commission on Accreditation of Hospitals (now known as the Joint Commission on Accreditation of Healthcare Organizations) was formed as a voluntary entity to establish quality-of-care standards for hospitals and to accredit those facilities adhering to the standards. In the 1980s, the National Commission on Quality Assurance was formed to accredit managed-care organizations.

No similar self-regulatory structures have gained equal prominence in public health regulation. For the most part, elected officials play that oversight role. In Michigan, for instance, the public health officer needs approval from the local board of health (politically elected) to take regulatory actions. Several organizations have emerged to monitor certain aspects of public health practice. These organizations might stimulate changes in public health practice and management that will influence regulatory policy. For example, the National Association of City and County Health Officers conducts surveys and offers a forum for public health officials. The National Association of Local Boards of Health (NALBOH) provides similar functions for elected officials with public health oversight responsibilities.

Although based on a regulatory model, the public health system has been slower to adopt performance assessment systems than the private health care system. In recent years, however, NALBOH has developed a National Public Health Performance Standards Program based on a self-assessment instrument.[8] The instrument measures compliance with standards established for 10 essential public health services, including workforce development and identification of health hazards in the community. Meeting these standards will require regulatory policies.

One of the most important and unique functions of public health agencies is assessing the status of a community's health and ability to control outbreaks and prevent the spread of disease. This assessment is commonly achieved through population-based surveillance. No academic institution or other government agency is positioned or authorized to conduct disease surveillance. Generally, state legislatures authorize the institution of disease surveillance, and regulatory agencies determine what diseases are assessed and how.

For reportable or notifiable diseases for which there is a public health response to each reported case, such as tuberculosis (TB), every case must be counted. Until the 1980s, reporting in most states was based exclusively on a physician's diagnosis. Redundant, overlapping reporting systems were developed in the 1980s to overcome delays and/or absence of reporting by physicians. These systems required reports not only from physicians but also from hospitals and laboratories. For example, 1985 Colorado Board of Health regulations not only required physicians and hospitals to report cases of acquired immunodeficiency syndrome (AIDS) but also required laboratories to report persons with positive scrologic tests for human immunodeficiency infection (HIV). Sometimes prevalent cases are required to be reported (as with infections caused by HIV or hepatitis C) because such infections, even though asymptomatic in the host, are contagious. Reporting may also involve secondary data sources, such as a hospital discharge data set (e.g., severe traumatic brain injuries in Colorado). Hospital discharge data may be transmitted to an intermediate agency, such as a hospital association, which uses the data for proprietary purposes in addition to facilitating reporting by hospitals. This private, intermediary role may be modified by new federal HIPAA regulations, especially if named data are collected.

LEGAL AUTHORITY

Debates over the role of government in the private sector date back to the emergence of the American market economy in the early nineteenth century. At that time, the Federalists, led by Alexander Hamilton, argued that a governmental presence was needed to guarantee property, enforce contracts, and encourage the nascent entrepreneurial ethos.[9] In contrast, the Jeffersonians argued against intrusive government and in favor of self-reliance. This debate continues today over the proper regulatory oversight of health-care delivery and public health.

Federalism

The U.S. system of government is based on the concept of dual sovereignty between the states and the federal government, known generally by the term *federalism*. In a federalist system, states and the federal government share sovereignty over domestic policy.[b] One of the enduring tensions in American political history is the shift between the two for control over policy. Before the New Deal era of the 1930s, states' rights dominated public policy. From the 1930s through the 1970s, the federal government was in control. Now the pendulum has shifted again, with states dominating the policy arena, although federal funds continue to support state and local public health activities.

Under the Constitution, certain rights and responsibilities, such as preparing for the common defense and conducting international affairs, are reserved to the federal government. Before the twentieth century, this grant of authority was interpreted narrowly, thus greatly limiting the involvement of the federal government in health-related legislation. Indeed, the Tenth Amendment reads, "The powers not delegated to the United States by the Constitution, nor prohibited by it to the states, are reserved to the states respectively, or to the people." This was intended to ensure that the federal government would not encroach too heavily on the autonomy of the state governments and would maintain a federalist structure of government, which is to say a government comprising different autonomous levels. Although the Tenth Amendment expressly limits federal power, it still allows the federal government to control different areas of law without dependence on the states.

Thus, activities such as overseeing public health are traditionally within the states' authority. Before the enactment of Medicare and Medicaid in 1965, health-care regulation was almost exclusively left to the states.[10,c] Using the police powers (i.e., the inherent right of a sovereign government to protect the health and welfare of the state's citizens), states have taken responsibility for regulating how public health services should be defined, organized, and delivered; how they should be monitored; and how the public and private sectors should interact regarding public health services.

Preemption

An important aspect of the balance between federal and state authority and between state and local primacy is the concept of preemption. Preemption means that the superior government unit can block the inferior government entity from regulating a particular area. The rationale is to provide national uniformity in certain areas. When Congress legislates in an area and reserves power to the federal government, states may not regulate. For example, the federal government has exclusive authority for regulating nuclear power—an authority that precludes, or preempts, any state or local attempt to regulate this field. At the state and local levels, preemption laws prevent local authorities from enacting restrictions that are more stringent than, or at variance with, the state laws. In tobacco control, for instance, many state laws specify that local ordinances may not be stronger than the statewide law.[d] Preemption is an important strategy used by various industries to avoid more stringent local regulation.

Many preemptive laws have actually diminished the levels of protection afforded by local regulations in instances when the local regulations were more stringent than the state laws. Beyond preventing localities from enacting ordi-

the agency's response to the comments is included. Then, the final regulation is incorporated into the Code of Federal Regulations (C.F.R.). At the state level, either the public health code or the state's administrative procedures act specifies the requirements that an agency must meet before a regulation becomes valid. States differ as to when and how the proposed regulations must be made available, but few states make agency regulations as accessible as the C.F.R.

At the federal level, a regulatory impact analysis must be submitted to the Office of Management and Budget. In addition, the concept of a negotiated regulation between industry and government has become increasingly popular. In the so-called neg-reg process, the regulatory agency meets with members of the affected industry to develop a regulatory approach that is acceptable to each side to avoid contentious and time-consuming litigation.[g] Some states have a similar requirement or process. In Colorado, for example, a regulatory analysis is required with any proposed regulations. Agencies must engage as many potential stakeholders as possible to discuss the proposed rule before the public hearing is held.

Industry groups opposed to the regulation will often challenge it as being beyond the agency's scope of authority. In tobacco-control regulations, for example, affected industry groups (including the tobacco industry and retail merchants) may argue that a local regulation is invalid because it is preempted by state law or because the legislature has not granted or delegated sufficiently broad regulatory authority to the local agency. Although most of these challenges lose, some have succeeded[11,14] and may effectively delay the regulation's start date. Thus, public health practitioners need to work with their agency's attorneys to clarify the nature of their regulatory authority before issuing a proposed regulation.

Public health practitioners should view the public hearing as an opportunity to engage the public and gather support for the regulation. This process also can offer an opportunity to defuse opposition and to generate public support. Coalitions of supporters may form in ways not previously anticipated because the hearing offers them an opportunity to participate. Such public support is important in an era of general distrust of government and for moving aggressively into controversial areas.

Challenging Regulations

Once the regulations go into effect, additional opportunities exist to challenge their application. Just as state public health codes specify what must be done enact regulations, the codes also specify actions to be taken to enforce Again, the key is to maintain due process notions.

Suppose, for instance, that a local health department enacts a regu garding restaurant inspections for compliance with food and sanit

nances that address community-specific needs, preemption reduces the amount of debate over local policies. A local debate helps to educate the community about the potential dangers of a particular public health problem (such as a debate with a city council about exposure to tobacco smoke in restaurants and other public places). Thus, communities lacking the ability to participate in local debates over public health decisions may be less attentive to the dangers involved and less aware of ways to address the problem.

Regulatory Authority

Regulatory agencies derive their authority from the legislature. Thus, agencies must act within the bounds set by the legislature. At the federal level, affected industries have challenged regulations on the basis that Congress has unconstitutionally delegated authority to the regulatory agencies. The industries argue that Congress has not provided adequate guidance to the agencies but has instead inappropriately transferred its legislative authority to the agencies. Although a few such challenges have been successful, courts have not been overly receptive to unlawful delegation challenges.

At the state level, the delegation doctrine has not raised any problems. In most states, public health legislation amounts to a broad grant of authority to enact regulations and policies to protect the public's health. Within that broad delegation of authority, agencies are expected to exercise discretion based on their technical knowledge and expertise. For the most part, agency exercise of discretion is uncontroversial, but it remains a source of potential challenge. In *Boreali v. Axelrod*,[11] for example, the court ruled that the state health department went beyond its authority to create a separate council to issue tobacco-control regulations. The court held that, because these issues were stalled in the legislature and because the council decided economic and social policy issues that are normally within the legislative sphere, the agency exceeded its authority. Likewise, the Supreme Court recently refused to uphold the Food and Drug Administration's authority to promulgate tobacco-control regulations, arguing that Congress had never clearly delegated such authority to the agency.

Constraints on Authority: Personal Liberties

An important constraint on regulatory authority is the belief that intrusion into individual liberties must be limited and reasonable. The phrase "least restrictive alternative," used by the judiciary in analyzing a law, captures this sentiment. Many public health actions, ranging from tobacco control to vaccination requirements, restrict an individual's Fourteenth Amendment liberty interests. When determining whether the regulation intrudes too much into personal freedoms, courts attempt to balance the agency's legitimate need to protect the public's health with the individual's right to freedom from excessive government interference in personal lifestyle choices. Agencies must, therefore, weigh the nature of the public health benefits against the nature and extent of the encroachment into individual liberties.

For example, suppose a public health agency determines that a person with cavitary pulmonary TB is not compliant with directly observed therapy being administered in the agency's TB clinic. When considering how to address the state's legitimate interest in preventing transmission of *Mycobacterium tuberculosis*, the agency needs to consider a number of actions it could take. The agency's response may depend on the likelihood that the bacterium is multidrug resistant, the risk that the patient is now contagious, the reasons the patient has not complied with therapy, and the options available under existing state law. The agency could issue an administrative quarantine or isolation order confining the patient to home until he or she is no longer contagious, could seek a court order confining the patient to a locked hospital ward until he or she is no longer contagious, or could seek a court or administrative order requiring him or her to complete a full course of therapy. The risk to the public could be greatest if the bacterium is multidrug resistant because of the difficulty and cost in treating active or latent infection in this instance.

The tension between protecting the public's health without unduly infringing on individual liberties animates some of the most difficult public health policy challenges. In particular, agencies must protect the public's health without invading personal privacy, which is not always easy. For instance, some agencies want detailed data on individual HIV and AIDS cases in order to conduct contact tracing, but others assert that making such information available will discourage the very reporting needed both to identify infected persons and to understand prevalence trends.

RULE-MAKING AUTHORITY

One of a public health agency's most important functions is to issue regulations and then enforce them.[e] Someone opposing a department's regulations or regulatory authority has two opportunities to challenge any regulations—when they are first promulgated and then when they are applied.

Issuing Regulations

Gathering information

When considering what regulations to adopt, public health agencies need to gather appropriate information to assess the scope and content of the regulations. Agencies generally have authority to gather needed information. Agencies also

may choose to conduct a public hearing solely to explore specific problems and elicit input from the public. Another way is to gather data through routine inspections and investigations.[f] More often, agencies will conduct a hearing after issuing a proposed regulation.

The data-gathering process is essential for successful regulatory activity because it forces the agency to examine the justification for the regulation and the availability of supporting documentation. It also forces the agency to assess alternatives and to anticipate objections to the regulation, and it exposes any need for additional data collection.

Once the authority to act is established, the important considerations are to determine whether and why to regulate. It is up to the health officer to persuade those politicians with authority to act and the public that regulation is needed. To do so, the agency must conduct a full investigation into the problems that the regulation will address and how the proposed regulations will improve the public's health. Any supporting documentation should be presented at the public hearing, along with the rationale for the rule. To minimize challenges to or lack of compliance with the rule, compelling rationale is necessary for why the regulation is needed and how it will address a serious public health problem.

The process

The administrative process is rooted in ideas of due process and fairness and in the belief that the public should have an opportunity to review and comment on the regulations. If statutorily mandated procedures are not strictly followed, courts will rule that the regulation has not been appropriately issued. The procedures guiding agency actions are set forth in administrative procedures acts.

The key process requirements are to provide notice to the public and to solicit public input. These requirements can sometimes be suspended to respond to an emergency, but the ordinary process will include notice and an opportunity to be heard. Most state codes specify the requirements regarding the time and place of a hearing and the subject matter. For instance, Michigan permits both the state and local public health agencies to promulgate rules "necessary or appropriate to implement" the department's functions.[12] Before adopting such rules, the department must hold a public hearing to allow any person to present data and arguments for or against the regulation. A notice of the hearing must be published "not less than 10 days before the public hearing and not less than 20 days before adoption of the regulation."[13]

At the federal level, the Administrative Procedure Act determines the process of promulgating regulations. With exceptions only for emergency situations, all regulations must first be issued as a Notice of Proposed Rulemaking and published in the *Federal Register*. As part of the process, interested citizens are given a certain time period for submitting comments. The agency then reviews the comments. When the final regulation is published in the *Federal Register,*

During a routine inspection (or in response to a formal complaint), the investigator uncovers evidence that the proprietor violated the regulation. The investigator may issue a summons for a fine of $50 for a first offense. At that point, the proprietor can either pay the fine or contest it. If the owner contests it, he or she is entitled to a fair hearing before an impartial administrative law judge (ALJ).

Before a particular case can proceed, the defendant must be informed of what the charges are so that he or she can prepare an adequate defense. Although the rules of evidence are not as strict as for a judicial proceeding, the violator is entitled to a full and fair hearing. Due process protections permit the defendant to be represented by an attorney (if desired—defendants are certainly allowed to represent themselves), to present witnesses and evidence, and to cross-examine the government's witnesses. The entire hearing is be recorded, with the full record being available on appeal.

At the conclusion of the hearing, the ALJ must write a formal opinion. The opinion must set forth the ALJ's finding of facts and the reasons for reaching the decision. In Michigan, the health department reviews the opinion and can affirm, dismiss, or modify the decision. If a fine or other sanction is imposed, the violator can request that the local board of health review the decision. If still dissatisfied with the decision, the proprietor can appeal to the local courts. Before the violator can seek judicial review, he or she must exhaust all available administrative remedies. This may include appealing first to the chief health officer and then to the local board of health. The full range of appropriate administrative remedies is set forth in the public health codes.

Judicial Standards of Review

An important aspect of public health practice is the interplay between legislation and regulation. Regulatory authority is delegated by the legislature. Once regulations are enacted or applied, courts may be asked to rule on their validity. In one sense, judicial standards of review are fairly easy to describe. In reality, however, they are notoriously difficult to apply. Two general principles of the judicial standard of review are important to public health practitioners.

First, courts should generally defer to the regulatory agency's expertise in reviewing the regulations. Under the Supreme Court's *Chevron* doctrine,[15] as long as the regulatory record, when viewed as a whole, supports the agency's determination, courts should not intervene, even if a court might have reached a different decision on the basis of the same facts. Because the expertise, the ability to collect and analyze data, and the ability to conduct further studies all rest with the agency, courts are reluctant to overturn a regulation.

Second, courts defer to the agency's findings based on the agency's factual review of all pertinent aspects of the regulation. As with appellate review of a jury verdict in a civil case, the appellate courts depend on the written record and justification provided by the agency. The agency's findings should be overturned only if they are arbitrary and capricious (i.e., not based on facts in the record), when the authority to act is not clear, or when the agency omits analyses required by the legislature.

Courts are generally less deferential when reviewing the agency's interpretations of its regulations, which agencies often do through subsequent policy statements. In part because the policy statements are not issued on the basis of public comment and review, courts tend to be considerably less deferential when reviewing an agency's policy interpretation of its regulations. This is important for enforcement. If the violation is clear from the regulations, courts will usually side with the agency. However, if the public health agency relies on a policy statement to find a violation, courts may not necessarily uphold the agency, particularly if the agency has not disseminated the policy statements to potential violators.

ADMINISTRATIVE STRATEGIES AND REMEDIES

Much of the art of public health practice is deciding what actions to take in response to a public health code violation. A public health agency has a broad range of remedies for enforcing its regulations. Should states with referral authority for criminal activities seek a criminal punishment, or is a civil fine sufficient? Should the agency seek fines or try to enjoin the activity? Deciding on which remedy to pursue requires knowledge of the range of potential sanctions as well as the trade-offs involved. Each state's public health code is likely to specify the range of permissible sanctions and remedies.

Civil Strategies and Remedies

Civil sanctions involve a range of options, from monetary penalties to injunctions. The purpose of civil fines is simply to provide an inducement to comply with the regulations. Failure to comply can be costly.

Most public health codes specify the amount of money that a violator will pay. A civil fine is usually graduated based on the number of violations, with repeat violators paying successively higher amounts. For example, a statute regulating noise levels may specify a $50 fine for the first offense, $100 for a second, and $500 for a third violation.

Another civil remedy is to use the licensure authority to ensure compliance and to deter violations. Many activities affecting public health require a license from the state or from the local authorities. For example, tobacco and alcohol vendors are licensed. If they sell tobacco or alcohol to minors, their vendor's license can be suspended following an appropriate hearing. License suspension is particularly valuable for enforcing restrictions on the sale of tobacco and alcohol to minors. Although the investment in enforcing these laws is not trivial, vendors may respond more positively to losing their license than to a simple fine (which they may treat as just the cost of doing business). From a practical standpoint, licensing fees (along with fines paid for violations) may well sustain an aggressive enforcement effort.[16]

A related use of licensing authority deals with state oversight of health-care facilities. All states license both health-care facilities and providers. States and local authorities can use the licensure process to ensure that these facilities comply with local health and safety codes.

Injunctions are an important component of local public health practice. An injunction is a court order requiring an actor to stop a defined activity that is prohibited by law. For example, if a firm or individual violates noise pollution ordinances, the public health department can either cite the violator for civil penalties or ask a court to enjoin the activity. Injunctions are issued when a violation of the law is ongoing (such as an ongoing exposure of the public to a disease risk), monetary damages are not available, and irreparable harm would occur if the injunction were denied. For example, an injunction might be used to close a restaurant until the outbreak of salmonellosis has been identified and eliminated. Courts must balance the equities between the need to continue the activity and the public's health.

A controversial use of injunctions has been to enjoin HIV-infected persons who, despite counseling, continue to expose others to the virus. The purpose of the injunction is to stop the risky behavior, but, because of the manner in which HIV is usually transmitted, that is, by unsafe or unprotected sexual activity and by sharing contaminated needles, compliance with the injunction is difficult to monitor. Degrees of evidence of noncompliance exist: Having a sex partner of the index patient diagnosed with an acute sexually transmitted disease, such as gonorrhea, is stronger evidence of unsafe behavior than having a sex partner assert that he or she was not informed of the HIV infection in the index patient and that unprotected sex occurred.

HIV is a lifelong infection, and, even if virus is not detected in serum, the infected person may still be contagious. Therefore, an injunction could be enforced indefinitely or until a treatment exists for HIV infection that renders the person noncontagious. Furthermore, whether unsafe sex between two consenting adults, of whom one or both are HIV infected, represents a public health threat or an ongoing violation of the law is controversial. In this context, the injunction could be viewed as one of several types of therapeutic intervention designed to protect the public health. Its value in comparison to repeated, intensive behavior counseling and social therapy must be individually evaluated. Little long-term experience exists to guide agencies or the courts in this area of public health practice.

One strategy to consider is using the taxing authority. Almost all states, for instance, tax cigarettes and alcohol. Some states authorize taxing at the local level as well. In an era of anti-tax fervor, public support for new taxes is difficult to generate. However, the public generally supports the concept of taxing alcohol and cigarettes, even if the public disagrees about the optimal taxing levels.

A related civil strategy is litigation. This is a controversial approach that has met with limited success in high-visibility areas. States succeeded in using litigation to compel a settlement with the tobacco industry over the costs to state Medicaid programs of tobacco-related disease. Localities have tried a similar strategy against gun manufacturers for failing to monitor the distribution of their products. So far, these suits have been limited or thrown out altogether in the appellate courts, despite some initial success among jurors. In addition, some states have responded to local agency lawsuits by enacting laws that allow only the state to sue, thereby preempting such litigation.

One advantage of litigation is that it may result in settlement negotiations that an industry might not otherwise be willing to join. However, a disadvantage is the cost of litigation and the potential for the state legislature to enact laws preempting such litigation.

Criminal Strategies and Remedies

Many public health statutes provide for both civil and criminal fines. Because agencies and courts are generally reluctant to characterize a public health violation as a criminal matter, most fines sought are civil. For instance, most statutes for code violations, such as for nuisance or pollution, are defined as misdemeanors (minor crimes) subject to a criminal or civil fine. Agencies usually ignore the criminal aspect and simply seek a civil fine. In some instances, however, a violation is so severe as to warrant a criminal sanction. The most obvious case is when a firm dumps toxic and hazardous wastes into the environment and ignores an agency's or court's order to cease the activity. At that point, a civil fine may be viewed as an insufficient penalty, and the firm's actions may justify a criminal indictment. For both political and legal reasons, the evidence must be strong and the activity must be egregious to support a criminal trial. Unlike a civil action, the state in a criminal trial must show that the defendant intended to violate the laws and did so beyond a reasonable doubt. This is a high standard, and support for criminal investigations has been slow.

Traditional Public Health Strategies and Remedies

Some of the most difficult decisions a public health agency must make include when to exercise traditional public health remedies to halt the spread of disease. Agencies usually attempt to impose the least restrictive method to outbreak control. For example, when a case of measles occurred in a child attending school, public health agencies often issued a school exclusion order rather than requiring all undervaccinated children to be vaccinated. The exclusion order meant that nonvaccinated or undervaccinated children were sent home and could not be readmitted to school until the outbreak was over, which was generally 2 to 4 weeks after the onset of illness in the last reported case. However, the excluded children were not required to be vaccinated. The effect on disease control of such an order was to remove potentially susceptible children from contact with infectious or incubating cases, thereby preventing a subsequent generation of disease. At a time when fear and distrust of vaccinations are increasing among the U.S. population, a public health remedy that does not require vaccination but effectively stops disease transmission is useful. Measles, however, is now rare in the United States, and this remedy may not be as effective with other communicable diseases, such as varicella, or in nonschool settings such as child-care centers and adult workplaces.

Two areas that would seem to be receptive to the use of traditional public health strategies but raise surprising complications are the distribution of needles to injecting-drug users who have HIV infection or AIDS and disease reporting requirements. In the former situation, many states have criminal statutes preventing the exchange of clean needles—but how can a public health agency develop and implement a needle-exchange program without violating the laws against distribution? In the latter case, agencies need to collect a wide range of data to monitor disease-prevalence trends—but increasing concern for individual privacy and confidentiality enhances the risk that individually identifiable data could be disclosed.

Public health agencies also have the power to conduct screening examinations for various diseases. These are useful for monitoring disease prevalence trends. For instance, several states track reports of prenatal substance exposure (PSE) and HIV exposure to monitor disease trends.[17] The controversial aspect of these prevalence tracking efforts is whether to identify individuals for contact tracing in the case of HIV infection and for referral to child welfare authorities in the case of PSE. Some states mandate screening for certain populations or diseases. Colorado mandates HIV screening for prisoners. Other states, including Wisconsin, mandate screening and reporting to detect PSE.[15]

Education is another traditional public health strategy that must be viewed as complementary, but also integral, to the regulatory process. Education has had some stunning successes, particularly in conjunction with regulatory activity. For example, the designated driver advertising campaign has dramatically reduced drunk-driving fatalities. Although less dramatic (and somewhat more contentious), the accumulated information from education campaigns about the dangers of tobacco use has contributed to reduced adult and teen smoking rates over time.

Trade-Offs in Selecting Remedies

As the above discussion suggests, public health agencies must often make trade-offs when deciding which remedies to pursue. At a very general level, regulations must be written to protect the community without unduly burdening the individual freedoms that the law preserves. At a more specific level, agencies must always be concerned about how its scarce resources will be allocated. Retaining public support is critical in securing this balance.

Some of the inherent trade-offs are obvious. For instance, speed of securing a fine as opposed to the heightened administrative burden of seeking an injunction or a criminal sanction is one such consideration. Another is to be concerned with political feasibility. In many instances, the public health code will require a final decision from an elected official (such as a local board of health) before the public health action can be undertaken.

As a general proposition, public health agencies need to consider the targets of the proposed regulation; data available to support the regulation; anticipated interest group opposition; the cost of the chosen strategy; its potential effectiveness (in terms of both achieving the desired goal and reaching a large number of people); and the equities involved in pursuing the regulation. Another factor to consider, similar to what physicians face in the private health system, is that public health officials no longer control the flow of information as they once did. The availability of information over the Internet and the speed with which information and rumors (such as the relation between autism and the measles-mumps-rubella vaccine [MMR]) can spread clearly complicates the process of promulgating and enforcing public health regulations.

FUTURE CHALLENGES

In terms of the public health regulatory environment, state and local public health policy makers should be prepared to address several challenges. These challenges range from technical concerns (e.g., cost–benefit analysis) to conceptual concerns (e.g., public health as a collective enterprise).

Cost–Benefit Analysis

Two factors strongly suggest that some form of cost–benefit analysis (CBA) (i.e., cost-effectiveness analysis, risk-utility analysis) will become standard practice for issuing state and local public health regulations. First, the federal government is increasingly using some form of CBA in issuing its regulations. Sooner or later, this will lead to expectations that state and local regulations will also incorporate this analysis. Second, public pressure for more efficient government will force state and local officials to justify the cost of each and every regulation in terms of benefits to the community.

The problem at the local level will be that it can be time-consuming to gather and analyze cost–benefit data, especially if staff have not been trained to do so. Defining the intangible benefits is always difficult. On the negative side, this will slow down the regulatory process and force agencies to choose between competing regulations. More positively, those regulations issued with a solid CBA will be easier to justify to the public.

Regulatory Takings

Under the Fifth Amendment, the government cannot confiscate private property without paying just compensation. For example, when a local government condemns a property to construct a road under eminent domain, the government must pay the owner the property's fair market value. Until the mid-1980s, the takings doctrine only applied to an actual condemnation of the property. Regulations were generally exempt from this doctrine. Starting in the early 1990s, the Supreme Court expanded the meaning of the takings clause to include partial regulatory takings.[18] If, for instance, the U.S. Environmental Protection Agency declares part of a property a protected wetland, diminishing the value of the entire parcel but only regulating a portion, the owner could request compensation under the Fifth Amendment.

The implications of this doctrinal shift for public health regulation are profound. Although the takings doctrine has not yet interfered with the government's ability to enact zoning, rent control, or environmental regulations, the takings doctrine acts as a limitation on the range of regulatory strategies the government can pursue. At a minimum, public health agencies may need to think twice about taking certain actions. For instance, regulatory takings issues may be raised for ordering herds of deer and elk to be killed if they live in a region with chronic wasting disease (a transmissible spongiform encephalopathy). Likewise, ordering sheep to be killed if they originate from a farm where scrapie (another transmissible spongiform encephalopathy) has been detected may result in a takings challenge.

Public–Private Partnerships

Public health practice at the beginning of the twenty-first century must take into account certain fundamental policy shifts. In particular, the health-care system is increasingly competitive based on market principles, and the public seems less willing to support investments in public health. As a result, public health agencies must develop alternative strategies to regulation that involve public–private partnerships. Most state codes permit public health agencies to contract with the private sector for goods or services. Perhaps the most dramatic of these public–private arrangements is Medicaid managed care. State Medicaid agencies use their contracting authority to solicit bids from the private sector to provide Medicaid services. The private sector is also more actively engaged in providing prevention services for its members.

The use of public–private partnerships to provide public health services presents both opportunities and challenges. The opportunities are to use such partnerships to achieve public health goals without issuing regulations or going through contentious litigation challenging the regulations. By using the contracting mechanism, public health agencies can specify the terms of engagement and set the expectations for how the programs will be monitored. However, serious challenges need to be confronted. First, the resources to monitor the contracts adequately may not be available. Second, contractual terms that reflect public health goals need to be negotiated. A more serious concern is that shifting public health services to the private sector will call into question the need for the public health system altogether.

New Public Health Concerns

The public health regulatory model is based on controlling communicable diseases. For many future activities, this model will still be appropriate and effective. Public health concerns, however, are not limited to communicable diseases, and a different regulatory strategy may be needed for issues that do not fall within that approach. Take, for example, questions surrounding youth violence and genetics technologies. Are these public health issues? Does legal authority exist for public health department attempts to regulate in these areas? If so, what types of regulatory strategies might be considered?

Even the old verities will arise in different ways. When *Jacobson v. Massachusetts* was decided, few people refused the smallpox vaccination. Now, every state has a statute exempting individuals from vaccination on the basis of religious or medical criteria, and 15 states allow an exemption on the basis of personal or philosophic objections to vaccination. Add to this the concerns about neurologic effects of pertussis vaccine, fears about MMR autism and hepatitis B vaccine causing multiple sclerosis, and the real association of the original rotavirus vaccine and intussception. A health department is thus likely to confront a growing number of people who choose not to have their children vaccinated. They may base their decisions on personal concerns about the risks of vaccination and do not understand that the cumulative effect of many such personal decisions is to increase each unvaccinated child's risk of acquiring a particular communicable disease.

At a time of general public distrust for government and a declining investment in public health resources, public health agencies need to be cognizant of alternative strategies to achieve public health objectives. One approach is to use the media to advocate for such goals. Another is to rely on moral suasion to convince the public that certain actions need to be taken. One might view this as similar to an education strategy, but it needs to be thought of in broader terms than simply trying to educate the public. Instead, it means using local media to make the case for public health and using the moral high ground to advocate for public health strategies.

Public Health as a Collective Enterprise

Public health regulations are based on population data and are designed to achieve the greatest good for the greatest number. Yet that collective goal conflicts with the ethos of individualism now dominating social policy. It also raises problems with the increasing number of people unwilling to submit voluntarily to vaccination programs. Because of well-publicized (though unfounded) fears of developing autism from MMR, many states have enacted legislation permitting medical or religious exemptions from vaccination requirements for children entering school. Public health agencies must balance between their mandate to protect communities from the spread of contagious diseases without unduly burdening individuals who do not want to be protected (i.e., vaccinated). That is, the uninfected have an individual right to remain uninfected and to take advantage of the vaccination exemption. However, this is never just an individual decision because serious public health implications exist for society if an individual contracts and communicates the disease to others. Therefore, representing both interests simultaneously is challenging.

Notes

[a] For an examination of these arrangements, see Nicola RM, Berkowitz B, Lafranza V, eds. Issue focus: the turning point initiative. *Journal of Public Health Management and Practice* 2002; 8.

[b] The Tenth Amendment reads, "The powers not delegated to the United States by the Constitution, nor prohibited by it to the states, are reserved to the states respectively, or to the people." This was intended to ensure that the federal government would not encroach too heavily on the autonomy of the state governments and to maintain a federalist structure of government.

[c] Article 1, Section 8, of the Constitution provides federal jurisdiction over health matters to promote the general welfare.

[d] Not all preemption provisions are alike. Massachusetts' preemption only applies to the sale of cigarette rolling paper, while other states (i.e., Florida) preempt local jurisdictions from enacting any clean indoor air restrictions.

[e] In rare circumstances, an agency with public health functions may not be a regulatory agency. For example, the Centers for Disease Control and Prevention has enormous public health responsibility, but it does not issue or enforce regulations.

[f] For a thorough summary of information gathering techniques, see chapter 14 in FP Grad, *The Public Health Law Manual*, 2nd ed. Washington, DC: American Public Health Association, 1990: pp. 265–87.

ᵍ It would be naive to think that affected industries were ignored in regulatory policy before "reg-neg," but the explicit inclusion of the industry in the regulatory process is substantially different.

References

1. Gostin LO. *Public Health Law: Power, Duty, Restraint.* Berkeley: University of California Press, 2000.
2. *Black's Law Dictionary.* Abridged 6th ed. St. Paul, MN: West Publishing Co, 1991.
3. Act of July 31, 1789, ch. 5, *Stat.* 29 (p. 44) (1789).
4. *Jacobson v. Massachusetts,* 197 U.S. 11 (1904).
5. Smillie WG. *Public Health: Its Promise for the Future. A Chronicle of the Development of Public Health in the United States, 1607–1914.* New York: Macmillan Co., 1955.
6. Jost TS. Oversight of quality medical care: regulation, management or the market? *Arizona Law Rev* 1995;37:825–68.
7. Arrow KJ. Uncertainty and the welfare economics of medical care. *Am Economic Rev* 1963;53:941–73.
8. The National Association of Local Boards of Health. *National Public Performance Standards Program: Local Public Health Governance Performance Assessment Instrument* (Version 4.0, Final Draft), April 13, 2001. Available at http://www.nalboh.org/perfstds/perfstds.htm. Accessed December 11, 2001.
9. Sellers C. *The Market Revolution: Jacksonian America, 1815–1846.* New York: Oxford University Press, 1991.
10. *Dukes v. U.S. Healthcare, Inc.,* 57 F.3d 350, 357 (3d Cir. 1995).
11. *Boreali v. Axelrod,* 517 N.E.2d 1350 (N.Y. 1987).
12. Michigan Compiled Laws Annotated, Part 333, Sections 2233 and 2441.
13. Michigan Compiled Laws Annotated, Part 333, Section 2442.
14. *Brewery, Inc. v. Delaware City-County Board of Health,* No. 98CVH-12–413 (C.P. Delaware County, Ohio, July 22, 1999).
15. *Chevron, USA, Inc. v. Natural Resources Defense Council, Inc.,* 467 U.S. 837 (1984).
16. Jacobson PD, Wasserman J. Tobacco control laws: implementation and enforcement. *J Health Politics, Policy, Law* 1999;24:567–98.
17. Zellman GL, Jacobson PD, Bell RM. Influencing physician response to prenatal substance exposure through state legislation and workplace policies. *Addiction* 1997; 92:1123–31.
18. *Lucas v. South Carolina Coastal Council,* 505 U.S. 1003 (1992).

3

Ethics and the Practice of Public Health

PHILLIP NIEBURG, RUTH GAARE BERNHEIM,
AND RICHARD J. BONNIE

> Throughout human history, the major problems of health that men
> have faced have been concerned with community life. . . .
>
> George Rosen[1]

At the heart of public health practice and public health law is the complex relation, recognized throughout human history, between health and community life. The relation is deeply embedded with ethical questions, ranging from the community's role in shaping social norms about health-related behavior to the scope of the community's authority to suppress an individual's risk-taking behavior.

Understanding ethics—the study of what is right and good for humans—is central to understanding the relation between community and health and provides a way to critically evaluate public health policies. One goal of studying ethics is helping public health officials think systematically about reasons or justifications for specific policies or actions; these reasons are generally framed in terms of human welfare and universalizable norms that are explained and specified by particular community values.

Public health decisions usually are made by public officials purporting to act both *for the benefit of* and *on behalf of* the public. Justifications grounded in ethical reasoning are essential for understanding and evaluating public health practice and policies because the concepts of *benefit, harm*, and *risk* are value laden and because appropriately acting *on behalf of* the public requires an interactive process of identifying, interpreting, and informing public values on health and human good.

43

Our goal in this chapter is to familiarize practitioners of public health and public health law with the concepts and terminology of and approaches to public health ethics so that they can better characterize and respond to the ethical questions they encounter in their practices. We hope to thereby facilitate critical reflection on reasons—ethical justifications—for particular decisions and courses of action. We will (1) offer general observations about public health ethics, (2) describe several approaches to common ethical issues that arise in practice, and (3) offer some guidelines or perspectives for reflecting on public health interventions or policies.

PUBLIC HEALTH ETHICS

Exploring the different dimensions of the concept of "public" is helpful to understanding the special relation between public health and ethics. Around 600 BC, Hippocratic writings began to describe the causal connections between the environment and disease, and Greek communities began hiring municipal physicians to manage epidemics and investigate the soil before new colonies were established. Since then, "public" health usually has had at least three dimensions: (1) the "public" as the *population*, which focuses on the health status and characteristics of a particular group of people and its environment; (2) the "public" as *community*, with its unique culture, history, and ethical traditions; and (3) the "public" as *state*, which refers to the legal and governmental structures of the body politic. To this day, public health practitioners continue to work within and integrate all three dimensions of "public" health.

Although science can quantify a population's health and risks and political institutions can provide broad authority for government action, neither answers the two core ethical questions for the "community" and for public health practitioners: (1) When should a community authorize or constrain collective government action on behalf of the population's health? (2) What type of public health interventions ought to be undertaken? Underlying these questions are fundamental issues about the relationships between individuals and the state, the role of experts and scientific information, and the impact of political, economic, and social power.

Law and Ethics in Public Health

Public health law and public health ethics have different starting points for approaching these core questions. *Public health law*, as part of the political structure, examines the legal powers and duties of the state, as well as the limitations on the power of the state to constrain individual interests.[2] *Public health ethics*, grounded in the community, starts with a more basic and expansive question: In light of a community's values, norms, and metaphors, and given the current scientific understanding and contextual features of a particular problem or policy, what ought to be done, "all things considered"?

Although legal considerations are an important aspect of the ethical analysis and provide one source of guidance about the community's moral stance, the law is clearly not the sole source of moral authority. For example, substantive ethical analysis can provide a critique of current law, as well as justification for new or revised laws. In addition, because public health law is often broadly framed, leaving much room for administrative discretion, ethical analysis can help elucidate and interpret applicable law and provide additional justification and legitimacy for public health authority and action in a particular situation where more than one alternative course of action is legally permissible.

Sources for Reflection and Deliberation in Public Health Ethics

In our pluralistic society, where consensus is often lacking on substantive ethical questions, public health ethics often involves balancing or reconciling deeply rooted values. Because ethical reflection on any public policy issue takes place within a particular community with a unique history and culture, the starting point is a consideration of the insights and norms from the common morality, established legal traditions, professional public health practice, and previous public health cases. Because public health ethics focuses on decision-making about real-world cases in public policy, however, insight from other sources must be considered, including the moral claims and concerns of numerous individuals and groups affected by public health policies. In addition, formal ethical theories can provide a useful framework for reflection and conceptual clarity. Influential theories include those that focus on the outcomes of actions (e.g., consequentialism) and others that focus on rights, duties, or other intrinsic moral features of actions (e.g., deontology). Beauchamp and Childress, however, pointed out that individual theories and principles provide only general guides for conduct and that everyday moral reasoning blends "appeals to principles, rules, rights, virtues, passions, analogies, paradigms, narratives and parables."[3] In addition, justification for different policies in our community can change over time as our understanding of scientific, social, and political factors evolves.

Numerous ways exist to approach ethical deliberation. Some people would frame the analysis with a statement of general principles or values that captures the moral concerns at issue in a particular case, then discuss alternative policies in terms of those principles or clusters of values. Others find beginning with analogous cases or policies about which general moral consensus exists more useful, then analyzing the relevant similarities to and differences from the current case. Still another approach identifies the various stakeholders in a particular policy or case, then elucidates and balances the varying moral claims of each stakeholder group. In particular, this stakeholder approach implicitly acknowledges the fundamental partnership of public health professionals with individuals and particular groups in the community in understanding and assessing the value-laden benefits and harms. Although essentially utilitarian, it makes explicit the costs and benefits to different groups and recognizes the complex ongoing nature of the human relationships involved.

All of these approaches ultimately contribute important moral insight and are appropriately integrated into public health policy analysis. For example, public health policies on human immunodeficiency virus (HIV) and acquired immunodeficiency syndrome (AIDS) have been influenced by ethical guidance from numerous sources beyond the traditional ethical analysis that balances population harms and risks with individual liberties (i.e., balancing principles of beneficence and autonomy). Evolving U.S. public health responses were influenced by sources of moral insight such as reflection on personal narratives of those suffering or affected by HIV or those treating HIV-infected patients; assessment of empirical data about social harms such as stigma and discrimination; attention to varying cultural understandings about the meaning and experience of HIV infection, as understood through the use of metaphors in language; consideration of the impact of interventions on relationships, including on community trust; and, finally, public discussion of the perspectives of various stakeholders among people already infected with HIV, those not yet infected but considered "at risk," and other groups in the community.

Roles of Public Health Professionals in Ethical Reflection

Because the community is the source of moral authority and legitimacy for public health decision making, addressing ethical questions in public health requires dialogue, accountability, and transparency with the public. Nagel, for instance, highlighted the need to exercise public authority to reflect the moral understanding of the group in whose name any decision is being taken.[4] He suggests that because moral judgments, unlike scientific judgments, are "everyone's job," people making such judgments should justify and make them available in a way that the public will find persuasive.

Relationship between health professionals and the community

Public health ethics also increasingly acknowledges the partnership between public health professionals and the community in together defining goals and articulating values. This evolution is similar to the evolution in clinical medical ethics that occurred during the last half century, in which the doctrine of informed consent, based on respect for the autonomy of individual patients, established the patient as a partner in defining his or her treatment plan. With its focus on the population, the public health professional's partnership with the community suggests an analogous relationship in which the community takes an active role in defining its public health problems, collecting data and interpreting results, and designing appropriate interventions. This concept is based on respect for the roles of the community and its component individuals in determining values related to their own health, and it grows out of increasing evidence that this partnering process leads to more effective public health interventions.

Relationship between public health lawyers and the community

Public health lawyers can be confronted with ethical dilemmas that result from their dual ethical obligations as attorneys and as employees of a public agency that has as a primary goal improvement of population health outcomes. Although their roles primarily are to interpret law and regulations and to provide guidance on adherence to legal requirements, they may on occasion become aware of highly beneficial polices or actions that have been implemented without adequate legal authority. For example, information may become known to the lawyer that agency funding is supporting a project for which it was not explicitly intended and about which community support is divided. An example might be a community group using local government funds to provide clean syringes and needles to drug users to curb the spread of HIV infection. A decision to act on this information requires complex balancing of the following types of considerations: (1) the lawyer's professional responsibility to ensure that public funds are expended according to law, (2) the lawyer's obligation as a public servant and as a citizen to support policies that enhance the health of the population in general and of a vulnerable subgroup of the population in particular, and (3) the possibility of bringing the agency into compliance with the law without imperiling the continuation of the program. Lawyers working in public service have a complex obligation as trusted agents of the community to help the agency conduct its important mission while also ensuring that the agency operates within the boundaries of its legal authority.

As with other law officers in government, counsel for public health agencies can differ significantly in their conceptions of their role. To put the issue most cleanly: is their job to help the agency implement its policies (i.e., find ways to avoid legal obstacles and develop best possible arguments when the law is in doubt), or is their job to serve as a quasijudicial guardian of the law? In an office where the instrumental conception prevails, lawyers would be inclined to take some legal risks to help the agency accomplish its goals. On the other hand, in an office where the quasijudicial role prevails, lawyers would tend toward more conservative interpretations of legal authority and would not be viewed by their clients as partners in strategic planning. Although neither conception is ethically preferable, individual lawyers may be more comfortable, ethically speaking, in one role or the other. An explicit acknowledgment of the particular role played by the lawyer may provide an important contextual feature for an ethical analysis of what should be done in any given situation.

Public health perspectives and values

In general, public health practitioners tend to refer to and use as guideposts values and perspectives fundamental to contemporary conceptions of public health. These values and perspectives, which must also be reflected in any sensible understanding of the ethical foundations of public health practice, include the following:

1. A *population-based perspective* on preventing harms and promoting benefits, grounded not only in theory but also in the methods of the field (e.g., epidemiology) and the services offered.[2]
2. An *emphasis on prevention*, which is implicit in the Institute of Medicine's description of the mission of public health as "fulfilling society's interest in assuring the conditions for people to be healthy."[5] Also implicit within this description is the concept that primary prevention, that is, preventing the acquisition of disease in individuals or in populations, is preferable to secondary and tertiary prevention, focusing on ameliorating disease impact once disease has occurred, although the importance of providing services and support to persons already affected by disease is also recognized.
3. A *commitment to social justice*, including attention to a fair distribution of benefits and burdens and to the protection of those at greatest risk for harms.[3] This conception of justice acknowledges the public policy constraints on resources.[6]
4. A *commitment to community participation* in public decision making about health as a way of understanding and influencing its health-related collective values. An expanded role for participation by community groups is increasingly recognized in both the policies and ethics of public health. For instance, in 2000, the Institute of Medicine called for partnership in research (i.e., conducted *by* rather than *on* communities) as well as interventions guided by the community's voice.[7] This approach implies that, whenever possible, public health practitioners should facilitate public dialogue intended to elicit and incorporate community values.
5. Recognition of the importance of earning and *sustaining community trust* through transparency, promise keeping, and accountability. Most public health practitioners in the United States are employed by one or another level of government. To the extent that these practitioners function according to rules determined by the organizational guidelines and policies for that level of government, trust in government will be sustained.

Human rights and public health

Certain tensions between individual rights and public health are inescapable. Public health laws sometimes impose burdens on people that they would rather not bear, such as requiring vaccination or the use of protective devices (e.g., helmets or seatbelts). People must sometimes submit to procedures for screening, such as employee drug testing, and public health surveillance systems may compromise individual privacy and lead to discrimination. Despite these tensions, however, human rights and public health are concordant in many important ways. Both human rights and public health are concerned with promoting and protecting human welfare, and both increasingly recognize the vital role that social and environmental conditions play in achieving this goal. As pointed out in a recent World Health Organization publication, "A health and human rights approach can strengthen health systems by recognizing inherent differences among groups within populations and providing the most vulnerable with the tools to participate and claim specific rights."[8]

The complementary and sometimes conflicting ways in which the human rights and public health disciplines view the world have been noted, as has the importance of bridging the differences between the two.[8,9] For example, by putting the individual rather than the collective at the center of health policies or activities, human rights analyses may not always explicitly capture some important collective goals of public health. Nevertheless, human rights concepts do provide an extremely helpful strategy for public health practitioners to consider and use in addressing fundamental determinants of health.

A Guide to Considering the Ethical Issues in Public Health Practice

No simple formulas exist for considering the ethical aspects of newly emerging public health issues (or for rethinking existing problems). Table 3–1 provides a brief framework that can guide practitioners' reflections on the ethical aspects of public health decisions in a way that reduces the chance of omitting a major consideration.

The framework moves sequentially through four steps: (1) assessing the health problem itself and the positions of the various stakeholders, (2) identifying ethical considerations embedded in the problem, (3) identifying and analyzing possible solutions, and (4) evaluating both the process itself and its outcome to help practitioners consider ways to improve current and future practice.

Ethical reflection in public health policy making is not only rigorously analytic but also imaginative. Imagination is helpful for understanding the complex dimensions of a problem from many perspectives (provided by stakeholder approaches); for developing creative partnerships and solutions to issues; and for explaining and justifying policies with rhetorical strategies that build community

TABLE 3–1. A Guide to Framing Ethical Aspects of Public Health Decision Making*

Assessing the Public Health Problem

What is the public health issue of concern? What are the indications for acting? . . . for *not* acting?

What role does the community need to play in assessing this situation? Are issues of collective health interest involved? Have opinions been publicly expressed already? Can more opinions be elicited?

Are commercial interests at stake? Which other groups, organizations, or persons are stakeholders in this issue? What specific issues are at stake for each of them? Is each of these groups aware of the issues at stake for themselves and for the others?

Do any stakeholders have conflicts of interest? Conflicts of obligation?

Do any issues of power exist in the interactions between stakeholders that need to be acknowledged or addressed?

Do relevant laws or regulations exist that help frame or bound the issue?

Identifying and Recognizing Ethical Issues and Considerations

What specific ethical values are involved in the decision(s)? Specifically, what are the harms or burdens and benefits for individuals and harms or burdens and benefits for society?

What are the moral claims of the various stakeholders?

What are other ethically relevant considerations in this situation?

Have similar cases or situations occurred that could serve as precedent? Are these documented in the public health or ethics literature?

Are any institutional policies relevant to the situation?

Do any public health or other professional groups or associations provide guidelines or recommendations on this type of situation?

Identifying Options and Making and Implementing Public Health Decisions

What are the ethically acceptable options for resolution? What are the politically acceptable options?

What ethical justifications can support each option?

What are the appropriate roles for government in resolving this issue?

What are the various roles that the public health practitioner might play in resolution (e.g., teacher, mediator, advocate, policy drafter)?

How can the issue be satisfactorily resolved?

Would a legal opinion be necessary or helpful for moving toward a resolution?

Is an external ethics consultation desirable? If so, how should its role in any resolution be framed? Who should participate in creating that frame?

Later: Evaluating the Resolution(s)

How might the process of coming to the decision have been managed better?

Does the resolution satisfactorily address the problem? If not, why not?

Should the decision now be revisited?

*Adapted from reference 10.

support and trust. In the sections that follow, we describe some cases and approaches to analysis as examples of the kinds of ethical issues likely to be encountered in practice and as examples of useful ways of framing those issues.

COMMON ETHICAL ISSUES IN PUBLIC HEALTH: EVOLVING APPROACHES

Autonomy, Coercion, and Beneficence

Much traditional ethical analysis of public health has focused on coercive or mandatory government action and has typically been framed as a "balancing" of individual rights or interests against potential harms and risks to particular others or to the public in general. Analysis usually focuses on scientific assessment of the severity and type of harm and the degree of risks, as in the claims of individuals for exemption to vaccination requirements or in decisions to quarantine or otherwise detain infectious individuals.

Balancing interests and principles in ethical reflection about public health activities

Beauchamp and Childress[3] have thoroughly described the process of balancing *prima facie* principles or norms that express morally relevant values for a given situation and have cited six conditions necessary to justify infringement of one *prima facie* norm in favor of another in this type of conflict:

1. Better reasons can be offered to act on the overriding norm than on the infringed norm (e.g., if persons have a right, their interests generally deserve a special place when these interests are balanced against the interests of persons without a comparable right).
2. The moral objective justifying infringement must have a realistic prospect of achievement.
3. The infringement is needed because no other morally preferable actions can be substituted.
4. The infringement selected must be the least possible infringement, commensurate with achieving the primary goal of the action.
5. The agent must seek to reduce any negative effects of the infringement.
6. The agent must act impartially; that is, the agent's decision must not be influenced by morally irrelevant information about any party.

MANDATORY HIV TESTING. Beauchamp and Childress[3] also provided a helpful example of conflict between the principles of individual autonomy and beneficence (i.e., in this case, preventing harm to others) in the public debate about mandatory HIV testing in the early response to the HIV epidemic. They reasoned that, although these two *prima facie* principles conflicted, to justify overriding respect for autonomy it was necessary to demonstrate that mandatory testing both (1) was required to prevent harm to others and (2) had a reasonable chance of preventing that harm. They pointed out that, even if mandatory HIV testing could meet these requirements, the testing policy would still need to meet the two other conditions of least infringement (No. 4 above) and reducing negative effects (No. 5 above, i.e., the consequences to individuals from testing). On the basis of this analysis, the authors concluded that most forms of mandatory HIV testing were not justifiable because other approaches would have an equal or greater chance of success with less infringement of autonomy.

COERCION AND THE CONTROL OF URBAN TUBERCULOSIS. During a period of increasing morbidity from tuberculosis (TB) during the early 1990s, New York City updated its health code to facilitate the use of legal action to ensure treatment compliance of TB patients.[11] Briefly, patients who were considered noncompliant with treatment regimens could be issued legal orders requiring directly observed therapy for TB or, if noncompliant with that intervention, requiring mandatory detention in a locked hospital ward. Although TB program goals were met, as measured by the reduction of both new TB disease and drug-resistant TB cases, the program was criticized for two reasons. First, the mandatory detention could be invoked for people who might be "expected" by observers to fail to adhere to less restrictive interventions rather than those documented to have already failed to adhere to the intervention. That is, incarceration was based on perceived noncompliance with a TB treatment regimen rather than on the infectiousness—and thus immediate risk to the public—of TB patients.[12,13] Second, incarceration could continue until the entire treatment course had been completed, even though the period of infectiousness would have ended well before completion of TB treatment.

On the basis of factors described by Beauchamp and Childress[3] and cited earlier, concern about several of the conditions they thought necessary to justify infringement of a *prima facie* norm, in this case the autonomy of TB patients facing incarceration, clearly is at the heart of the expressed criticisms. For example, the possibility of using less restrictive approaches to ensure compliance (No. 4) may not have received sufficient attention, particularly because assessment of future compliance with treatment[12] and future risk to the public from TB patients rendered noninfectious by partial treatment is not an exact science.[13]

PRIVACY IN CONTACT TRACING AND PARTNER NOTIFICATION. In the United States, programs to control sexually transmitted diseases, TB, and selected other infectious diseases that occur in epidemic form (e.g., meningococcal disease) often conduct activities to notify the close contacts of infected persons that they, the contacts, may be at risk for disease by virtue of their exposure to the infected person or to a common source. Elicitation of this contact information is almost always done as a voluntary activity during the process of investigating and treating infected patients themselves. Successfully recruiting the contacts into the public health-care and treatment system depends on contacts' consenting to diagnostic testing or prophylactic treatment, depending on the disease in question. This contact tracing and partner notification activity has become a well-established component of public health, one necessary to accomplish societal disease control goals. However, this activity has sometimes been viewed by members of the public as an invasion of privacy, especially by the infected persons themselves and, perhaps even more important, by the persons whose identities as a contact are revealed by others as part of the public health disease investigation process. This privacy concern of course increases when the disease in question (e.g., HIV or another sexually transmitted infection) involves sexual or other private behaviors or is considered to be stigmatizing.

Conflict Between Beneficence and Non-Maleficence: Childhood Vaccination

Another *prima facie* principle described by Beauchamp and Childress[3] is non-maleficence, defined as refraining from actions that inflict harm. These authors distinguish between beneficence and non-maleficence and, in addition to the direct infliction of harm, include in non-maleficence the concept of not exposing others to *risks* for harm. Having said this, conflicts can occur in public health law and ethics between principles of beneficence and non-maleficence. A clear example of this type of conflict is the issue of laws and regulations requiring vaccination of school children. In this example, the laws are beneficently intended to encourage attainment of societal disease-prevention goals of reducing the morbidity burden associated with these diseases by reducing the number of persons at risk of acquiring and transmitting them. Although most children benefit from this public health policy, a small number suffer serious adverse effects of vaccines during the vaccination process and apparently might have been better off as individuals if not vaccinated.

An ethical analysis of this conflict can begin (but not end) with the idea of *utility*. A utility analysis for the population indicates that the best overall result is clearly achieved by continuing to vaccinate children. That is, many more children are benefitted than harmed by the vaccination process. However, this conflict also allows for an analysis using the somewhat more sophisticated ethical principle of *double effect,* which has been invoked to address the idea that a single act with two outcomes, one bad (maleficent) and one good (beneficent), may be morally acceptable.[3]

Justification for carrying out an act with double effect requires satisfying four conditions:

1. The *nature* of the act: The act itself must be good, or at least morally neutral.

2. The agent's *intention*: A good effect or outcome from the act must be intended.
3. A distinction between *means* and *effects*: The bad effect of the act must *not* be a means to its good effect.
4. *Proportionality* between good and bad effects: The act's good effect must outweigh its bad effect.

Applying these conditions of double effect to mandatory school vaccination laws, we see that (*1*) the vaccination process is good in and of itself, (*2*) a good effect is intended, (*3*) the adverse effect is not required to accomplish the good effect, and, finally, (*4*) at the population level, the disease-prevention effects of childhood vaccination outweigh its adverse effects. As with the utility analysis, this analysis also leads to a conclusion that mandatory vaccination is not morally prohibited even though it may directly result in harms to some persons.

Paternalism, Rights, and Public Health Benefits

Ethical and legal justifications for the state's authority to regulate individual behavior to protect the health of the population are well established. In 1905, the landmark Supreme Court case *Jacobson v. Massachusetts*, expressed the philosophical underpinnings for state collective action in terms of the social compact or covenant, citing the "manifold restraints to which every person is necessarily subject for the common good." Public health authorities historically have justified exerting control over individuals by demonstrating that burdens on individual liberties are outweighed by reasonable evidence of harm or risk of harm, usually from infectious disease, to the health of others.

More controversial, however, are public health interventions aimed at individual behaviors that do not directly or immediately threaten the health of third parties. With increasing evidence that causes of mortality and morbidity in industrialized countries are linked to behavioral and social factors such as smoking, diet, and injuries, some public health interventions, such as motorcycle helmet laws, seek to promote the population's health by reducing the behavioral risks of individuals. Such government regulation often is challenged as paternalistic in that autonomous individuals' known preferences or actions are restricted or overridden not because of a threat to the health of others, but to benefit the very individuals whose preferences or actions are overridden.

Paternalistic interventions are deeply suspect in liberal democracies that greatly value individual rights and liberty. Philosophical support for the anti-paternalism principle is found in John Stuart Mill's argument that society should allow autonomous individuals to live according to their own beliefs, as long as they do not interfere with a like freedom of others or cause significant harm.[14] Public health interventions that benefit those considered unable to decide for themselves, such as children, are universally accepted as a justifiable form of paternalism (usually called "weak" or "soft" paternalism). Public health interventions for the benefit of competent adults, however, such as seatbelt requirements, continue to be debated. Some have argued that these laws represent an example of justified paternalism because they demonstrably enhance individual welfare with only a trivial loss of freedom. Others have argued that these requirements are not really paternalistic at all because they increase net social utility or reduce collective social costs. Costs may include direct costs (e.g., medical costs), indirect costs (e.g., lost productivity or earnings), or emotional costs (e.g., psychological distress of others witnessing individual harm resulting from particular risk-taking behavior).

Other liberty-restricting interventions that produce both individual and collective health benefits, such as water fluoridation, also have been challenged as paternalistic. Whether these interventions actually restrict "liberty" in any meaningful sense can be questioned; but even if we assume that putting fluoride in the water supply restricts the liberty of a person who does not want to consume the fluoride, we can argue that water fluoridation, because it provides the most practical and cost-effective way to achieve legitimate public goals, justifies the burdens imposed on the minority. Justifications for this and similar public health actions have been framed in terms of cost-sharing, collective action, economy of scale, or efficiency.

Benefits and burdens in public health settings in which paternalism is a concern must be balanced against the values of justice and of sustaining trust with members of the community. For example, important considerations sometimes include whether legislation benefits or unduly burdens a vulnerable minority; whether it singles out one risk behavior, such as motorcycling without helmets, and not other similar behaviors, such as bicycling without helmets; whether individuals most affected by the intervention have had sufficient opportunity to voice their concerns; and the potential for unintended consequences and social costs of the intervention, such as stigmatization or discrimination.

Ethical Aspects of Choosing a Policy Instrument

Government public health professionals have many policy instruments available for influencing individual behavior, from education and information management (e.g., health promotion campaigns), to direct regulation (e.g., compulsory screening of newborn infants), to taxation. Public health policy activities can be sorted into six general categories: (1) regulating or otherwise influencing the conditions under which goods or services are available—which encompasses prohibitions as well as various forms of regulated access; (2) regulating the presence of health-enhancing or health-reducing substances or conditions in the physical environment; (3) regulating or otherwise affecting the flow of information and messages relating to health and behavior; (4) prescribing sanctions or loss of privileges to deter undesired behavior and require desired individual behavior; (5) using noncoercive incentives and disincentives for individual behavior—which include taxes and other mechanisms to affect the price of target behaviors; and (6) influencing social norms (including attitudes and beliefs) about health and behavior.[15]

The relevant ethical considerations differ markedly across the categories. The third category, for example, affecting information flow, raises substantial questions about the justifications for suppressing the free flow of information, whereas use of sanctions to coerce compliance accentuates concerns about paternalism and the tensions between public health and individual liberty. Three factors, each of which raises its own ethical concerns, are particularly important for deciding which approach to use when individual rights are implicated: (1) whether the intervention is the least restrictive of individual rights, (2) whether efforts have been made to reduce any negative effects of the infringement, and (3) whether the intervention's burdens do not disproportionately affect a minority or vulnerable population. Aside from tensions between liberty and public health, other prominent ethical concerns relate to the proper thresholds for identifying risks as a matter of public concern in environmental health and safety regulation and the proper scope of public health efforts to shape social norms.

Government public health interventions can include both health education and social marketing campaigns designed to encourage individuals to change health behaviors for their own good and at the same time to encourage a change in the social norms in the population. Smoking, alcohol abuse, drunk driving, and seatbelt use have each been the focus of health promotion campaigns that have led to changing social norms. Although health education programs that communicate factual information about health and behavior are usually justified on the basis that their goal is enhancement of individuals' choices to lead healthier lives, some health promotion and social marketing campaigns that use persuasive strategies to encourage behavior change raise questions about the appropriate role of government in directing social values and individual lifestyles. Faden provided a useful framework for analysis of health promotion campaigns in relation to individuals, distinguishing between persuasion, which includes appeals to reason that enhance the autonomy and decision-making capacity of individuals, and manipulation (both manipulation of information and psychological manipulation), which undermines an individual's capacity for autonomous behavior.[16] Although autonomy-enhancing public health programs seem ethically preferable to interventions that restrict individual liberty, a more complex ethical analysis would be warranted to assess the appropriate role of health campaigns designed to change social values over time. Important considerations would be the degree of community involvement in a decision to focus on certain risk behaviors, the degree of involvement of all stakeholders, the types of information or marketing materials used, and whether persons targeted by the campaign were informed of its goals.

Distribution of Benefits and Burdens—Control of Urban Lead Poisoning

Lead poisoning is a good example of the difficulties involved in balancing benefits and burdens among many stakeholders in public health. In many U.S. urban areas, paint in older houses remains a large and important cause of lead poisoning in young children, a condition that can result in, among other things, permanent neurodevelopmental impairment. Although abatement of this problem by removal of old paint and by other approaches is technically feasible, it is a costly process. Key decisions in the process of preventing urban lead poisoning include which individuals or organizations (e.g., local government, owner, resident, paint company) will pay for lead removal. Lead abatement typifies the challenges of removing old environmental health hazards. These interventions often involve government-mandated measures imposing economic cost on businesses or using public funds to improve the health of subgroups of the population who are often poor. The ethical questions include deciding which individuals and organizations should bear the potentially large costs of lead abatement, the degree to which *public* resources should be allocated to address the issue, and which stakeholders should be involved in decisions about how to intervene. In some cases, local laws requiring paint removal from rental properties by landlords have been passed and implemented. One problem with this solution is that the consequent burdens on landlords can lead them to withdraw from the market in the old city neighborhoods, raising the possibility of reduced availability of affordable housing. This concern shows the need for a communitywide planning process.

This type of public health problem raises complex ethical issues of substantive and procedural justice. For example, recent lawsuits seek damages from companies associated with lead paint manufactured more than 50 years ago. One public comment on this issue questioned the justice involved in attempting to punish paint companies whose current stockholders were unlikely to "have held stock at the time of any improper conduct."[17] A full discussion of the ethics of the use of litigation as a public health tool is beyond the scope of this chapter, but we refer the interested reader to Parmet and Daynard's thorough review of this topic.[18]

THE PUBLIC HEALTH PRACTICE AND POLICY ARC

Consideration of the ethical dimensions of actions (or decisions not to act) by public health practitioners should include an examination of the broad spectrum of these potential actions and decisions as they commonly occur in public health practice. Our goal in this section is to increase awareness of—rather than provide answers to—the relevant issues by considering the steps to contemplating, creating, and evaluating public health interventions.

Recognizing the Existence of a Problem

The involvement of public health practitioners in an actual or perceived public health-related problem or event often begins with a concern about a threat to the community. That initial concern may be based on information from a reportable disease surveillance system, from a disease registry or other data source, or entirely on anecdote. An initial practitioner decision may be how to respond to the potential existence of a problem, at least to the extent of acting—or declining to act—to obtain additional data. The threshold for such recognition can be set in a variety of ways (e.g., statistical, intuitive, supervisor's mandate) and may therefore have one or more ethical components. Alternatively, sometimes a decision to obtain additional information before acting or responding could be perceived as contributing to a delay in implementing an effective response, thus contributing to the occurrence of additional morbidity. Obviously, those who make decisions about the need for additional information should not have any personal conflict of interest that could affect their willingness to acknowledge the problem.

Collecting Additional Information

Assuming a decision is made to obtain more information either to confirm a problem's existence or to better characterize it, additional collection efforts can be undertaken using one or more of several partially overlapping methods (e.g., outbreak investigation, community survey, additional active surveillance activity). Decisions about which individuals or groups should be sources for information or specimens and how the information or specimens will be collected can have ethical dimensions, for example, targeting the information collection effort so that it is representative and fair in terms of distributing the information collection burden and so that any stigma and dignitary harms caused by that collection effort are minimized. The mechanics of obtaining these additional data can also have ethical dimensions in terms of the amount of attention paid to issues of informed consent and to privacy and confidentiality concerns (e.g., considering informed consent issues in outbreak investigation situations; minimizing statistical bias in the information collection process).

Research or practice

Debate is sometimes heard about whether data-collection aspects of surveillance, outbreak investigations, health services research, program evaluation, or other standardized information-collection activities carried out by local, state, or federal public health authorities represent research or public health practice. If considered research, such activities fall under the U.S. Code of Federal Regulations (45 C.F.R. 46), which guides research ethics and thus requires the involvement of the institutional review board (IRB) process. If considered practice (i.e., nonresearch), these activities do not fall under the extant federal research regulations.

This difference in labeling an activity as research or nonresearch may be less important from an ethical perspective than from an administrative one. When the issue under consideration is the type and amount of ethical review a government data collection activity should undergo, we consider the most important question to be whether significant risk related to that activity exists for members of the public. At the outset of any such activity, the risk issue should be explicitly addressed by a responsible individual or group. A determination of "no significant risk" should be documented in some accountable way. If risk (e.g., to privacy, to confidentiality, to dignity) is—or might be—involved, then a more thorough review of risks and benefits should be conducted by a publicly accountable group or individual, even if no IRB involvement is formally required. Which groups or individuals conduct that review may become relevant.

Specific ethical issues in legally sanctioned disease surveillance and outbreak investigations

Surveillance for diseases for which reporting is mandated by law and investigation by competent government authorities of outbreaks of diseases of public health importance are activities for which individual consent is not explicitly required. However, the nonconsual nature of these data-collection processes means that attention to privacy and confidentiality concerns should be paramount in the data and specimen-collection and storage processes. In addition, any invasion of privacy can be minimized—and more easily justified—by collecting only the identifying information clearly needed for subsequent disease-control efforts and by removing identifying information from data and specimens once the information is no longer useful.

Privacy and confidentiality, although partially overlapping concepts, are not identical.[3] *Privacy* refers to the individual's interest in limiting access to his or her body (or to specimens) or to personal information. *Confidentiality,* which sometimes is considered a subset of privacy, refers to the *redisclosure* of private information originally disclosed to others in a confidential (e.g., patient–doctor) relationship.

Outbreak investigations may be ethically complicated for other reasons. For example, some public health practitioners consider epidemic illness of uncertain origin in members of the public as sufficient justification for expecting the cooperation of ill people (or the cooperation of family members) in outbreak investigations without having to conduct formal and explicit informed consent procedures. However, that rationale becomes less helpful when persons not directly affected by disease are involved in outbreak investigations. For example, the justification for not routinely obtaining standard explicit informed consent from persons serving as uninfected controls (e.g., randomly selected, unaffected neighbors or co-workers) in outbreak-related case-control studies is a more complex informed consent issue.

Analyzing and Presenting Information

Analysis and presentation of the additional collected information may be straightforward but also may have subtle ethical dimensions. For example, how rigidly or loosely a statistical threshold is set for determining a problem ($p < 0.05$? $p < 0.001$?, $p < 0.10$?) can determine whether a problem's existence is identified or missed. How information in a written or oral report is framed or portrayed can determine whether the report's conclusions about a disease or its risk factors will stigmatize certain individuals or groups. Whether reports reach in a timely fashion the representatives of groups contributing information to the data collection process can have an impact on subsequent levels of trust by affected communities.

Formulating a Response or Intervention

Once the existence of a problem is confirmed or at least strongly suspected, a response is likely to be contemplated. An appropriate public health response can take many forms and have several ethical dimensions. For example, the New York City TB situation described earlier involved a decision about whether the response should be the more traditional health promotion role or should involve the government's health protection role—in that case, the use of public health's police powers. Resource allocation decisions provide other potential problems. The principle of justice requires either that intervention programs allocate resources to ensure sufficient coverage of vulnerable populations or, if sufficient resources are not available for complete coverage, that they create and maintain an equitable and transparent system for rationing resources.

Evaluating the Public Health Response

As with other individuals directing the use of public resources, public health practitioners are obligated to ensure through informal or formal evaluation the effective and efficient use of resources.[5] Enough new information about subsequent disease occurrence must be collected after an intervention is applied to document accomplishment of these goals or to indicate how an intervention could be improved to accomplish them. Information collection may take the same form as the original data-collection process (and involve similar ethical concerns), or, as sometimes happens, a specific program evaluation effort can occur.

Often, these evaluation activities must take place without specific informed consent for each data extraction step. In fact, in many settings such as evaluation of quality of health services, the routine obtaining of informed consent is considered infeasible. Despite the absence of a formal individualized consent process, however, privacy and confidentiality issues still are likely to be of some concern to persons whose information is being used, and evaluation activities should be conducted with such concerns in mind. Such program evaluation activities sometimes offer the possibility of removing identifying information from data files before or as they are extracted for evaluation. In any case, the minimum amount of identifying information should be obtained, and the identifying information obtained should be removed at the earliest possible moment.

CONCLUSION

Although concerns about balancing benefits and burdens between communities and individuals have been expressed throughout recorded history, public health ethics per se is a new and evolving focus. Current discussion in the field focuses on the ways in which discourse and reflection about ethics can be incorporated into public health education and public health practice (e.g., whether a formal code of ethics should be created to guide the actions of practitioners). Heightened awareness of principles, precedent-setting cases, and stakeholder claims will enrich public health practice so that practitioners and officials can continue to give thoughtful attention to moral, as well as to scientific and political, justifications for public health activities.

References

1. Rosen G. The origins of public health. In: *A History of Public Health.* Expanded edition. Baltimore: Johns Hopkins University Press, 1993: pp. 1–5.
2. Gostin L. A theory and definition of public health law. In: *Public Health Law: Power, Duty, Restraint.* Berkeley: University of California Press, 2000: pp. 1–22.
3. Beauchamp TL, Childress JF. *Principles of Biomedical Ethics,* 5th ed. Oxford: Oxford University Press, 2001.
4. Nagel T. Moral epistemology. In: Bulger RE, Fineberg HV, eds. *Society's Choices: Social and Ethical Decision Making in Biomedicine.* Washington, DC: National Academy Press, 1995: pp. 201–14.
5. Institute of Medicine. Summary. In: *The Future of Public Health.* Washington, DC: National Academy Press, 1988: pp. 1–18.
6. Lamm RO. Redrawing the ethics map. *Hastings Center Rep* 1999; pp. 29:28–9.

 7. Institute of Medicine. *Promoting Health: Intervention Strategies from Social and Behavioral Research.* Washington, DC: National Academy Press, 2000.
 8. World Health Organization. *A Human Rights Approach to TB: Stop TB Guidelines for Social Mobilization.* Geneva: World Health Organization, 2001.
 9. International Federation of Red Cross and Red Crescent Societies, Francois-Xavier Bagnoud Center for Health and Human Rights. Human rights: an introduction. In: Mann JM, Gruskin S, Grodin MA, Annas GJ, eds. *Health and Human Rights: A Reader.* New York: Routledge, 1999: pp. 21–8.
10. Miller FG, Fletcher JC, Fins JJ. Clinical pragmatism: a case method of moral problem solving. In: Fletcher J, Lombardo P, Marshall MF, Miller F, eds. *Introduction to Clinical Ethics.* 2nd ed. Hagerstown, MD: University Publishing Group, 1997: pp. 21–38.
11. Gasner MR, Maw KL, Feldman GE, et al. The use of legal action in New York City to ensure treatment of tuberculosis. *N Engl J Med* 1999;340:359–66.
12. Campion EW. Liberty and the control of tuberculosis. *N Engl J Med* 1999;340:385–6.
13. Coker R. Tuberculosis, non-compliance and detention for the public health. *J Med Ethics* 2000;26:157–9.
14. Mill JS. "On Liberty," chs 1 and 3. In: *Collected Works of John Stuart Mill.* Toronto: University of Toronto Press, 1977.
15. Bonnie RJ. The efficacy of law as a paternalistic instrument. In: Melton GB, ed. *The Law as a Behavioral Instrument.* Lincoln: University of Nebraska Press, 1985: pp. 131–211.
16. Faden RR. Ethical issues in government-sponsored public health campaigns. *Health Educ Q* 1987;14:27–37.
17. Rodberg S. Lead paint as a public nuisance. *Am Prospect* 2001;12:11.
18. Parmet WE, Daynard RA. The new public health litigation. *Annu Rev Public Health* 2000;21:437–54.

4

Criminal Law and Public Health Practice

ZITA LAZZARINI, SARAH SCOTT, AND
JAMES W. BUEHLER

This chapter introduces the unique characteristics of criminal law, provides a broad overview of the many substantive areas in which criminal law and public health law interact, and discusses in depth three specific areas: use of public health research and investigation techniques that can characterize crimes that are subsequently prosecuted by the criminal justice system; criminalization of exposure to or transmission of communicable diseases; and the role of the local medical examiner's (ME's) office in both public health and the administration of criminal justice.

Definitions and Goals

A good legal definition of a *crime* is "an act performed in violation of duties that an individual owes to the community. It includes both harmful conduct (*actus reus*) and a culpable state of mind (*mens rea*)."[1] *Public health* can be defined as "what we, as a society, do to create the conditions in which people can be healthy."[2]

Broadly defined, the goal of the public health system is to protect the public health. Specifically, this emphasizes an approach to preventing disease and promoting health for the entire population of a specified area rather than for a single patient, as in traditional medicine. A good public health system includes methods for identifying patterns and sources of disease, assessing risk for disease, adopting the most appropriate measures to prevent and control disease, promoting healthy behaviors for individual members of society, and educating the public and policy makers about health risks and health benefits.

The goals of the criminal justice system are to protect the public safety and welfare through preventing, detecting, investigating, and prosecuting crime. Criminal prosecution and its sanctions aim to punish violators, deter future crime, and impose a measure of retribution against the offender on behalf of society that is roughly commensurate with the perceived seriousness of the crime.

Society, through its lawmakers, has determined that some behavior with public health implications is so dangerous that it merits criminal sanctions. At times, health officials support such sanctions; in other situations, they may prefer noncriminal solutions. Public health officials may be able to harness aspects of the criminal justice system to achieve public health goals. Similarly, scientific techniques used in public health investigations and cutting edge scientific knowledge can also be used in the criminal justice system. Although the objectives of public health and criminal justice overlap in significant ways, efforts to use the criminal justice system as part of public health efforts may have unintended or contradictory effects, and use of techniques developed for population-level health studies may require special oversight and privacy guarantees when applied in the criminal justice system.

Differences and Similarities

Both criminal law and public health provisions derive their authority from related duties of government. Public health authorities must protect the public's health and welfare, while law enforcement seeks to protect the peace, welfare, and morals of society. The *police power*, defined as the residual power held by the states to make legislation and regulations to protect the public health, welfare, and morals and to promote the common good, underpins both public health and criminal provisions. Moreover, enforcement of public health measures and transgressions of the criminal law often involve the same mechanisms and even common sanctions.

The sources of criminal law and public health law can differ. Most public health law is articulated in statutes (adopted by the legislature) and regulations (promulgated by state or federal agencies on the basis of the authority of the executive). Courts review and interpret public health-related legislation and produce "case law"—bodies of legal opinions that guide the application of the law. Criminal law is also codified in statutes and regulations. Criminal law (and to a lesser degree public health law) also owes much of its basic structure to the "common law"—judge-made law that is modified case-by-case over generations.

For example, most jurisdictions now have statutes defining the varying degrees of homicide, assault, battery, and burglary. However, most of these distinctions are closely tied to generations of common law decisions in which judges defined and distinguished the elements of the different crimes and the types of intent required for conviction. In public health, the common law roots are more deeply buried, but familiar public health concepts such as "nuisance" have common law origins.[3]

Finally, although public health law and criminal law begin with the same source of government power and similar duties, their articulated goals diverge in important ways. Both try to protect the public's health and welfare. Criminal law, however, also explicitly seeks to punish and exact retribution for wrongs done to society.[1,4] Public health and criminal law share similar roots of authority, yet criminal law retains distinguishing characteristics with which public health practitioners should be familiar.

Power of the state

In a criminal prosecution, the government's interest is usually represented by a prosecutor who argues the case on behalf of the people of the state or commonwealth. The prosecutor implements government intent expressed in particular criminal laws by seeking sanctions against a defendant accused of violating that law. The defendant (usually a person, although in some instances an incorporated entity may be criminally charged) is represented by his or her own attorney. The fact that the government has permanent staff to investigate and prosecute violations of criminal law and has regularly budgeted funds from the taxpayers to carry out these prosecutions highlights an important aspect of criminal law—the potential imbalance of power between the two sides. On one side of the case, the state has substantial resources to pursue a conviction against an individual. On the other side, the defendant, an individual, may lack education, sophistication, or even a thorough understanding or the ability to gain a thorough understanding of the issue being litigated and usually cannot match the government's extensive resources.

The public health arena usually lacks the overt drama of the courtroom (except in rare occurrences of epidemic disease), yet the power of public health authorities also extends deeply into individuals' lives through regulation of a wide range of commercial, personal, and daily activities. Although rarely used, the coercive powers of public health can be as drastic as depriving individuals of liberty. Less intrusive actions on behalf of public health can still have weighty consequences. Public health authorities can condemn property; regulate access to food and medicines; restrict the import and export of products; and control the flow of intensely sensitive personal information. None of these powers should be taken lightly, and the potential impact of each on individuals can have long-term consequences, as can involvement with the criminal justice system.

Due process

Offsetting the power of the government against a criminal defendant is a series of important rights that attach to a prosecution. Many of the rights are derived from interpretations of the U.S. Constitution. Both the Fifth and Fourteenth Amendments to the U.S. Constitution guarantee due process when an individual is to be deprived of his or her liberty or property. Due process in criminal cases guarantees clear notice of the charges brought against a defendant, the presumption of innocence until guilt is proven beyond a reasonable doubt, a right to a hearing, the opportunity to present evidence and to cross-examine witnesses at that hearing, the right to appeal the decision on the basis of an accurate written record, and the critical right to the appointment of counsel for defendants who cannot afford one.

In public health, due process rights also apply to any person whose liberty or property rights are threatened by public health actions. Where public health authorities seek to deprive individuals of liberty (e.g., confinement for disease control or civil commitment), due process guarantees protections similar to those in criminal prosecutions. For lesser intrusions on rights (e.g., disease surveillance, mandatory physical examinations, or testing), courts have interpreted the Fifth and Fourteenth Amendments as demanding fewer procedural protections. In determining what degree of protection accrues in individual cases of public health action, courts will consider (*1*) the nature of the interest or liberty subject to limitation, (*2*) the risk for erroneous decision-making, and (*3*) the fiscal and administrative burdens of applying additional procedural protections.[5] Overall, courts will impose much more extensive protections when the right or interest involved is important, the risk for erroneous deprivation of the right is real and substantial, and the burdens of providing that protection are not disproportionate to the benefits.

Burden of proof

"Burden of proof" refers to the allocation of responsibility to demonstrate that a matter alleged in a court is factually true and to the level of confidence in the allegation required in that particular setting (sometimes also called "standard of proof"). Generally, the prosecution (in criminal cases) or the plaintiff (in civil cases) bears the burden of proof for all the major elements of a case. For example, to convict a defendant of violating a law against exposure or transmission of human immunodeficiency virus (HIV) infection, the prosecution (under most statutes) would have to prove that (*1*) the defendant knew he or she was HIV infected and (*2*) he or she knowingly exposed another person through sexual intercourse, sharing of injection equipment, or other behavior prohibited in the statute. Without the prosecution's proof, the defendant does *not* have to prove his or her innocence, although he or she would clearly want to refute any prosecution evidence of the key elements.

In contrast to civil law (dealt with elsewhere in this book and including torts, contracts, and property law), criminal law demands the highest standard of proof for conviction before punishment can be imposed—proof of guilt of violating the law "beyond a reasonable doubt." In general, public health proceedings require findings to be based only on a "a preponderance of the evidence," meaning that the evidence presented indicates that an event most likely occurred or a fact is most likely true. When, however, public health authorities seek to confine an individual who poses a danger to the public health (such as to isolate a person with infectious tuberculosis [TB]) or seek to impose other significant burdens on individual liberties (such as court-ordered directly observed therapy [DOT]), due process demands that the findings be based on "clear and convincing evidence"—a higher standard than preponderance of the evidence but somewhat less stringent than "beyond a reasonable doubt."[6,7]

Some legal authorities have endeavored to assign numerical values to the different standards of proof with varying degrees of success. The easiest standard to translate into numerical probabilities is "by a preponderance," which is widely agreed to mean a probability of greater than 50% ($p > 0.50$) that the facts, as asserted by the public health authorities, are true. Assigning probabilities to "clear and convincing evidence" and to "beyond a reasonable doubt" is more problematic.[8] In fact, one state supreme court reversed a lower court ruling where the trial court had instructed the jury that "beyond a reasonable doubt" was about "seven and a half" on a scale of one to 10 ($p > 0.75$). The Nevada Supreme Court held that "reasonable" is an inherently qualitative concept and should not be reduced to numbers.[9]

Penalties

Violations of the public health code (i.e., specific orders of a commissioner of health or of a local board of health) may be punishable as a misdemeanor. Traditionally, misdemeanors were punishable by a fine of up to $500, imprisonment for up to 1 year in the county jail, or both. Specific other public health measures may also indicate that a violation is a misdemeanor.[10] Violations of public health regulations and public health-related offenses, such as violating environmental regulations or breaching mandated confidentiality, may also be felonies, which traditionally are punishable by a prison term of 1 year or longer and higher fines. A felony conviction will result in more serious and long-term significance for the record of the defendant.

Many public health-related misdemeanors and felonies are codified in statewide public health statutes or local health codes. However, a state penal code itself may contain miscellaneous specific provisions that reflect public health goals, including laws punishing intentional exposure to or transmission of a particular disease, child abuse and neglect provisions, and drug-control laws (Table 4–1).

Administrative courts and criminal law

In more populous jurisdictions, administrative courts or other civil tribunals may adjudicate less serious violations of the local health code or other local public health measures. These courts hear less serious violations that tend to occur frequently and require regular imposition of fines or abatement orders to maintain the public safety or health. The New York City Health Code, for instance, allows closure of buildings that pose a condition dangerous to life or health (New York City Administrative Code, sections 17-142–17-159, concerning a public nuisance). The New York Board of Health, an appointed administrative body, hears many of these cases and assesses penalties for nuisances and can order closure of buildings. Although administrative law courts are often characterized as a lower form of proceeding than ordinary civil courts, these administrative bodies can have enormous powers in imposing sanctions (i.e., closing an establishment harmful to the public health) or ordering abatement measures (i.e., draining standing water that can harbor mosquitos and clearing away debris that attract vermin).

An excellent illustration of the congruence of civil, criminal, and administrative law is provided by comparing and contrasting the administrative procedures for handling unhealthy conditions in housing under the New York City Health Code and the more formal civil procedures for handling public safety nuisances in housing that can also affect the public health. The New York City Administrative Code allows closure of housing if residents have been convicted of prostitution two or more times; have conducted an unlicensed business in the building; have violated alcoholic beverage–control laws; or have been convicted of three or more violations of drug-control laws; or if the condition of the housing is "inimical to the public health," as defined by the New York City Health Code. (sections 7-701–7-714). Under these procedures, an attorney acting on behalf of the City of New York must obtain an injunction in civil court to close the building. Obviously, in this scheme, a record of *criminal* convictions in the areas of prostitution or violations of the drug-control laws help establish a civil *prima facie* case (i.e., "the plaintiff's production of enough evidence to allow the fact-trier to infer the fact at issue and rule in the plaintiff's favor") for closing housing.[11]

Whether a case is prosecuted criminally or handled in a regular civil or an administrative court depends on how the state and locality have defined jurisdiction for their courts. The person framing the case, whether a civil lawyer or a prosecutor, will have in mind the most important sanction (e.g., closure, fine, imprisonment) and will most likely steer the case into the forum that can most efficiently impose that sanction. Civil law sets the range of fines that each level of court can assess, and civil law will delineate the forms of relief in the civil

TABLE 4–1. Examples of State Public Health Provisions with Criminal Penalties and Criminal Provisions Related to Public Health Problems

PUBLIC HEALTH PROBLEM	PENAL CODE SECTION	PUBLIC HEALTH CODE	GENERAL STATUTE	PENALTY OR LEVEL OF OFFENSE
Preventing alcohol sales to minors			Conn. Gen. Stat 30–86: Prohibits sales of alcohol to minors	Fine of not more than $1500 or imprisonment up to 18 months or both
Preventing tobacco sales to minors	Cal Pen Code 308: Prohibits sale of tobacco or smoking paraphernalia to minors, permits criminal or civil action			Criminal action: Misdemeanor Civil action: First offense, $200; second, $500; third, $1000
Control of paraphernalia used to inject illegal drugs			M.G.L.A. (Mass.) 94C 27: Requires a prescription for purchasing or possessing syringes	M.G.L.A. 94 C 38: First offense punishable by imprisonment for not more than 1 year or by a fine up to $1000 or both. Second offense punishable by imprisonment for 2 years or fine up to $2000 or both
Reducing tobacco consumption by taxing tobacco			Conn. Gen. Stat 12–330f: Prohibits manufacturing, acquiring, possessing, or selling tobacco and tobacco products where no tax has been paid	Fine of $500, imprisonment for 3 months, or both

(continued)

TABLE 4-1. Examples of State Public Health Provisions with Criminal Penalties and Criminal Provisions Related to Public Health Problems—Continued

PUBLIC HEALTH PROBLEM	PENAL CODE SECTION	PUBLIC HEALTH CODE	GENERAL STATUTE	PENALTY OR LEVEL OF OFFENSE
Reducing drunk driving			Cal Veh Code § 23550: Enhances penalties for multiple offenses of driving under the influence of drugs or alcohol	Imprisonment for 180 days to 1 year and fine of $390 to $1000
Child abuse and neglect	NY Penal Law 260.10: Criminalizes endangering the welfare of a child			Class A misdemeanor
Control of paraphernalia related to drug use	NY Penal Law 220.45: Criminalizes possessing a hypodermic instrument	NY Public Health Law 3381: Requires prescription for sale and possession of hypodermic needles		Class A misdemeanor
Sale and distribution of adulterated food		410 ILCS 620/3.1: Illinois public health statute prevents sale of adulterated or misbranded food and cosmetics	Florida 500.04	(Florida) 500.121: The Department of Public Health can impose fines up to $5,000 for violation and suspension and revocation of permits (Illinois) 410 ILCS 605/3: Class A misdemeanor.

Transmission of HIV by persons who know they are infected	ILCS 5/12/16.2: Criminal transmission of HIV: Prohibits many specific acts that could expose anther to HIV	Class B felony
Confidentiality of medical records and public health information	Arkansas Code Ann. 20-7-307	Misdemeanor punishable by a fine or by imprisonment
Improper disposal or use of hazardous waste	415 ILCS 5/44: Environmental Protection Act	Level of offense depends on category of criminal act (misdemeanor to felony)
Case investigations of sexually transmissible diseases (including HIV), need to protect confidentiality of contact information	410 ILCS 325/5.5: Authorizes the Department of Public Health to investigate risks for transmission of HIV and to notify contacts of the risk when the situation warrants	Section(d) establishes a confidentiality of information requirement. Violation of confidentiality is a Class A misdemeanor

and administrative courts in terms of compelling or prohibiting actions that affect the public health.

OVERVIEW: HOW CRIMINAL LAW IS RELEVANT TO PUBLIC HEALTH PRACTICE

Although this chapter cannot describe in detail all the nuances of criminal law and public health interaction, this section aims to give a brief overview of the intersection of the two disciplines in many areas. The following section describes several such areas in greater detail.

Scientific Methods Used by Both Public Health and Criminal Investigations

Public health authorities and criminal investigators can use many scientific techniques—from basic epidemiology to increasingly sophisticated genetic analyses. For example, genetic analyses are used in public health investigations to track the spread of specific strains of infectious diseases (e.g., different strains of *Mycobacterium tuberculosis,* hepatitis virus, or HIV), while criminal investigators use similar molecular biology techniques to include or exclude individuals as suspects in a case where biologic evidence has been collected. Whether a particular laboratory test is used as a part of an epidemiologic study, individual patient care, or a criminal investigation, adherence to proper technique in collecting, transferring, processing, and reporting results is essential. The consequences of the same test can vary profoundly depending on the context in which it is used, and different safeguards may be appropriate under different circumstances. For example, in a broad, population-level assessment of the prevalence of a specific gene or strain of infection in a specific population, maintaining an accurate link to the identity of the individual from whom the biologic sample was taken may not be necessary. In fact, it may be undesirable or even prohibited by research protocol or by law. In contrast, if the results of a laboratory test will be used to implicate a person in a criminal investigation, then everyone handling the sample must be able to demonstrate that it is, and has been, identified as coming from the person in question to be admissible and probative in court. This is known as "maintaining the chain of custody" of the evidence.

Criminal Law Theories in Relation to Public Health Goals

Law plays many roles in public health practice. Law expresses the mission or agenda of public health agencies, and although it provides authority for action, it also sets limits on that authority. The law can act as a direct tool of disease and injury prevention and health promotion. The law can also educate the public and policy makers about important public health issues.[5] Criminal sanctions in public health are usually intended as a tool to change or avoid unhealthy behavior. To a lesser degree, such laws function as a means to educate the citizenry of the parameters of acceptable behavior. At least two theories about how criminal law can change individuals' behavior are worth mentioning: deterrence and norm setting.

The theory of deterrence suggests that people obey the law primarily because they fear they will be caught and punished.[12,13] For example, deterrence supposes that persons who otherwise would not wear motorcycle helmets (and, in fact, still think it is "cool" not to wear one) will change their behavior to avoid an expensive ticket. The theory that law sets or reflects community norms suggests, instead, that individuals obey the law because the law has influenced or reflects what they and their peers believe is "right," regardless of the availability or likelihood of punishment.[14,15] In practice, norm setting suggests that where most members of a community believe that driving drunk is wrong, most will obey the law against driving under the influence regardless of the likelihood of being caught or punished. In reality, both motivations probably influence individual behavior, and people may obey or disobey different laws for different reasons, or they may be motivated by a combination of fear of punishment and a desire to be seen as "normal" or "upstanding" by adhering to community norms. It cannot be ignored that the citizens' perceptions of reasonableness or their grasp of the importance of the law at issue affects their motivation and behavior. The degree to which law affects behavior becomes important when we look more closely at specific kinds of criminal laws and the behavior they seek to prevent or change.

Public health practitioners should be aware of the wide variety of public health laws that potentially invoke criminal penalties. These include laws that specifically criminalize behavior that endangers the public health (e.g., sexual exposure or transmission laws), health and safety code requirements that carry criminal penalties for violations, and laws that directly target unhealthy individual behavior. For example, one powerful way that occupational safety and health codes are enforced is through prosecution of violators for criminal misconduct.[16,17] Health and safety regulations aimed at the general public may also carry criminal penalties such as New York City's regulations mandating window guards on all upper-story residences occupied by children (Section 17-123[d] of the New York City Administrative Code). Laws with public health objectives that carry criminal penalties include provisions mandating the use of protective devices such as child safety seats in cars, seatbelts, and bicycle and motorcycle helmets; prohibitions of the sale of tobacco or alcohol to minors; and restrictions on the time and place of alcohol sales to adults (Table 4–1).

Public Health-Related Activities Within the Criminal Justice System

The United States incarcerates a higher proportion of its population than does any other western democracy. An estimated 2.8% of the adult U.S. population is incarcerated or under court supervision at any one time.[18] Prison and jail populations have doubled and even quadrupled during the past 20 years in many places, in large part because of increased arrest and incarceration of persons accused of drug-related offenses (percent of federal prisoners sentenced for drug offenses, 1970: 16.3%; 1980: 25.6%; 1990: 52.2%; 2000: 56.9%).[19] Minorities are disproportionately likely to be arrested and incarcerated in most state and the federal prison systems.[20,21] Women and juveniles tried as adults are the fastest growing segments of the correctional population.[22]

Prisoners generally have more health problems than nonincarcerated people. Rates of TB, HIV infection, hepatitis, and mental illness are many times higher among incarcerated than nonincarcerated individuals, with HIV infection rates 12 to 17 times higher in prisons and jails.[23] The high number of women in prisons means increased need for basic and specialized gynecologic, obstetric, and pediatric care in correctional facilities. Prison health problems are public health problems not only because of the high prevalence of communicable diseases traditionally associated with public health but also because prisoners disproportionately represent populations underserved by health services. Incarceration provides one opportunity to use public health interventions to improve health and, by extension, the health of the communities to which they belong. Almost 500,000 prisoners are released from state and federal prisons each year, and many more are discharged from city and county jails.[24] Failure to address their health needs is a lost opportunity for improving public health.[25,26]

Efforts to address health problems in correctional institutions take many forms. In some jurisdictions, efforts to prevent transmission of communicable diseases during incarceration have led to mandatory testing of detainees or inmates for TB, sexually transmitted diseases (STDs), and HIV infection. In some situations, such as in the control of TB in New York City, the introduction of comprehensive testing and treatment programs was driven by lawsuits against the correctional system on behalf of those incarcerated. In contrast, mandatory HIV testing in some systems was opposed by prisoner advocates, while other groups of prisoners went to court seeking testing and segregation of infected prisoners.[25]

Public health programs often target groups deemed to be at high risk for specific health problems. Approaches that involve education, voluntary testing, assurances of confidentiality, and offers of treatment change profoundly when focus shifts from nonincarcerated to incarcerated populations. For example, the prison setting may make it impossible for health officials to protect confidentiality to the degree possible in the community. Prison regulations may mandate reporting of certain information to authorities, and prisons themselves are closed societies in which information about who receives medical care, who takes medicine, and who attends special programs often becomes common knowledge. When voluntary measures become mandatory for a prison health program, the additional emphasis on imposing control on the individual raises the question of whether the focus on control is primarily to meet public health or correctional goals.

Coercive laws have both beneficial and harmful effects. For example, many states' statutes permit testing of criminal defendants for HIV in sexual assault cases before or after conviction. When this information is used to provide data about risk for infection to survivors of sexual assault, it can serve important individual and public health purposes, allowing for informed decisions about the use of postexposure prophylaxis and for education to reduce the risk for transmission to partners of the survivor.[27] When, however, it becomes part of the case against the accused, numerous opportunities exist for prejudice to be expressed overtly or covertly by judges, prosecutors, and juries.

Increasingly, as discussed above, advances in molecular biology are also being used in criminal cases. DNA testing of biologic evidence to support claims of guilt or innocence of a specific defendant are becoming widespread. Every state in the United States has some form of a "DNA data-banking" law, mandating that a biologic sample be obtained from prisoners convicted of specific felonies, which vary from state to state. The convicted offender's sample is analyzed and the results entered into a data bank for future reference. From a public health perspective, use of such banked information to rapidly identify repeat violent offenders could reduce the incidence of future violence.

The vast majority of U.S. courts will admit evidence obtained by standard molecular biology techniques. The use of molecular biology in this context is commonly referred to as "DNA evidence" or "DNA testing." Many prisoner advocates argue that failure to permit or require testing where biologic evidence exists but has not been previously analyzed or used may result in the frequent miscarriage of justice and even the execution of innocent individuals.[28,29] Other proposals, however, create different concerns. For example, should law enforcement agencies be allowed to conduct nationwide efforts to match evidence obtained from a crime scene against all stored and tested DNA samples to identify suspects in a case? These samples could include those obtained by the military, in prisons, or by other law enforcement agencies or samples that an individual has given to exclude himself or herself from suspicion of another crime. Use of molecular biology techniques of identification combined with personal information that may have been collected for noncriminal justice purposes raises significant privacy concerns and deserves careful scrutiny to ensure that Constitutional rights are protected.

Laws that Act as Barriers to Public Health Practices

Sometimes lawmakers enact laws to address public health or criminal justice problems that eventually become barriers to effective public health efforts as circumstances change. In the course of the epidemic of HIV infection and acquired immunodeficiency syndrome (AIDS), two areas of policy and practice emerged that illustrate this dilemma: laws governing access to sterile syringes and needles and police practices and policies concerning condoms.

In the early 1990s, virtually all states had in place drug paraphernalia laws that criminalized the sale, purchase, and possession of syringes with the intent to use them to inject or ingest illegal drugs. A smaller number of states also had specific laws that required a valid physician's prescription for all sales of syringes and needles. An intermediate number of states had pharmacy regulations that discouraged the sale of syringes to persons without a valid medical purpose. These provisions had been adopted in response to earlier "epidemics" of drug use, specifically the 1960s and 1970s (drug paraphernalia laws) and the early 1990s (syringe prescription laws).[30] Beginning in the late 1980s, numerous studies indicated that the re-use of contaminated syringes by injection drug users (IDUs) contributed significantly to the spread HIV, hepatitis B and hepatitis C, and other bloodborne diseases. Injection drug users use contaminated injection equipment in part because of the scarcity of sterile syringes created by the criminal provisions described above. In 1995, a scientific panel of the National Academy of Sciences, Institute of Medicine, concluded that legal barriers to purchase and possession of syringes were contributing to epidemics of bloodborne disease and should be rescinded.[31]

The original laws sought to discourage drug use by making syringes more difficult to obtain. This created a dilemma for policy makers who then faced a new, yet pressing, public health crisis: how to prevent the spread of HIV and other bloodborne diseases. Many federal (Centers for Disease Control and Prevention [CDC], Health Resources and Services Administration, National Institute on Drug Abuse, Substance Abuse and Mental Health Services Administration), national (American Medical Association), public health (Association of Sate and Territorial Health Officers, National Alliance of State and Territorial AIDS Directors), legal (American Bar Association), pharmaceutical (American Pharmaceutical Association), and pharmacy (National Association of Boards of Pharmacy) groups and agencies have issued recommendations emphasizing the need for access to sterile syringes for IDUs who continue to inject drugs.[32,33] The prohibition on use of federal funds to support syringe-exchange programs remains in place, and most states still criminalize sale or possession of syringes for use with illegal drugs. At the same time, however, state, local, and private organizations continue to support syringe exchanges in all major cities and in many localities. In addition, several states have deregulated the sale of syringes (Connecticut, Maine, New York, New Hampshire, Rhode Island) or removed them from the definition of prohibited paraphernalia (Oregon, Wisconsin).[30,34]

Prostitution (i.e., "sex work") remains illegal in 49 of 50 states, and those engaged in such work have often been targets of coercive public health and law enforcement activities.[35] Policy and practices originally meant to discourage sex work can directly interfere with HIV prevention efforts. For example, the practice of some police departments of seizing and destroying condoms found on persons suspected of commercial sex activity or using possession of condoms as probable cause to arrest individuals on related charges effectively discourages sex workers from possessing or using condoms, which could prevent HIV and other STDs.[36] Although many of these police practices related to condoms are now rare, some advocates argue that maintaining criminal provisions against sex work makes the conduct more dangerous for the sex workers and the clients and should be revisited.

THE ROLE OF EPIDEMIOLOGY IN PUBLIC HEALTH AND CRIMINAL LAW

Epidemiology—the science of health and disease in populations—can characterize health problems arising from criminal activity because the basic approach of epidemiology in seeking clues to the cause or source of disease does not depend on the specific etiology or mode of becoming ill. Insights gained from such investigations can be used to inform public policy, as in the epidemiologic assessment of alcohol use as a "risk factor" for homicide.[37] The techniques of field epidemiology traditionally used by public health agencies to investigate outbreaks of disease can also be applied to situations in which disease clusters result from suspected criminal activity, as in the study of victims in a series of child murders in Atlanta during 1979–1981[38] or in clusters of illness or death in hospitals or other health-care settings where staff have been suspected of intentionally harming patients.

Clusters or outbreaks of disease in hospitals are not uncommon and usually result from unintended breakdowns in procedures for preventing the spread of infectious diseases or errors in administration of medications. Rarely, medication errors result from acts by health-care workers who intentionally seek to harm patients, and in several instances the CDC has contributed to investigations of disease clusters in health-care facilities where such intentional harm was suspected. In these instances, the techniques of the investigation have been modeled after standard epidemiologic approaches.[39] These steps include

- Documenting that an outbreak has indeed occurred. This usually involves determining that an increase in a specific disease has occurred during a defined period of time in excess of rates that would be expected on the basis of prior trends.
- Characterizing the "cases." Who has been affected by the problem in question? A description of the affected persons, including an initial assessment of their commonalities, can yield important clues about the cause or source of an outbreak.

• Developing and testing various hypotheses about the cause or source of the problem. Often this is an iterative process as various hypotheses are tested and either rejected or accepted and as the investigation becomes increasingly focused and specific.

In many respects, these steps, particularly the latter two, are not unlike those in a criminal investigation, and epidemiologists who investigate outbreaks have been popularly described as "disease detectives."

In a hospital outbreak, the iterative process of testing different ideas may involve

• An assessment to determine whether any procedural changes in the hospital were associated temporally with the outbreak, such as introduction of a new product or staffing changes
• A comparison of exposures (e.g., care by specific staff, administration of specific medications, performance of specific diagnostic procedures) among those with or without the disease in question
• A comparison of disease rates between individuals with or without specific exposures

An example of an investigation that used each of these steps is the epidemiologic evaluation of an outbreak of unexplained deaths on the cardiology ward of a children's hospital in Toronto, Ontario, Canada.[40] A nurse was arrested and accused of intentionally administering fatal overdoses of digoxin, a commonly used heart medication, to four infants. Suspicion had been aroused among the cardiology staff about several deaths that had occurred during the weeks preceding her arrest. In one instance, an extraordinarily high level of digoxin had been detected in the blood of an infant who had not been prescribed this medication. The hospital notified legal authorities, and the police conducted a rapid investigation that led to the arrest. After a highly publicized preliminary hearing, all charges against the nurse were dismissed, and she was exonerated by the presiding judge. The hospital subsequently invited the Ontario Ministry of Health and the CDC to conduct an epidemiologic investigation of the deaths during the time in question. The staged scientific investigation yielded the following information:

• During a 9-month period, a distinct fourfold increase in death rates occurred on the cardiology ward compared with earlier time periods, ending abruptly with the nurse's arrest. No other comparable increase in deaths was observed elsewhere in the hospital. An extensive review of possible reasons for the increase in deaths on the cardiology ward did not account for the observed trends.
• Children who died on the cardiology ward during the 9-month "epidemic period" were more likely than children who died during previous or subse-

quent months to be 1 year of age, have an intravenous line in place, have a pattern of death that suggested digoxin toxicity and a timing of death inconsistent with their clinical status as judged by an independent expert in pediatric cardiology, and suffer sudden clinical deterioration between midnight and 6 A.M. For a few children, laboratory data were sufficient to indicate that a fatal overdose of digoxin had been administered shortly before death, and none of them received a *prescribed* dose of digoxin during this time frame.

• A review of staffing schedules indicated that deaths were more than 60 times more likely to occur when a particular nurse was on duty than they were at other times; this nurse typically worked during the night shift and was not the person originally arrested.

A subsequent year-long "Royal Commission of Inquiry" reviewed both the conduct of the police investigation, including the original arrest, and possible reasons for the increase in deaths. This review included testimony from the team that conducted the epidemiologic investigation. The presiding judge concluded that 8 deaths, and possibly 15 additional deaths, resulted from digoxin toxicity and that none of these deaths resulted from an accidental medication error. However, in the absence of any more direct evidence implicating a hospital staff member, a second arrest was never made.

Two investigations involving the CDC that occurred after the Canadian investigation used similar approaches. Key to all of these investigations was the role of expert clinical consultants who assessed whether the timing of death or cardiac arrest was consistent with the clinical course of the patients or whether the pattern of morbidity or mortality fit with the toxic effect of particular medications.

When evaluating a cluster of approximately 30 excess deaths and cardiopulmonary arrests that occurred during a 10-month period among patients in the pediatric intensive care unit of a large hospital in San Antonio, Texas, investigators from the Texas Department of Health and the CDC were not able to explain conclusively the increase in adverse events.[41] Again, the duty time of one nurse was strongly associated with deaths and cardiopulmonary arrests. In this instance, the nurse was eventually convicted of intentionally harming one child who did not die but suffered bleeding as the result of having been administered excessive doses of heparin, a drug that inhibits blood clotting. At the trial, the lead epidemiologist provided testimony describing the overall pattern of mortality and morbidity and the findings of the epidemiologic study. The epidemiologist's testimony bolstered more direct testimony about the one case of the nonfatal injury that was the subject of the nurse's eventual conviction (G.R. Istre, personal communication, December 7, 2001).

A third investigation involved a review of cardiac arrests during a 14-month period in an intensive care unit at a large urban hospital in Maryland.[42] In 88 instances of cardiac arrest that occurred during a particular shift, one nurse was the assigned caregiver for 57 of the patients, and the risk of suffering a cardiac arrest was over 40 times greater for patients of this nurse than for patients of other nurses. In this cluster, overdoses of potassium, a commonly used supplement in intravenous fluids, was suspected. The epidemiologic investigation was used by the police to focus attention on specific hospital staff. Upon initial questioning, the implicated nurse confessed to intentionally harming patients. During her trial, the initial confession was withdrawn. In the absence of more direct eyewitness evidence linking the nurse to intentional acts of harm, the presiding judge dismissed all charges on the grounds that no firm evidence existed that a crime had been committed and that unintentional errors in medication administration could not be excluded.[43]

A common theme in each of the above investigations is the seemingly long period (9 to 14 months) during which increases in morbidity or mortality occurred before abnormal patterns were recognized and brought to the attention of public health or law enforcement authorities. In response, each of the above studies recommended improvements in ongoing monitoring of adverse events in the hope that any increases in morbidity or mortality, regardless of the source or cause, would be detected sooner. Other recommendations focused on improving procedures for administration of medications to decrease opportunities for either intentional or unintentional mishaps.

The studies also demonstrated that, despite the strong statistical association between duty times of individual hospital staff and adverse patient outcomes in these cases, such associations were viewed as circumstantial in the context of the criminal legal proceedings. Thus, the epidemiologic data were deemed useful in framing the criminal investigations, but they did not provide definitive evidence that crimes had been committed or that individuals were responsible for having committed crimes.

Epidemiologic studies, when combined with more direct eyewitness evidence, can contribute to conviction in criminal cases. An epidemiologic investigation conducted by the Office of the Chief Medical Examiner of Suffolk County, New York, during 1985–1987 resulted in the conviction of a nurse responsible for at least four deaths and possibly for 31 more. In that case, the successful conviction was based on three factors: (1) one witness survived and remembered being injected by an unfamiliar male nurse before losing consciousness; (2) epidemiologic evidence; and (3) toxicologic evidence from four of the suspected victims who were exhumed. The epidemiologic evidence indicated that a patient was 35% more likely to die during the shift of the particular nurse than during the shift of any other staff member. This supported orders of exhumation for 35 bodies. The nurse was suspected of administering succinyl choline, a muscle relaxant used in anesthesia, which is difficult to detect post mortem. However, four of the exhumed victims showed traces of Pavulon (pancuronium bromide), another muscle relaxant that is detectable in the body for a period of time; and none of these former patients had had Pavulon prescribed for them during life. On the basis of the evidence of the four victims with traces of Pavulon, the nurse was convicted.

The difficulties in using epidemiology to meet the rigorous standard of proof in criminal cases is in sharp contrast to the role and use of epidemiology in class action product liability cases tried in civil courts. Civil courts have been far more receptive to the use of epidemiologic studies as evidence. For example, the plaintiffs used epidemiologic studies in the cases involving the putative association between Bendectin (an antinausea drug commonly prescribed for pregnant women) and the risk for birth defects[44]; the putative association between silicone breast implants and autoimmune diseases[45]; and the putative association between paternal exposure to Agent Orange and birth defects.[46] The term *putative* is used deliberately because in each of these cases, although the epidemiologic data figured prominently in civil judgments in favor of the plaintiffs, the strength of the epidemiologic evidence was tentative or seriously questioned in subsequent analyses. This demonstrates that juries and judges may interpret epidemiologic data differently from most scientists.

THE MEDICAL EXAMINER'S OFFICE: OVERLAPPING PUBLIC HEALTH AND CRIMINAL JUSTICE FUNCTIONS

In some instances criminal and public health functions are woven into the mission and practice of a single agency. The critical task of the ME is to ascertain the cause and manner of death. The ME's office usually includes investigators, administrators, and staff specially trained in forensic pathology. To aid in determining cause of death, MEs depend on the resources of a forensic toxicology laboratory or access to one for key tests. In most jurisdictions, the ME is authorized or required to investigate all cases of sudden or suspicious death and report the results. For example, New York City mandates reporting of deaths from all forms of child abuse and neglect; unexpected deaths in health-care facilities of all types; deaths that may have resulted from medical malpractice, whether in a doctor's office or in a hospital; deaths suspected to have resulted from a reaction to a medication; deaths in which a medical device may have malfunctioned or been misused; deaths from fires; deaths while a prisoner is detained in legal custody; deaths from the use of a consumer product (which is then reported to a national program); and deaths from "casualties," including industrial accidents and deaths of children falling out of unguarded windows (Sec. 557[f] New York City Charter). By accurately determining the cause of death, this unusual government agency, which is both "semi-public health" and "semi-criminal," serves public health, clinical, and criminal objectives.

Public Health Objectives

As part of the public health infrastructure, MEs are the diagnosticians of dispossessed persons and sign a death certificate if no private doctor has treated an individual before death. In this function, MEs evaluate trends in drug abuse; identify and report fatal child abuse or neglect; diagnose and report infectious diseases; investigate suicides and accidents; independently evaluate medical treatment provided by jails, prisons, and nursing homes; and autopsy unexpected fatalities in hospitals, providing relevant information to review panels.

The ME also can investigate clusters of untimely deaths to identify an emerging threat to public health. In 1993, the state ME for New Mexico noted three deaths in previously healthy young Navajos. Complete forensic autopsies were performed on each decedent, and an investigator from the ME's office was assigned to work with the state epidemiologist. On the basis of these efforts, the CDC was able to release the first public information about isolation of hantavirus.[47] In New York City, other examples of the ME working closely with public health officials and collecting vital public health data include a program for confidential partner notification for persons who died without knowing that they were infected with HIV and case confirmation and description of basic disease pathophysiology for cases of suspected West Nile virus.

Clinical Objectives

Medical examiners are also critical to maintaining high clinical standards. With the decline in the United States of hospital-performed autopsies, the value of the ME autopsy has increased because it is often the only source of reliable feedback on the accuracy of diagnoses made during life.[48] Medical examiners issue death certificates that are completed correctly with an etiologically specific underlying cause of death. Doctors in regular practice are not necessarily trained in the proper completion of death certificates, and the ME's office instructs its colleagues about how to discharge this important responsibility. Accurate determination of causes of death and accurate completion of death certificates serve clinical and public health goals by helping to standardize one facet of vital statistics data, which are a bedrock source of data on public health trends.

Criminal Justice Objectives

Finally, the ME provides crucial evidence within the criminal justice system. A modern ME's office can combine epidemiology, toxicology, and postmortem results to determine whether criminal activity produced an epidemic of premature death. Thus, autopsy reports list the manner of death as accident, suicide, homicide, therapeutic complication of medical treatment, or undetermined. The definition of a homicide for the purposes of a ME is generic: Did the decedent die at the hands of another? The ME leaves the question of responsibility to the criminal justice system.

Medical examiners have long known that both hospitals and cemeteries are filled with people whose illness resulted from injury rather than disease.[49] The CDC began the National Center for Environmental Health and Injury Control in the early 1980s, followed by the Medical Examiner and Coroner Sharing Program in 1986, and finally the National Center for Injury Prevention and Control in 1990. Concern about people injured intentionally or unintentionally is clearly pertinent in the ME's office: "Another vast area of great concern to public health [and the ME] is the study of violence and its handmaiden, substance abuse, or vice versa."[49] Identification of deaths from injuries produces data directly relevant to public health authorities, law enforcement personnel, and often both.

Independence

Because of the multiple roles the ME plays, autonomy—similar to that of the historic coroner—helps protect the office from influence or political pressure. In New York, the independence and autonomy of the ME has been of great civic concern. In a 1980 report, a New York state senator stated that "Because of its unique responsibilities this office must not be perceived as subservient to or controlled by any other branch of government."[50] Similar recommendations were contained in a 1967 Report by the Committee on Public Health by the New York Academy of Medicine.[51]

ROLE OF LAWS THAT CRIMINALIZE BEHAVIOR THAT HARMS THE PUBLIC

Public health codes traditionally allowed prosecution of individuals for a misdemeanor for failure to adhere to disease-control laws. Violations could include failure to report a notifiable disease, breaches of confidential information, and maintenance of unsanitary premises. For food or health-care establishments or residences that pose a danger to the public health, failure to follow a "public health order" issued by the commissioner of health can result in closure of the facility. Violators usually incurred the mildest of misdemeanor sentences, up to $500 or 6 months in jail.[10]

The emergence of the HIV/AIDS epidemic led to use of criminal law to impose more serious penalties. These efforts have been motivated, in part, by public concern over highly publicized cases of frightening or morally reprehensible conduct on the part of a few HIV-infected individuals, such as a father who injected his son with an HIV-infected syringe to avoid paying child support[52] or a young man, knowing of his HIV infection, who had unprotected intercourse with at least 47 young women without disclosing his HIV infection.[53]

Prosecutors have used two broad types of criminal provisions in these cases. In some, prosecutors used common law crimes, usually attempted murder, assault, aggravated assault, or reckless endangerment. These common law offenses require both a culpable state of mind (intent for attempted murder and assault; willful disregard of risk for reckless endangerment) and a wrongful act for conviction. Proving intent can be difficult, especially where the activity, such as having sexual intercourse, is otherwise legal and nonviolent. In an increasing number of states, prosecutors have the option of HIV-specific exposure and transmission laws for prosecution of these activities. Most HIV-specific laws do not require intent to cause harm, only knowledge that one is HIV infected and proof of the prohibited act for prosecution.

Recent research has uncovered 316 cases of prosecution of individuals in the United States during 1986–2001 for willful exposure to or transmission of HIV.[54] Of these cases, at least 184 resulted in a conviction based on some HIV-related charge. A total of 211 cases involved charges of sexual exposure. A significant number of prosecutions were for actions that were unlikely to cause infection, including 75 cases involving spitting, biting, or scratching and 10 involving other activities (e.g., throwing a blood-soaked towel, throwing feces, or licking). Five others involved selling blood, and 12 involved actual or threatened injection with a syringe; in two, the mode was unknown or uncharged. Although not available for all the cases, data on penalties reinforce earlier studies that suggest that judges are willing to impose harsh sentences in such cases, even in cases involving little or no real risk for transmission.[55–57]

The particular characteristics of HIV-specific exposure and transmission laws vary significantly around the county. By the end of 2001, at least 26 states had at least one law specifically criminalizing HIV exposure in certain circumstances. Fifteen states had statutes criminalizing exposure or transmission of HIV through sexual intercourse, intimate contact, or exposure to bodily fluids. Eight states' laws criminalized use of needles, syringes, or other injection equipment that could transmit HIV, and 12 others prohibited donation of blood, organs, or tissue by persons with HIV. Three states' laws criminalized behavior that poses little risk of infection, including spitting, biting, or smearing or throwing blood, saliva, semen, urine, or feces. In four states the person with HIV must have had the specific intent to infect another person for a crime to have occurred. For example, California's statute requires intent to infect:

Any person who exposes another to the human immunodeficiency virus (HIV) by engaging in unprotected sexual activity when the infected person knows at the time of the unprotected sex that he or she is infected with HIV, has not disclosed his or her HIV-positive status, and acts with the specific intent to infect the other person with HIV, is guilty of a felony punishable by imprisonment in the state prison for three, five, or eight years. *Evidence that the person had knowledge of his or her HIV-positive status, without additional evidence, shall not be sufficient to prove specific intent* [emphasis added].[58]

Some states (e.g., Michigan and Illinois) define prohibited sex acts and other activities that could transmit the virus while others (e.g., Florida) are very general. Michigan's statute provides that

(1) A person who knows that he or she has or has been diagnosed as having acquired immunodeficiency syndrome or acquired immunodeficiency syndrome related complex, or who knows that he or she is HIV infected, and who engages in sexual penetration with another person without having first informed the other person that he or she has acquired immunodeficiency syndrome or acquired immunodeficiency syndrome related complex or is HIV infected, is guilty of a felony.
(2) As used in this section, "sexual penetration" means sexual intercourse, cunnilingus, fellatio, anal intercourse, or any other intrusion, however slight, of any part of a person's body or of any object into the genital or anal openings of another person's body, but emission of semen is not required.

Illinois's statute[59] includes the following specific language and definitions:

A person commits criminal transmission of HIV when he or she, knowing that he or she is infected with HIV:
(1) engages in intimate contact with another;
(2) transfers, donates, or provides his or her blood, tissue, semen, organs, or other potentially infectious body fluids for transfusion, transplantation, insemination, or other administration to another; or
(3) dispenses, delivers, exchanges, sells or in any other way transfers to another any nonsterile intravenous or intramuscular drug paraphernalia.

[The statute goes on to define HIV, intimate contact with another, and intravenous or intramuscular drug paraphernalia.]

Florida provides a more general prohibition:

It is unlawful for any person who has human immunodeficiency virus infection, when such person knows he or she is infected with this disease and when such person has been informed that he or she may communicate this disease to another person through sexual intercourse, to have sexual intercourse with any other person, unless such other person has been informed of the presence of the sexually transmissible disease and has consented to the sexual intercourse.[60]

Fifteen states have also adopted laws applying to specific populations or imposing enhanced sentences under certain circumstances. Ten states have laws regarding prostitution involving HIV-positive individuals. Three states allow prosecutors to use HIV status to enhance penalties for other crimes, including sex offenses, and five states have special provisions for assaults against law enforcement officials.

Laws also differ on whether they include consent of the other person (12 states) or use of condom (2 states) as an affirmative defense. When these defenses are not included, or implied by interpretation, such laws effectively prohibit HIV-infected persons from engaging in a wide range of sexual activities for life. From a public health perspective, such laws reflect an unrealistic expectation and may be unenforceable.

Congruence of Prosecution with Public Health Goals

Use of criminal law to prevent or deter behavior that endangers others provides some advantages over use of civil law. According to constitutional standards, criminal law is required to clearly define prohibited activity, provide fair procedures to defendants, and fix terms of punishment. It has clear goals: deterrence, punishment, incapacitation, and rehabilitation.[1] The process of making criminal law should also be transparent and public enough to allow public objection to laws widely perceived as unfair. Criminal law, by its public nature, can also set clear standards for what society considers unacceptable and thus bolster normative standards of conduct. Most of these characteristics are congruent with public health goals and ideally could reinforce public health efforts in other areas. Moreover, even those who oppose widespread application of these laws may assert that some statute is necessary as a public sanction to punish egregiously reckless or intentional acts of exposure or transmission.

Divergence of Prosecution from Public Health Goals

Use of criminal law to punish individuals for exposure or transmission of HIV or other STDs raises important issues of fairness and practicality in the field of public health. Many HIV-infected individuals have engaged in some activity that could transmit the virus to another, without first disclosing their HIV status to that person.[61–63] If law criminalizes behavior that is common or otherwise legal, enactment of the law may do little to provide actual notice to those it affects of its existence or possible consequences for its violation.[1] Without effective notice, the law cannot serve either its deterrent or its norm-setting functions. Also, if many of the most highly publicized cases involve nonsexual behavior, even publicity around the prosecutions may not signify to most HIV-infected persons that their sexual conduct is covered by the law.[54]

If prosecutors use the law to punish behaviors that are highly unlikely to result in transmission (e.g., spitting, biting, scratching) and to seek harsh punishments, such prosecutions also raise fundamental issues of fairness. These prosecutions are, by their nature, "exceptional," and those punished justifiably believe that they have been singled out for some reason unrelated to either law enforcement or public health goals. From a practical perspective, widespread enforcement of these provisions would create an incentive for intrusive surveillance of highly personal activities such as sexual relationships and drug use. This level of invasion into personal behaviors is unacceptable to most Americans, and thus consistent enforcement of criminal provisions is unlikely.

Given the relatively small number of overall prosecutions for all types of exposure or transmission since the beginning of the HIV epidemic, the laws also appear to be selectively enforced. Selective enforcement raises the specter of abuse of discretion or prejudice on the part of those reporting, prosecuting, and adjudicating these cases. Enforcement of criminal law provisions that is motivated by prejudice or fear, rather than by legitimate efforts to protect society, "corrupts both citizenry and police and reduces the moral authority of the criminal law, especially among those portions of the citizenry—the poor and subcultural—who are particularly likely to be treated in an arbitrary fashion."[63] Finally, because all common law and HIV-specific criminal prosecutions depend on the defendant knowing his or her HIV status, enforcement of these statutes could deter individuals who know they are at risk for infection from being tested. It could also deter those who test positive from revealing the names of their sex or needle-sharing partners for fear that one of them might become subject to criminal prosecution.[1,65] In these ways, use of criminal prosecutions may diverge from public health goals.

CONCLUSION: UTILITY OF THE LAW IN RELATION TO PUBLIC HEALTH PRACTICE

Overall, little empirical evidence exists on how and whether criminal law influences behavior in the public health field. Collection and analysis of these data should be a priority of future work.

Certain characteristics stand out as probable indicators of where the law works. Where criminal enforcement is part of an overall strategy that involves a well-regulated system of relatively public activity—such as operation of food establishments, workplace safety regulations, driving, and public sale or consumption of dangerous products—criminal law may function best in supporting public health objectives. Such a system usually includes established monitoring systems, well-known standards for compliance, and the absence of highly intrusive monitoring. Other characteristics emerge that might make criminal enforcement less effective. Vague or broadly defined prohibited conduct, poor dissemination of information about the illegal nature of the conduct, and the need for highly intrusive monitoring to detect violations all suggest that criminal enforcement will be rare, selective, or potentially biased against already disfavored individuals or populations. However, even in some situations where laws could be abused, they may have symbolic or normative value that operates benignly. The normative impact and its characteristics and scope need to be explored, using empirical methods wherever possible. The symbolic importance of the laws needs to be weighed against their potential harms or unintended consequences.

Science has far outstripped the law in the speed of scientific discoveries and advances. The HIV/AIDS epidemic has highlighted many stresses in the joining of criminal law and public health law. Molecular biology technology systematically used for criminal justice purposes has the potential to eliminate the anonymity of rape, assault, and murder improving the apprehension of serial criminals and exonerating those falsely accused, but it also poses serious philosophical and privacy questions for which no one has easy answers.

When the practitioner reviews the public health and criminal laws of his or her state, many incongruities become evident. Many of the public health laws need revision to reflect changing priorities in public health, and many of the criminal laws affecting public health need to be modified to accommodate due process and avoid unfairly selective use. Laws empowering MEs need to be reviewed to make sure that the ME's authority is sufficient to discharge his or her important responsibilities in detecting crime and protecting public health. Properly regulating powerful technologies has never been easy because science is an intellectual activity that requires room for experimentation and exploration; nevertheless, fair regulation of scientific areas affecting public health and safety must be undertaken if appropriate safeguards do not exist.

Finally, when considering use of the criminal law in any area related to public health, policy makers and practitioners should be aware of the risk of unintended consequences. Examples of unintended actual and possible consequences abound, including those discussed in this chapter, such as the impact of syringe prescription and drug paraphernalia laws on the spread of bloodborne diseases among IDUs. Another controversial area that should be studied carefully is whether exposure and transmission laws create resistance to voluntary testing during the HIV epidemic. In the roil of human events, the search for ways to control public health brings imperfect solutions; yet sensitive study, analysis, and empirical experience may be able to minimize the undesirable unintended consequences of modern public health measures.

References

1. Gostin LO. *Public Health Law: Power, Duty, Restraint.* Berkeley: University of California Press, 2000.
2. Institute of Medicine. *The Future of Public Health.* Washington, DC: National Academy Press, 1988.
3. *Bamford v. Turnley*, 3 B.&S 67, 122 Eng. Rep. 27 (Exch. Ch. 1862), summary of which appears in Dobbs DB, Hayden PT, eds. *Torts and Compensation: Personal Accountability and Social Responsibility for Injury*, 3rd ed. St. Paul, MN: West Publishing Co., 1997.
4. Pincoffs EL. The problem of punishment. In: *Philosophy of Law: A Brief Introduction.* Belmont, CA: Wadsworth Publishing Co., 1991: pp. 9–19.
5. Gostin LO, Burris S, Lazzarini Z. The law and the public's health: a study of infectious disease law in the United States. *Columbia Law Rev* 1999;99:59–128.
6. *Greene v. Edwards*, 263 S.E.2d 661 (W. Va. 1980).

7. *Addington v. Texas*, 441 U.S. 418 (1979).
8. Saltzburg SA, Diamond JL, Kinports K, Morawetz TH. The nature and structure of criminal law. In: *Criminal Law: Cases and Materials*, 2nd ed. New York: Lexis Publishing, 2000: pp. 1–67.
9. *McCullough v. State*, 657 P.2d 1157 (Nev. 1983).
10. Grad FP. *Public Health Law Manual*, 2nd ed. Washington, DC: American Public Health Association, 1990.
11. Garner BA, ed. *Black's Law Dictionary, Pocket Edition*. St. Paul, MN: West Publishing Co., 1996.
12. Zimring FE, Hawkins GJ. *Deterrence: The Legal Threat in Crime Control*. Chicago: University of Chicago Press, 1973.
13. Becker G. Crime and punishment: an economic approach. *J Political Economy* 1968; 76:169–217.
14. Kuperan K, Sutinen JG. Blue water crime: deterrence, legitimacy, and compliance in fisheries. *Law Society Rev* 1998;32:309–37.
15. Tyler TR. *Why People Obey the Law*. New Haven, CT: Yale University Press, 1990.
16. Rabinowitz RS, Hager MM. Designing health and safety: workplace hazard regulation in the United States and Canada. *Cornell Int Law J* 2000;33:373–434.
17. Magnuson JC, Leviton GC. Policy considerations in corporate criminal prosecutions after *People v. Film Recovery Systems, Inc*. Notre Dame Law Rev 1986;62:913–39, note 14 and text.
18. Bureau of Justice Statistics, U.S. Department of Justice. Prison and jail inmates at Midyear 1999. *Bureau Justice Statistics Bull* NCJ-181643, 2000. Available at http://www.ojp.usdoj.gov/bjs/abstract/pjim99.htm. Accessed November 27, 2001.
19. Bureau of Justice Statistics. Sourcebook of criminal justice statistics Table 6.51: Federal prison population, and number and percent sentenced for drug offenses (United States 1970–2001). Available at http://www.albany.edu/sourcebook/. Go to section 6, Corrections, and find listed table. Accessed December 15, 2001.
20. Freeman A. HIV in prison. In: Burris S, Dalton HL, Miller JL, eds. *AIDS Law Today: A New Guide for the Public*. New Haven, CT: Yale University Press, 1993: pp. 263–94.
21. Bureau of Justice Statistics, U.S. Department of Justice. Sourcebook of criminal justice statistics online. Table 6.312: Rate (per 100,000 U.S. resident population in each group) of sentenced prisoners under jurisdiction of State and Federal correctional authorities. Available at http://www.albany.edu/sourcebook/. Go to section 6, Corrections, and find listed table. Accessed December 15, 2001.
22. Bureau of Justice Statistics, U.S. Department of Justice. Jail populations, by age and gender, 1986–99. Available at http://www.ojp.usdoj.gov/bjs/glance/jailag.htm. Accessed September 24, 2001.
23. U.S. Department of Justice. 1994 Update: HIV/AIDS and STDs in correctional facilities. In: *Issues and Practices in Criminal Justice*. Washington, DC: National Institute of Justice, 1995. Available at http://www.ncjrs.org/pdffiles/hivaid94.pdf. Accessed December 20, 2001.
24. Bureau of Justice Statistics, U.S. Department of Justice. Sourcebook of criminal justice statistics Table 6.68, p. 534. Available at http://www.albany.edu/sourcebook/1995/pdf/t668.pdf. Accessed October 5, 2001.
25. Burris S. Prisons, law and public health: the case for a coordinated response to epidemic disease behind bars. *Univ Miami Law Rev* 1992;47:291–335.
26. Hammett TM, Rhodes W, Harmon P. HIV/AIDS and other infectious diseases among

correctional inmates: a public health problem and opportunity [abstract 571]. *National HIV Prevention Conference*, Atlanta, GA, August 1999. Available at http://www.cdc.gov/hiv/conferences/hiv99/abstracts571.pdf. Accessed December 20, 2001.

27. Gostin LO, Lazzarini Z, Alexander D, Brandt AM, Mayer KH, Silverman DC. HIV testing, counseling and prophylaxis after sexual assault. *JAMA* 1994;271:1436–44.

28. Christian K. And the DNA shall set you free: issues surrounding postconviction DNA evidence and the pursuit of innocence. *Ohio State Law J* 2001;62:1195–241.

29. Ryan GH. "Innocent execution prevention." Testimony of Illinois Governor, George H. Ryan, before the U.S. House Judiciary Crime Subcommittee, Chair Henry Hyde, on June 20, 2000. Federal Document Clearing House (2000 WL 19304891).

30. Gostin LO, Lazzarini Z. Prevention of HIV/AIDS among injection drug users: the theory and science of public health and criminal justice approaches to disease prevention. *Emory Law J* 1997;46:587–696.

31. Normand J, Vlahov D, Moses LE, eds. *Preventing HIV Transmission: The Role of Sterile Needles and Bleach*. Washington, DC: National Academy Press, 1995.

32. CDC, Health Resources and Services Administration, National Institute on Drug Abuse, Substance Abuse and Mental Health Services Administration. *HIV Prevention Bulletin: Medical Advice for Persons Who Inject Illicit Drugs*. Washington, DC: U.S. Department of Health and Human Services, Public Health Service, 1997.

33. The American Medical Association (AMA), the American Pharmaceutical Association (APhA), the Association of State and Territorial Health Officials (ASTHO), the National Alliance of State and Territorial AIDS Directors (NASTAD), and the National Association of Boards of Pharmacy (NABP). *Joint statement encouraging state-level action to reduce the legal and regulatory barriers that currently restrict access to sterile syringes in nearly every state*. Includes summary of (and link to) American Bar Association letter expressing similar support for reducing barriers. Available at http://www.ama-assn.org/ama/pub/category/1808.html. Accessed December 15, 2001.

34. American Bar Association. *Report on Deregulation of Hypodermic Needles and Syringes as a Public Health Measure: A Report on Emerging Policy and Law in the United States*. Available at http://www.abanet.org/irr/aidsproject/publications/needles.pdf. Accessed May 25, 2001.

35. Brandt AM. *No Magic Bullet: A Social History of Venereal Disease in the United States Since 1880*. New York: Oxford University Press, 1987.

36. International Committee for Prostitutes' Rights. Health: "our first concern." In: Pheterson G, ed. *A Vindication of the Rights of Whores*. Seattle: Seal Press, 1989: pp. 109–31.

37. Goodman RA, Mercy JA, Layde PM, Thacker SB. Case–control studies: design issues for criminological applications. *J Quant Criminol* 1988;4:71–84.

38. Blaser MJ, Jason JM, Weniger BG, et al. Epidemiologic analysis of a cluster of homicides of children in Atlanta. *JAMA* 1984;251:3255–58.

39. Gregg MB. Conducting a field investigation. In: Gregg MB, ed. *Field Epidemiology*. New York: Oxford University Press, 1996: pp. 44–59.

40. Buehler JW, Smith LF, Wallace EM, Heath CW, Rusiak R, Herndon JL. Unexplained deaths in a children's hospital, an epidemiologic assessment. *N Engl J Med* 1985;313:211–6.

41. Istre GR, Gustafson TL, Baron RC, Martin DL, Orlowski JP. A mysterious cluster of deaths and cardiopulmonary arrests in a pediatric intensive care unit. *N Engl J Med* 1985;313:205–11.

42. Sacks JJ, Stroup DF, Will ML, Harris EL, Israel E. A nurse-associated epidemic of cardiac arrests in an intensive care unit. *JAMA* 1988;259:689–95.
43. Weaver C. The chilling case of nurse 14. *Regardies* 1988;8:93–144.
44. Brent RL. Bendectin: review of the medical literature of a comprehensively studied human nonteratogen and the most prevalent tortogen-litigen [review]. *Reprod Toxicol* 1995;9:337–49.
45. Angell M. Shattuck lecture—evaluating the health risks of breast implants: the interplay of medical science, the law, and public opinion. *N Engl J Med* 1996;334: 1513–8.
46. Stephenson J. New IOM report links Agent Orange exposure to risk of birth defect in Vietnam vets' children [Medical News and Perspectives]. *JAMA* 1996;275:1066–7.
47. CDC. Outbreak of hantavirus infection—southwestern United States, 1993. *MMWR* 1993;42:441–3.
48. Lundberg GD. Low-tech autopsies in the era of high-tech medicine: continued value for quality assurance and patient safety. *JAMA* 1998;280:1273–4.
49. Hirsch CS, Chief Medical Examiner of the City of New York. *Forensic Pathology and Public Health*. Maude Abbott Lecture to the United States and Canadian Academy of Pathology. Orlando, Florida, March 4, 1997. [Unpublished; copies available through the Office of Chief Medical Examiner, 520 First Avenue, New York, NY 10016.]
50. Goodman R. *New York State Senate Investigations Committee Report*, No. 1057. 1980.
51. New York Academy of Medicine. *Report by the Committee on Public Health*, Vol. 43, Bulletin, No. 3. New York: New York Academy of Medicine, 1967: pp. 241–9.
52. Associated Press. Father is accused of injecting son with HIV-infected blood. *Los Angeles Times* 1998 (April 24):Part A, p. 13.
53. CDC. Cluster of HIV-positive young women—New York, 1997–1998. *MMWR* 1999;48:413–6.
54. Lazzarini Z, Bray S, Messing N, Burris S, Blankenship K. Criminal law and HIV transmission: an analysis of criminal law as a structural intervention to regulate behavior. National HIV Prevention Conference, Atlanta, August 13–15, 2001, Poster No. 873.
55. Strader K. Criminalization as a policy response to a public health crisis. *J Marshall Law Rev* 1994;27:435–47.
56. *State v. Smith*, 621 A.2d 493 (N.J. Super. Ct. App. Div.), cert. denied, 634 A.2d 523 (N.J. 1993) (defendant convicted of attempted murder for biting a correctional officer).
57. *Weeks v. Scott*, 55 F.3d 1059 (5th Cir. 1995) (defendant convicted of attempted murder and sentenced to life in prison for spitting at a correctional officer).
58. California Health and Safety Code, Chapter 4, Sec. 120291(a).
59. Michigan Statutes. Sec. 333.5210; Illinois Compiled Statutes Annotated. Chapter 720. Criminal Offenses. Sec. 5/12–16.2 Criminal transmission of HIV.
60. Florida Statutes Annotated. Title XXIX Public Health. Sec. 384.24, Unlawful Acts.
61. Hays RB, Paul J, Ekstrand M, Kegeles SM, Stall R, Coates TJ. Actual versus perceived HIV status, sexual behaviors and predictors of unprotected sex among young gay and bisexual men who identify as HIV-negative, HIV-positive, and untested. *AIDS* 1997;1:1495–502.
62. Singh BK, Koman JJ 3rd, Catan VM, Souply KL, Birkel RC, Golaszewski TJ. Sexual

risk behavior among injection drug-using human immunodeficiency virus positive clients. *Int J Addict* 1993;28:735–47.
63. Niccolai LM, Dorst D, Myers L, Kissinger PJ. Disclosure of HIV status to sexual partners: predictors and temporal patterns. *Sex Transm Dis* 1999;26:281–5.
64. Kadish SH. The crisis of overcriminalization. In: *Blame and Punishment: Essays in the Criminal Law*. New York: Macmillan, 1987: pp. 21–35.
65. Dalton H. Law and responsibility lecture series. Shaping responsible behavior: lessons from the AIDS front. *Washington Lee Law Rev* 1999;56:931–52.

5

International Considerations

DAVID P. FIDLER, TONY D. PEREZ, AND
MARTIN S. CETRON

Public health literature in the 1990s frequently referred to the "globalization of public health."[1,2] How experts define this phenomenon varies, but the basic idea is that public health challenges transcend borders. The transnational nature of public health problems is not novel. Infectious disease specialists have long argued that "germs do not carry passports." Although the globalization of public health has long-standing importance, the analysis of public health law has neglected international aspects of public health. Public health law texts in the United States from the twentieth century, including those by Tobey (1939),[3] Wing (1990),[4] and Grad (1996),[5] contain little or no discussion of international considerations. Even Gostin's recent *Public Health Law* (2000)[6] does not deal with the global context of U.S. public health law.

In this chapter we seek to remedy the neglect of international considerations in the analysis of U.S. public health law. The first section focuses on the legal structure and sources of public health law viewed from an international perspective. The analysis concentrates on the legal structures created by the U.S. Constitution and international law. Next is a review of U.S. participation in international health diplomacy. This analysis looks at international health organizations and legal regimes to demonstrate that these efforts are important to U.S. public health. This section mentions other international legal regimes relevant for public health in which the United States has played or is playing a leading role.

The next two sections look at the law relevant to public health problems that U.S. public health officials and practitioners may face in their work: public health threats that (*1*) originate outside the United States but that, through people, animals, or goods, can be brought within the United States; and (*2*) flow out of the United States toward other countries. We also address emerging public health controversies that result from the U.S. pursuit of liberalization in international trade and foreign investment through international law.

The chapter concludes with thoughts on the future importance of international considerations in U.S. public health law. Not only is international law becoming more important in thinking about public health in the United States, but globalization is also generally affecting how U.S. public health will evolve in the coming decades. We call for public health lawyers and experts to increase attention on the international features of U.S. public health and the law that serves the public's health.

LEGAL STRUCTURES AND SOURCES FOR U.S. PUBLIC HEALTH LAW IN THE INTERNATIONAL CONTEXT

International relations experts argue that anarchy—the lack of any supreme, central power—characterizes international politics. Independent, sovereign states interact in this condition of anarchy. This "anarchical society"[5] of sovereign states creates a legal structure through which states pursue public health and other objectives. Within the sovereign state, national law guides the pursuit of public health. If states desire to cooperate on public health problems, then international law becomes the mechanism through which anarchy is structured to reflect public health concerns.[5] For U.S. public health practitioners, understanding the international context of U.S. public health law requires appreciation of (*1*) federalism and the U.S. constitutional structure—how public health law is organized within the United States; and (*2*) the structure of international law—how sovereign states legally cooperate in the international system.

U.S. Constitutional Structure and Domestic Sources of Public Health Law in the International Context

Scholars of U.S. public health law frequently note that federalism and the U.S. constitutional system leave most public health powers to the individual states of the Union. While the federal government has enumerated powers, such as the powers to tax and spend and regulate interstate commerce, that can be exercised for public health purposes, the states retain a great deal of sovereignty over public health. In the international public health context, however, the federal government has supreme power because of its constitutional monopoly in foreign affairs.

Under the Constitution, the federal government has the power to regulate commerce with foreign nations, to determine the conditions for immigration into the United States, and to make treaties with other countries. None of these powers is expressly a public health power; but the federal government uses these powers to achieve public health objectives, such as protecting the nation from the importation of food-borne pathogens, prohibiting the entry of immigrants with certain infectious diseases, and concluding agreements with other nations to achieve mutual public health goals.

The federal monopoly on foreign affairs powers means that the primary source of public health law in U.S. international relations is federal law. Statutes, codified in the United States Code (U.S.C.), and regulations, found in the Code of Federal Regulations (C.F.R.), are important sources of public health law. In the public health context, Congress often passes legislation that delegates authority to the Executive Branch, which then promulgates regulations to implement the law. The Executive Branch's handling of public health can be confusing because many executive agencies are involved in implementing statutory law. For example, the Department of Health and Human Services is responsible for federal quarantine; the Department of Agriculture inspects imported food; and the Food and Drug Administration regulates pharmaceutical imports. Because the federal government exercises numerous federal powers for public health purposes through multiple executive agencies, federal law affecting public health is scattered across the U.S.C. and C.F.R. in ways that make it difficult to see the composite picture.

The structure of the U.S. constitutional system also makes the judicial branch an important source of public health law in the international context. U.S. federal courts have interpreted treaties, statutes, and regulations in cases involving U.S. public health and foreign persons and products. Federal courts have also adjudicated cases involving the boundaries between state and federal public health powers in connection with health threats from other countries.

Structure of International Law and Public Health

International law constitutes the rules that regulate the relations among sovereign states and other actors (e.g., international organizations and individuals) in the international system. Many people think the rules of international law are not really "law" because they cannot be enforced the way domestic law is enforced. This attitude judges international law by the political conditions that characterize domestic law, which include a central government with a mandate to make and enforce laws. International law arises, however, in a political environment characterized by the absence of any central law-making or law-enforcing authority. International law should be judged not by the criteria of domestic governance but by the circumstances that characterize international relations.

The sources of international law are, therefore, different from the sources of domestic law. The classic sources of international law found in the Statute of the International Court of Justice (ICJ Statute) are (*1*) treaties; (*2*) customary international law, (*3*) general principles of law recognized by civilized nations, and (*4*) as supplementary means for determining rules of international law, judicial decisions of national and international tribunals and the teachings of the most highly qualified publicists of the various nations (ICJ Statute, Article 38[1]).

Treaties

Treaties are written agreements between sovereign states, the obligations of which are legally binding. Treaties do not bind states that do not ratify or otherwise accept them. Treaties have been analogized to contracts. Like treaties, contracts bind the persons involved but do not bind people who did not sign the contract. A large body of international law, now codified in the Vienna Convention on the Law of Treaties (1969), regulates the formation, implementation, interpretation, and termination of treaties. The treaty is a flexible instrument because states can use it for almost any purpose, and treaties can be bilateral or multilateral in their membership.

Customary international law

In contrast with treaties, customary international law (CIL) comprises unwritten rules that develop out of state interaction in the international system. A CIL rule forms when general and consistent state practice exists that is supported by the sense that following the practice is legally required.[6] General state practice means that the practice is widespread in the international system. Consistent state practice means that convergence in state behavior around a principle is discernible. The sense of legal obligation means that states follow the principle and practice because they believe they are required to do so under international law. Customary international law rules are binding on all states in the international system except on those that have persistently objected to the rules' formation.

Even though CIL is one of the most important sources of international law, it is problematic. Determining whether the criteria for CIL formation have been satisfied is fraught with difficulties.[7] Customary international law rules also tend to create general, ambiguous obligations about what states should do in specific situations. Some international lawyers argue, for example, that CIL imposes a duty on states to prevent, control, and reduce transboundary and maritime pollution.[8] Because this rule proves not very helpful, treaties are needed for states to craft more precise rules to reduce pollution.

General principles of law

The third primary source of international law is "general principles of law recognized by civilized nations," which are principles of domestic law that appear in national legal systems around the world. General principles of law have not been a robust source of international legal rules. International lawyers and tribunals dislike basing analysis on rules taken from domestic law. General principles of law have been used most frequently when international tribunals sometimes confront issues, such as the admissibility of circumstantial evidence, for which no international law exists. The tribunals refer to how domestic legal systems handle such issues in order to complete their analysis.

Judicial decisions and the writings of publicists

International lawyers use judicial decisions and the writings of scholars and practitioners to identify and interpret rules that arise from treaties, CIL, or general principles of law, which is why the ICJ Statute refers to them as "supplementary means" for determining rules of international law. However, sometimes these supplementary means are important in the creation and development of rules of international law. Historically, one drawback has been that decisions of international tribunals have been relatively few. As more international tribunals are established, like the Dispute Settlement Body of the World Trade Organization (WTO), the importance of judicial decisions of international tribunals will increase.

Sources of international law and public health

The bulk of international law that affects public health is found in treaties. One reason for this is that public health arose as an issue in international diplomacy only in the mid-nineteenth century. When sovereign states discussed infectious disease control in the second half of the nineteenth century, no CIL rules existed to guide cooperation because no general and consistent practice on public health matters had developed. Nor was reliance on general principles of law possible to sustain multilateral efforts on public health. In addition, because science informs public health policies, treaties are better suited to crafting scientifically appropriate rules than CIL or general principles of law.

Globalization and National and International Law on Public Health

The processes of globalization do not alter the national and international legal structures outlined above, but public health officials and legal experts believe that the law as traditionally produced has become anachronistic and requires reform. Much of the national and international law on controlling the international spread of infectious diseases, for example, developed during the time maritime commerce and travel were dominant and focuses on control at points of entry and exit. Although public health capabilities at exit and entry points remain important, the speed and volume of international trade, travel, and migration leave much of traditional national and international law on public health inflexible in facilitating responses to changing global public health conditions.

Individuals and goods that pose public health threats now typically enter society and commerce in the United States, bypassing border control systems and requiring more demanding public health action and cooperation among local, state, and federal governments (Box 5–1). Along with attention to traditional border strategies, public health experts perceive the need for regulatory approaches that deal with the threats to U.S. public health posed by mobile individuals, populations, animals, and goods.[9] This chapter mentions current efforts to revise national and international legal regimes to make the law more flexible and responsive in light of the challenges that globalization presents.

THE UNITED STATES AND INTERNATIONAL HEALTH DIPLOMACY

The United States has been involved in international health diplomacy since the late nineteenth century, and it remains a key player in global public health. This section looks at the United States' participation in international health diplomacy to indicate how important the global context is for U.S. public health law.

Beginning of U.S. Involvement in International Public Health Efforts

International cooperation on public health began in 1851, when European states convened the first International Sanitary Conference to discuss cross-border transmission of cholera, plague, and yellow fever.[10] The 1851 conference launched a series of international sanitary meetings and treaties that continued until the formation of the World Health Organization (WHO) in 1948. U.S. participation in this process started in 1881, when the United States hosted the fifth International Sanitary Conference. This conference marked the emergence of the United States as an important player in international efforts on public health.

The years immediately before and after the 1881 conference also saw the federal government adopt legislation aimed at public health threats originating in foreign countries. Congress passed the first national quarantine act in 1878, an action prompted by a yellow fever epidemic in the Western Hemisphere that reached the United States in 1878.[11] Congress enacted a statute in 1882 requiring the federal government to undertake medical inspection of aliens (defined as any person not a citizen or national of the United States [8 U.S.C. § 1101(a)(3)]) seeking admission to the country. These laws suggested that the federal government appreciated threats to U.S. public health from foreign products and persons

Box 5-1. Mobility and Infectious Disease Control

The speed and volume of international travel reached unprecedented levels in the later half of the twentieth century. The World Tourism Organization estimates annual international arrivals at close to 1 billion; meanwhile, the time needed to circumnavigate the globe has been reduced to 36 to 72 hours from 365 days at the turn of the twentieth century. High-speed and widespread international travel means that people and cargo move faster than the incubation periods for many infectious diseases, which no longer respect geographic borders. The burden of preventing importation and spread of communicable disease has therefore shifted beyond the sea ports of entry, as during the late nineteenth and early twentieth centuries. U.S. health-care providers face new challenges in recognizing, diagnosing, and treating previously "rare" infectious diseases once only found in the tropics or developing countries. In 1987, 2000, and 2001, outbreaks of meningococcal meningitis occurred among recent Haj pilgrims to Saudi Arabia and subsequently spread to their close contacts, causing meningitis outbreaks around the globe. West Nile virus first appeared in the Western Hemisphere in New York City in 1999 and has subsequently spread along the Atlantic states because of the mobility of vectors, humans, and animal reservoirs.

Medical screening of new U.S. immigrants and refugees has largely been shifted overseas to the countries' of origin or asylum. Much has been written about the challenges that foreign-born, new Americans pose to the U.S. public health system, especially in terms of tuberculosis (TB) elimination. Although all persons legally immigrating to the United States (ages $\geqslant 15$ years) are required by law to be screened for TB, limitations on screening tools, overseas laboratory capacity, and infrastructure constraints in many developing (as well as developed) countries result in some immigrants entering the United States with either undiagnosed or misdiagnosed TB; in some cases, latent TB is reactivated within the first year of immigration.

A recent TB incident illustrates the public health challenge that mobile populations can pose for federal, state, and local health departments, as well as the transportation industry. In May 2001, federal health officials received information from a state health department about a recent immigrant who had not presented for required TB treatment (directly observed therapy [DOT]). A quick investigation and interview of family members indicated that the immigrant had recently left the state to pursue employment in another state (secondary immigration is a particularly difficult issue for public health officials). The migrant took an 8-hour flight, stayed several days with family and friends, and took another flight (4 hours) to arrive at his destination. He then worked on a shrimp boat for several weeks before boarding a transcontinental bus and traveling cross-country for several days.

Clearly, the implications are staggering. First the host state health department was required to follow up all of the immigrant's contacts. Airline medical personnel were required to follow up with passengers and crew on the 8-hour flight. A second state health department was required to follow up those who may have come into contact with the man on board the shrimp boat and with his family and friends. Perhaps the most challenging, because bus companies do not routinely keep passenger information, were attempts to work with bus company officials to follow up on everyone who may have been exposed while the migrant rode cross-country.

Because of the speed, ease, and volume of modern travel, health officials increasingly face challenges to respond to public health incidents that require multijurisdictional coordination, multiagency participation, and a close working relationship between public health agencies and the private transportation industry.

and moved to improve public health defenses at points of entry into the United States. These exercises of federal legislative power occurred simultaneously with the beginning of U.S. participation in international health diplomacy.

U.S. Participation and Leadership in Regional and International Efforts on Public Health

Once engaged, the United States deepened its participation in international co-operation on public health and emerged as a leader in this area. The United States was instrumental in the establishment in 1902 of the first permanent international organization on public health—the Pan American Sanitary Bureau (PASB). The PASB supported hemispheric efforts to address infectious diseases through the development of important treaties, such as the Pan American Sanitary Code (1905, revised 1924) and the Pan American Sanitary Convention on Aerial Navigation (1928). The PASB also developed projects and activities in the first half of the twentieth century on other areas of public health, such as nutrition and noncommunicable diseases. The United States was also an original member state of the Office International de l'Hygiène Publique (OIHP), established in 1907 to support international efforts against infectious diseases. The OIHP became important for international law on infectious disease control because it was central to the flow of global epidemiologic information and was responsible for overseeing the main international sanitary treaties.

The U.S. refusal to join the League of Nations after World War I meant that the United States did not become a member of the Health Organization of the League of Nations (HOLN) in 1923. The United States played a leading role in the WHO's establishment in that it hosted the conference in 1946 that created the WHO. The United States pushed for the inclusion in the WHO Constitution of innovative powers for the WHO to adopt binding international legal regulations (WHO Constitution, Articles 21–22). The attachment of PASB member states to the PASB's independence meant, however, that the bureau was not absorbed by the WHO but instead retained its separate status while becoming the WHO's regional office for the Americas.

The United States and the World Health Organization

Even though U.S. influence can be seen in the development of both international health organizations and international law on public health from the late nineteenth century to the WHO's creation, the U.S. relationship with the WHO is complex and controversial. The United States has remained important to the WHO because it provides a significant portion of the WHO's budget, and U.S. experts have played important roles in the WHO, including, for example, in the global eradication of smallpox. But the relationship has often been contentious, especially when the WHO attempted to move beyond its technical and scientific roles into more political matters, such as connections between trade and public health. Against the advice and recommendations of U.S. public health officials, the United States opposed on trade-related grounds the WHO's efforts to (1) regulate the quality of pharmaceuticals moving in international commerce, (2) oppose corporate marketing of breast-milk substitutes in developing countries, and (3) develop the program on essential drugs and vaccines.[12] More recently, the United States and the WHO have clashed over the protection of intellectual property rights and strategies to increase access to drugs and vaccines in developing countries.

The relationship between the WHO and the United States involves many complicated factors. One of the most important is U.S. perceptions about international threats to U.S. public health. U.S. involvement in international health diplomacy from the late nineteenth century through the WHO's formation drew strength from the belief that international cooperation was essential to protecting U.S. public health. Advances in U.S. domestic public health in the first half of the twentieth century, and the development of antibiotics and vaccines after World War II, reduced the perception that the United States was vulnerable to imported infectious diseases—which were the central focus of international health cooperation from the mid-nineteenth century. International health diplomacy lost its appeal to U.S. self-interest. In addition, the United States engaged in a struggle for global supremacy with the Soviet Union that diverted resources in other directions, from bolstering free trade to managing nuclear deterrence. During the Cold War, public health was invisible as a matter of U.S. foreign policy.

Beyond the WHO: U.S. Influence on Global Public Health Through International Economics

U.S. power in global public health extends beyond the WHO. The United States probably has its greatest impact on public health globally through the liberalization of trade and foreign investment. The United States has led the development of international law on free trade now embodied in the WTO. World Trade Organization agreements now dominate areas traditionally in the WHO's province, such as food safety, the international spread of infectious diseases, and access to medicines (Box 5–2). In addition, through the exercise of U.S. power, institutions such as the World Bank and the International Monetary Fund wield influence in global public health because of their resources and willingness to demand that developing-country governments change policies in return for financial assistance. These indicators of U.S. power in global public health suggest

---

Box 5–2. General Agreement on Tariffs and Trade (GATT) / World Trade
Organization (WTO) Cases with Public Health Implications

- **Thai Cigarette Case (1990).** In a case brought by the United States, a GATT panel
  found that Thailand's ban on the importation of foreign-made cigarettes violated
  Article XI of GATT and could not be justified under Article XX(b) because the ban
  was not necessary to protect human health because it was not the least trade restrictive measure possible.
- **Beef Hormones Case (1998).** In a case brought by the United States and Canada,
  the WTO Dispute Settlement Body found that the European Community violated
  Article 5.1 of the Sanitary and Phytosanitary Measures Agreement because it had
  not based its import ban on meat raised with growth hormones on a risk assessment.
- **Canadian Patent Protection of Pharmaceutical Products (2000).** In a case
  brought by the European Community, the WTO Dispute Settlement Body ruled on
  aspects of Canadian patent protection for pharmaceutical products. The WTO upheld
  the Canadian regulatory review exception, under which competitors of a patent
  owner are permitted to use the patented invention, without the authorization of the
  patent owner during the term of the patent, to obtain government marketing approval
  for generic products, so they will have regulatory permission to sell in competition
  with the patent owner by the date on which the patent expires. The WTO struck
  down, however, the Canadian stockpiling exception, under which competitors could
  manufacture and stockpile patented goods before the patent expires, but the goods
  cannot be sold until after the patent expires.
- **Asbestos Case (2001).** In a case brought by Canada, the WTO Dispute Settlement
  Body upheld a French ban on the use of products containing asbestos because such
  products were not "like products" with substitutable nonasbestos containing products within the meaning of Article III(4) of GATT and because the ban was necessary to protect human health within the meaning of Article XX(b) of GATT.

---

that U.S. involvement in international health diplomacy involves protecting not
only U.S. public health but also how the exercise of U.S. power affects public
health in other countries.

PREVENTION AND CONTROL OF PUBLIC HEALTH THREATS
ORIGINATING OUTSIDE THE UNITED STATES

The traditional justification for federal activity in international public health—
to protect U.S. public health from threats originating outside the United States—
explains why the federal government enacted legislation to prevent and minimize the importation of infectious diseases through people, animals, and goods
and entered treaties to cooperate on infectious disease control. This section looks
at federal laws and international laws that connect with U.S. efforts to prevent

and control the impact on U.S. public health from threats originating in other countries.

General Principles on Protecting Domestic Public Health from Outside Threats

General principles of international law hold that a state has sovereignty over its borders; it alone determines what goods and people enter its territory. The only restrictions on this power are those the sovereign state imposes through constitutional or statutory law or accepts through treaties. To use an example explored below, the United States has agreed to comply with the WTO Agreement on the Application of Sanitary and Phytosanitary Measures in how it protects the U.S. population from foodborne pathogens. International law is used, thus, to discipline the exercise of sovereign power over human and commercial traffic crossing the state's borders.

Public Health Threats from People

Federal law on public health criteria for admission of aliens

Federal law requires that aliens wanting to be admitted into United States as refugees or immigrants be screened for public health purposes (8 U.S.C. § 1182 [a] [1]; 42 C.F.R. Part 34). Federal law also mandates medical examinations for public health purposes for aliens who want to change their immigration status from temporary to permanent residence (42 C.F.R. § 34.1 [d]).[13] Aliens seeking refugee status, immigrant visas, or adjustment of their immigration status are denied admission into the United States or a change in their immigration status on the following health-related grounds: (*1*) if they have a communicable disease of public health significance (currently, tuberculosis, human immunodeficiency virus [HIV], syphilis, chancroid, gonorrhea, granuloma inguinale, lymphogranuloma venerum, and Hansen disease [i.e., leprosy]); (*2*) if they fail to present documentation of having received vaccination against vaccine-preventable diseases (currently mumps, measles, rubella, poliomyelitis, tetanus and diptheria toxoids, pertussis, *Haemophilus influenzae* type B, and hepatitis B); (*3*) if they have or have had a physical or mental disorder and behavior associated with that disorder that may pose a threat to the property, safety, or welfare of the alien or others; and (4) if they are drug abusers or addicts (8 U.S.C. § 1182 [a] [1] [A]). The Attorney General has discretionary power to waive certain of these provisions in specific circumstances (8 U.S.C. § 1182 [g]). Aliens who seek entry into the United States through nonimmigrant visas (e.g., tourists) may be required to undergo a medical examination at the discretion of either U.S. consular officers overseas or U.S. immigration officers at the port of entry if these officers suspect that an inadmissible health-related condition exists.[14]

Recent U.S. experience with refugees suggests that enhanced health assessments of refugees before they depart for resettlement in the United States can improve refugee health and protect U.S. public health. The Centers for Disease Control and Prevention (CDC) developed in 1997 an enhanced health-assessment protocol for a portion of Barawan refugees from Somalia scheduled for resettlement in the United States.[15] In addition to the mandatory health assessment required by federal law, the CDC also screened a portion of the Barawan refugees for malaria, intestinal parasites, and schistosomiasis. The enhanced health assessment produced results that led the CDC to administer pre-embarkation therapy for malaria and intestinal parasites for all the resettling Barawan refugees to reduce refugee morbidity and mortality and to reduce the introduction of parasitic infections into the United States. The approach pioneered by the enhanced health-assessment protocol in the case of the Barawan refugees may provide a strategy to strengthen the traditional federal strategy to prevent the importation of diseases through aliens.

Federal quarantine law

The federal government has authority to apprehend, detain, examine, and conditionally release individuals entering the United States to prevent the introduction, transmission, or spread of certain infectious diseases from foreign countries into the United States (42 U.S.C. § 264; 42 C.F.R. Part 71). This power applies not only to aliens but also to U.S. citizens. Federal quarantine authority also exists to control infectious disease transmission between states of the Union (42 U.S.C. § 264; 42 C.F.R. Part 70). The infectious diseases against which federal quarantine powers can be exercised are determined by Executive Order; and currently the quarantinable infectious diseases include cholera or suspected cholera, diphtheria, infectious tuberculosis, plague, suspected smallpox, yellow fever, and suspected viral hemorrhagic fevers (Lassa, Marburg, Ebola, Congo-Crimean, and others not yet isolated or named; Executive Order No. 12452, 48 F.R. 56927, 22 Dec. 1983).[a] The federal government also has the statutory power to prohibit the introduction of persons from a foreign country when the Secretary of Health and Human Services determines that, by reason of the existence of any communicable disease in that country, serious danger exists of the introduction of such disease into the United States and the introduction of persons from such country increases this danger (42 U.S.C. § 265). State governments in the United States also possess quarantine powers in their respective public health laws.

In response to emerging and re-emerging infectious diseases and the threat of biologic terrorism, state and federal governments are re-evaluating their quarantine powers, which have not been exercised frequently during the twentieth century (Box 5–3). For example, the CDC is reviewing both interstate and

Box 5–3. Exercise of Federal Quarantine Authority

The exercise of federal quarantine authority during the last two decades has been limited to sporadic, isolated cases of disease or suspected disease on board airliners and vessels entering the United States from foreign countries. (The one noteworthy exception was the mobilization of federal quarantine staff and resources in response to a plague outbreak in Sarat, India, in 1994.*) Such exercises fall into one of the following three broad categories:

- **Isolation, quarantine, or both of a conveyance or passenger(s) to prevent the possible spread of a communicable disease**. For example, in an ongoing effort to eliminate measles in the United States, the CDC's the Division of Global Migration and Quarantine (DQ), National Center for Infectious Diseases, along with the National Immunization Program (NIP), established protocols to identify possible measles cases on board international flights and cruises. These protocols included isolation of possible cases, notification of passengers and crew, distribution of health and contact information, and coordination of the medical follow up of any such cases. Clearly, efforts to eliminate measles in the United States require effective response and notification protocols at ports of entry and surveillance systems.
- **The use of federal quarantine authority to stop a conveyance from moving passengers or cargo to prevent possible spread of communicable disease**. An example of this type of exercise of authority is the issuance of "No Sail Orders." From time to time, cruise ships on international itineraries visiting U.S. ports experience disease outbreaks on board (usually food-borne or water borne infections). By law, these outbreaks are to be reported to the CDC's Vessel Sanitation Program, National Center for Environmental Health, and the outbreaks addressed in a collaborative manner by the cruise ship line and the CDC. There are, however, exceptions.

  In July 2001, the CDC implemented an embargo on the importation of *Dracaena* shipments in standing water that could have introduced mosquito species not widely seen in the United States. The Los Angeles district office of the U.S. Department of Agriculture (USDA) notified the CDC that it had identified maritime cargo containers of "lucky bamboo" (*Dracaena* species), an ornamental plant, that were infested with mosquitoes. The CDC subsequently identified the Asian tiger mosquito (*Aedes albopictus*, a species previously not seen in California) and other species of mosquitoes associated with these cargo containers. *Dracaena* shipments in standing water appeared to pose a considerable risk of importing exotic mosquitoes into the United States. *Aedes albopictus* can transmit human diseases, such as western equine encephalitis, St. Louis encephalitis, and dengue viruses.
- **Preventing passengers from boarding a conveyance**. Such a case occurred in March 2000. Included among the immigration responsibilities of the DQ is that of monitoring the medical examinations performed by physicians overseas and the laboratories they use. In the last few years, this monitoring has included a systematic visit to those physicians (known as panel physicians) assigned by the U.S. Department of State to perform medical examinations to identify certain medical conditions in prospective immigrants and refugees destined for the United States. In March 2000, as part of this routine quality-assessment process, DQ staff visited several countries in sub-Saharan Africa. In one of these countries, 53 refugees ready to board an aircraft for the United States were not allowed to board because four

continued

continued

> had findings suggestive of active tuberculosis (TB) (CDC and WHO policy guidelines and regulations state that "persons with infectious TB must not travel by public air transportation until rendered non-infectious"). If these refugees had been allowed to board, medical follow up (including treatment and prophylaxis) of passengers and crew might have been required. Additionally, state and local health departments responsible for the medical follow up and resettlement of refugees would have encountered formidable challenges when attempting to identify refugees in need of TB follow up.
>
> *In September 1994, the DQ (the Division of Quarantine was officially redesignated as the "Division of Global Migration and Quarantine" in 2001) responded to an outbreak of bubonic and pneumonic plague in portions of India. Plague information was placed on the 24-hour Health Information for International Travel "hotline," both voice and fax mode, and a separate telephone number was designated for quick access to plague information. Advisory Memorandum number 107, "Plague in India," was published by the DQ and the Division of Vector-Borne Infectious Diseases, both in the National Center for Infectious Diseases. Special plague alert notices were prepared and distributed to all passengers arriving in the United States on direct flights from India, as well as to passengers on other flights that usually carry a substantial number of passengers whose travel point of origin was in India. Arrangements were made for distribution of health alert notice cards to all arriving international passengers at all U.S. ports of entry. Thirteen possible plague cases were identified among arriving passengers, none of which proved to be an actual case. As of October 19, 1994, the WHO considered the outbreak in India to be under control. The WHO recommended no restrictions for travelers visiting India. However, travelers to the affected areas in India were advised to seek medical attention for any illness that began within 6 days after their departure from India. No imported plague cases were detected in people in other countries, and no plague cases were reported among U.S. residents in India. The DQ discontinued the plague alert about 30 days after its implementation, as well as the distribution of plague alert notices. Other notices were subsequently cancelled or modified as appropriate.

foreign quarantine regulations with a view to producing revised regulations to modernize quarantine as a public health tool.

International law and public health criteria for admission of aliens

Four areas of international law relate to the exercise of U.S. public health sovereignty over the admission of aliens: (*1*) the International Health Regulations (IHR), (*2*) trade and investment treaties, (*3*) international human rights law, and (*4*) refugee treaties.

The IHR bind the United States because it accepted these international legal rules as a WHO member state. The IHR control public health measures taken at ports of entry in connection with persons infected with or suspected to be infected with cholera, plague, or yellow fever. The IHR prohibit, for example, making vaccination against plague a condition of admission of any person to a country's territory (IHR, Article 51). The IHR allow surveillance or isolation of persons infected or suspected to be infected with cholera for a period not to exceed 5 days from the date of disembarkation, but the IHR do not allow cholera infection to be a reason for refusing a person admission (IHR, Article 62). The measures to be taken against passengers on international voyages under the IHR are the maximum measures that a WHO member state may take against the three diseases subject to the IHR (IHR, Article 23). The IHR's limited disease coverage means that these regulations do not significantly discipline U.S. public health sovereignty in connection with treatment of persons.

The WHO is revising the IHR to address the problems that this international legal regime suffers because its approach to international infectious disease control has become outdated (Box 5–4).[16] During the revision process, the WHO seeks to move away from basing international infectious disease control on a list of specific diseases toward a global capability triggered by public health risks of urgent international importance. How the IHR revision will affect U.S. public health sovereignty in connection with the admission of aliens is unclear because the revision process is not complete and new concepts, such as "public health risks of urgent international importance" have yet to be clearly defined.

The United States has entered treaties that enable foreign business persons to live and work in the United States as part of the effort to liberalize trade and investment with other countries. These treaty provisions normally reserve to the United States the ability to deny temporary entry rights on the public health grounds provided in federal law. The North American Free Trade Agreement (NAFTA) provides, for example, that "[e]ach Party shall grant temporary entry to business persons who are otherwise qualified for entry under applicable measures relating to public health and safety and national secuity" (NAFTA, Article 1603). Thus, the United States could legitimately deny entry to a business person from Canada under NAFTA because the person has a communicable disease of public health significance, such as HIV infection and acquired immunodeficiency syndrome (AIDS).

The inclusion of HIV as a reason to deny aliens admission to the United States has been controversial. Experts have criticized the U.S. HIV-related immigration policy as a violation of human rights, which links this issue to international human rights law. Gostin and Lazzarini argued, for example, that "denying entry to individuals based solely on HIV infection fundamentally infringes on human rights."[17] However, the United States has not restricted its ability to deny entry to HIV-positive aliens in either treaty law or CIL. Whether denying entry to aliens with HIV makes public health sense remains controversial, but the United States does not violate international human rights law in denying aliens admission because they have HIV. Although legislated to protect public health, the HIV exclusion increasingly functions to prevent immigrants with HIV from becoming a "public charge," which is a different rationale for exclusion than public health (8 U.S.C. § 1182 [a] [4]). HIV-positive immigrants who can show that they have the financial resources and access to a health-care provider

---

Box 5–4. Revision of the International Health Regulations (IHR)

The IHR were originally adopted by the World Health Assembly (WHA) in 1951 as the International Sanitary Regulations. In 1969, the WHA changed the name to International Health Regulations. The IHR's objective is to ensure the maximum protection against the international spread of disease with minimum interference with world traffic. In 1995, the WHA instructed the WHO Director-General to revise the IHR in light of challenges mounting from emerging and re-emerging infectious diseases and globalization. The WHO Secretariat produced two drafts of the revised IHR, in February 1998 and in September 2000, for consideration by WHO member states. The current target date for the adoption of the revised IHR by the WHA is May 2003.

---

can receive waivers to the HIV exclusion rule. Refugees for whom "public charge" is not an exclusionary criteria per se can now more easily obtain waivers of the HIV exclusion rule.

The United States is party to the United Nations (UN) Convention Relating to the Status of Refugees (UN Refugee Convention, 1951), and it has enacted legislation to implement its obligations under this treaty (Federal Refugee Act, 1980). Basic disciplines required by the UN Refugee Convention are for parties to treat refugees no less favorably than they treat other aliens or their own nationals with respect to various public services and laws. The UN Refugee Convention requires, for example, national treatment for refugees in connection with public relief, labor laws, and social security, including provisions for occupational injury and disease, sickness, maternity, and disability (UN Refugee Convention, Articles 23–24). Thus, in applying public health laws to refugees, the United States has agreed to implement such laws in a nondiscriminatory manner.

Public Health Threats from Goods

Federal law

Federal quarantine law gives the U.S. government the power to prevent the introduction, transmission, or spread of communicable diseases from foreign countries or between states of the Union through the importation or interstate movement of property (42 U.S.C. §§ 264–265; 42 C.F.R. Parts 70–71). The U.S. Customs Service and Department of Agriculture are also empowered to prevent the importation of products believed harmful to human, animal, or plant health (e.g., cattle potentially infected with bovine spongiform encephalopathy or foot and mouth disease). These powers reflect Congress' exercise of its con-stitutional authority to regulate commerce with foreign nations and interstate commerce between states of the Union. Although the United States retains sov-ereignty over what goods from other countries enter its territory, international law affects this area more than it does the admission of foreign persons. The United States has played an influential role in the construction of international law that directly and indirectly affects U.S. efforts to keep health-threatening products out of the country.

International health regulations

The IHR regulate not only measures that WHO member states can take against people but also measures they can implement against goods in international commerce. The maximum measures that WHO member states may take under the IHR in connection with cholera, plague, and yellow fever include measures against goods. IHR provisions on measures against goods require WHO member states to apply measures that are appropriate scientifically and from a public health perspective. The IHR supports, for example, the WHO's position that trade bans and embargoes have no effect in stopping the spread of cholera and thus are excessive, irrational measures. The IHR's international legal effect on trade-restricting health measures is, however, limited because the regulations only deal with three infectious diseases.

The move away from a list of specific diseases toward public health risks of urgent international importance in the IHR revision will affect the IHR's impact on the exercise of U.S. public health sovereignty against foreign goods. Basing the revised IHR on public health risks of urgent international importance may mean that the revised IHR cannot contain specific maximum measures that may be taken against goods in connection with any specific disease. The WHO en-visions that identification and confirmation of public health risks of urgent in-ternational importance will be followed by WHO recommendations to member states about the appropriate public health measures to take. Whether the rec-ommendations will be legally binding on WHO member states is not clear and has not yet been the subject of serious negotiations.

International trade law

International trade law has broader application than the IHR because it is not limited to a short list of infectious diseases but instead affects a variety of trade-restricting health measures that states may take to protect public health from communicable and noncommunicable disease threats. This section focuses on the principles found in the system of international trade law within the WTO; but rules in regional trade agreements, such as NAFTA, follow the pattern dis-cernible in the WTO.

The General Agreement on Tariffs and Trade (GATT, 1994) contains rules that allow WTO member states to restrict trade for public health protection. The first set of rules in which public health considerations support trade restrictions relates to GATT's system of nondiscrimination created by the "most-favored-nation" (MFN) principle (GATT, Article I) and the national treatment (NT) principle (GATT, Article III). Under these principles, an importing GATT party cannot discriminate against imported products from another GATT party in favor of "like products" imported from another GATT party (MFN principle) or made within the GATT party importing the foreign product (NT principle). In the *Asbestos Case* (2001), the WTO Appellate Body ruled that health-threatening characteristics of a product could be considered in the "like product" analysis for purposes of applying the NT principle.[18] Thus, the Appellate Body held that products containing asbestos and products not containing asbestos were not "like products," even though consumers used the products for the same purposes, because asbestos fibers threatened human health. The same reasoning applies to the interpretation of the "like product" requirement in the MFN principle.

The second set of rules in GATT that relate to public health involve GATT's recognition that WTO member states may legally violate a GATT principle, such as the prohibition on quantitative restrictions (GATT, Article XI), if the measure is necessary for the protection of human health (GATT, Article XX[b]). For example, if the United States banned shipments of fruit from entering the U.S. market because the fruit was contaminated with highly infectious bacteria, viruses, or parasites, the ban would violate Article XI of GATT but would be justifiable under Article XX(b). This rule acknowledges the public health sovereignty of WTO member states but subjects such sovereignty to the disciplines of Article XX(b). This rule also applies to public health measures that restrict trade to protect against infectious and noncommunicable disease threats posed by goods, which gives GATT much wider public health significance in the trade context than the IHR.

If the trade-restricting health measure seeks to protect human health from risks arising from additives, contaminants, toxins, or disease-causing organisms in foods, beverages, or feedstuffs, then WTO member states have to comply with the WTO Agreement on the Application of Sanitary and Phytosanitary Measures (the SPS Agreement).[b] The SPS Agreement applies scientific and trade-related disciplines to trade-restricting food-safety measures. The scientific disciplines require that sufficient scientific evidence support the measures (SPS Agreement, Article 2.2) and that the measures be based on a scientific and policy risk assessment (SPS Agreement, Article 5.1). The SPS Agreement also mandates that WTO member states base their food-safety regulations on relevant international standards promulgated by competent international organizations, such as the Codex Alimentarius Commission (Codex) (SPS Agreement, Article 3.1). If a WTO member state applies measures more protective than applicable international standards, it may do so if it has a scientific justification for the more protective standard (SPS Agreement, Article 3.3). WTO member states must also accept the sanitary or phytosanitary measures of other member states as equivalent if the exporting member state can objectively demonstrate to the importing member state that its measures achieve the importing member state's appropriate level of protection (SPS Agreement, Article 4.1).

The SPS Agreement necessitates the involvement of public health experts and officials in various ways. The requirement for a trade-restricting health measure to be based on scientific evidence and a risk assessment calls for epidemiologic data. The importance of international standards, such as those developed by Codex, makes the standard-setting work of public health officials in WHO and elsewhere very relevant to the operation of international trade law. Litigation between WTO member states under the SPS Agreement will require scientific testimony and input from public health experts for the countries litigating the dispute. In addition, WTO dispute settlement panels may call on independent experts to help the panels evaluate scientific and technical evidence presented by the litigating parties (SPS Agreement, Article 11.2).

The WTO Dispute Settlement Body interpreted the SPS Agreement in a dispute between the United States and the European Community (EC) involving food safety in the *Beef Hormones Case* (1998).[19] In this case, the WTO Appellate Body held that the EC violated Article 5.1 of the SPS Agreement because it had not shown that its ban on the importation of beef raised with growth-promoting hormones was based on a risk assessment. Codex had previously determined that the hormones in question posed no threat to human health, but the EC imposed a ban on beef grown with such hormones. Although not technically part of the WTO's holding, the decision also suggested that the EC had no scientific basis for its total prohibition on the importation of hormone-raised beef.

Trade-restricting public health measures that do not fall into the food-safety category of the SPS Agreement may be subject to the disciplines of the WTO Agreement on Technical Barriers to Trade (TBT Agreement). Technical regulations set out product characteristics or their related processes and production methods that products must meet before being sold to consumers (TBT Agreement, Annex 1). The protection of human health is a legitimate objective for applying technical regulations to imported products (TBT Agreement, Article 2.2); but such regulations must be applied in a way that does not violate either the MFN or NT principle (TBT Agreement, Article 2.1) or create unnecessary obstacles to international trade (TBT Agreement, Article 2.2). The TBT Agreement requires that WTO member states use relevant international standards as a basis for their technical regulations, unless such use would be inappropriate or ineffective (TBT Agreement, Article 2.4). The WTO Appellate Body in the

Asbestos Case held that the French ban on the sale of products containing asbestos was a technical regulation that fell within the scope of the TBT Agreement and was subject to its disciplines.

The above paragraphs provide an overview of the complicated disciplines in international trade law and the WTO that apply to U.S. public health sovereignty. The basic message is that international trade law applies significant disciplines to the sovereign state's power to protect national public health from foreign products. Some experts have argued that the disciplines found in the WTO system and regional agreements such as NAFTA reduce the U.S. ability to protect itself from health-damaging foreign products in two respects: (*1*) the trade liberalization fostered by free trade agreements overwhelms the U.S. capacity to inspect foreign food products at the border for possible health-damaging chemicals and organisms; and (*2*) the disciplines used in the WTO and NAFTA to regulate public health sovereignty weaken the U.S. ability to protect the health of its population from dangerous foreign products.[20] The discourse between opponents and defenders of international trade law suggests, at the very least, that the debate is fundamental to how the United States will exercise its public health sovereignty in the years to come.

EXPORTATION OF PUBLIC HEALTH THREATS FROM THE UNITED STATES

The *Beef Hormones Case* involved not only whether the EC's exercise of public health sovereignty conformed to international trade law but also whether the United States exported a public health threat in the form of hormone-raised beef. This section looks at how U.S. federal law and international law address the exportation of public health threats from the United States.

General Principles on the Exportation of Public Health Threats

As a matter of constitutional law, Congress has authority under its power to regulate commerce with foreign nations to restrict or prohibit the emigration of persons who, or the exportation of products that, may cause public health damage in foreign countries. Whether international law contains rules that regulate the emigration of people for public health purposes or the exportation of dangerous products is more complicated. The United States can enter and has entered treaties that impose duties to prevent the disembarkation of persons with certain diseases (e.g., the IHR) and to regulate the exportation of dangerous products (e.g., Montreal Protocol on Substances that Deplete the Ozone Layer).

In addition, CIL holds that states must not allow their territory to be used in ways that cause damage inside the territory of another state. This rule has most often been invoked in connection with transboundary air or water pollution rather than in the context of the movement of people or goods. The reason for this is that, unlike with transboundary pollution, the state receiving refugees, immigrants, or tourists and importing goods has sovereign power and mechanisms to protect its public health from disease threats moving in international commerce. In other words, absent specific treaty obligations, the legal onus falls on the importing rather than the exporting state as a matter of international law. Public health practices do not, however, necessarily reflect this legal reality. Public health officials from different national governments cooperate and communicate to protect public health and do not restrict their collaborative efforts because, under international law, the legal onus to protect from threats falls on the importing state.

Exportation of Public Health Threats Through People

Federal law

Federal statutory law does not require the U.S. government to prevent people with diseases of public health significance from leaving the United States to travel to other countries. Such power exists in federal quarantine authority to prevent disease transmission between states of the Union (42 U.S.C. § 264; 42 C.F.R. Part 70), but existing federal quarantine law relating to foreign countries focuses on preventing the introduction of diseases into the United States and does not mention preventing the exportation of diseases from the United States (42 U.S.C. § 264; 42 C.F.R. Part 71).

International law

However, the United States has international legal obligations to restrict the movement of people from the United States to other countries under international law. The IHR requires WHO member states to take all practicable measures to prevent the departure of any infected person or person suspected of being infected (IHR, Article 30.1[a]). This obligation only extends to people infected with the three diseases that are subject to the IHR—cholera, plague, and yellow fever—so its legal impact on U.S. policies toward persons traveling to foreign destinations is limited. The IHR revision process proposes to allow the WHO to issue recommendations to countries after the identification and confirmation of a public health risk of urgent international importance. Presumably these recommendations could include preventing persons infected with, or suspected to be infected with, certain highly communicable diseases to be prevented from traveling to foreign countries. Whether such recommendations would be binding on WHO member states has not yet been decided in the IHR revision process.

Exportation of Public Health Threats Through Goods

Federal law

Congress has used its power to regulate commerce with foreign nations to restrict U.S. exports to foreign countries, mainly for reasons relating to national security. In the public health context, federal law contains provisions that regulate the exportation of products that might be harmful to public health in other countries. For example, a food, drug, device, or cosmetic that cannot be sold in the United States because it is adulterated[c] or misbranded can be exported if the product: (1) accords to the foreign purchaser's specifications, (2) does not conflict with the importing country's law, (3) is labeled that it is intended for export, and (4) is not sold or offered for sale in U.S. commerce (21 U.S.C. § 381 [e][1]).

Federal law also allows the exportation of drugs and devices not approved for sale or use in the United States if the drug or device complies with the laws of the importing country and has valid marketing authorization from the responsible government agency in that country (21 U.S.C. § 382[a]–[b]). For countries other than Australia, Canada, Israel, Japan, New Zealand, Switzerland, and South Africa and those in the European Economic Area, unapproved drugs cannot be exported unless the laws of the importing country also meet certain substantive requirements relating to oversight of drug safety and effectiveness (21 U.S.C. § 382[b][2][B]). Federal law also prohibits exportation of drugs and devices that, among other requirements, present an imminent hazard to the public health of the intended importing country (U.S.C. § 382[f][4][B]), a determination made by the Secretary of Health and Human Services in consultation with the appropriate public health official of the importing country. Neither the U.S. Export–Import Bank nor the federal government's Overseas Private Investment Corporation can under federal law support export or investment projects that may cause environmental or health damage in a foreign country (12 U.S.C. 635i-5[a][2]; 22 U.S.C. 2191[n]). Federal law does not, however, require that exported cigarettes comply with U.S. law on the manufacture, labeling, and packaging of cigarettes for domestic consumption (15 U.S.C. § 1340).

International law

Several treaties in international environmental law regulate the export of products deemed dangerous to human health and the environment, including the Montreal Protocol on Substances That Deplete the Ozone Layer (1987), Basel Convention on the Control of Transboundary Movements of Hazardous Wastes and Their Disposal (1989), the Rotterdam Convention on the Prior Informed Consent Procedure for Certain Hazardous Chemicals and Pesticides (1998), the Cartagena Protocol on Biosafety (2000), and the Stockholm Convention on Persistent Organic Pollutants (2001). Table 5–1 summarizes the export-related provisions of these agreements and the U.S. position on each.

TABLE 5–1. International Environmental Treaties and Export Controls on Substances Harmful to Public Health or the Environment

TREATY	EXPORT-RELATED PROVISIONS	UNITED STATES' POSITION
Montreal Protocol on Substances That Deplete the Ozone Layer	State parties must ban the export of certain ozone-depleting substances to nonstate parties	The United States has ratified the Montreal Protocol
Basel Convention on the Control of Transboundary Movements of Hazardous Wastes and Their Disposal	The treaty bans the export of hazardous wastes from OECD to non-OECD, to Antarctica, and to countries not party to the Basel Convention	The United States has signed but has not ratified the Basel Convention
Rotterdam Convention on the Prior Informed Consent Procedure for Certain Hazardous Chemicals and Pesticides	The treaty regulates the exportation of certain hazardous chemicals and pesticides from state parties through, among other things, the requirement of prior informed consent from the importing state party	The United States has signed but not ratified the Rotterdam Convention
Cartagena Protocol on Biosafety	The treaty applies an advanced informed agreement procedure to the exportation of living modified organisms	The United States cannot join the Cartagena Protocol because it has not ratified the Convention on Biodiversity and is unlikely in the near future to do so
Stockholm Convention on Persistent Organic Pollutants	The treaty prohibits states parties from exporting certain chemicals	The United States has signed the Stockholm Convention, and the Bush Administration has expressed support for its ratification

In the past, the United States also has used international law to open foreign markets for products that are harmful to human health. For example, the United States used federal law and GATT to open developing-country markets to tobacco exports from U.S. tobacco companies. In 1990, the United States prevailed against Thailand in a GATT case in which the panel held that Thailand's ban on the importation of foreign-made tobacco products was not necessary to protect human health within the meaning of GATT Article XX(b).[21] In the 1990s, however, the U.S. government and tobacco companies came under criticism through the WHO's effort to mount a global effort to reduce tobacco-related morbidity and mortality, an effort that includes crafting a framework convention on tobacco control (FCTC) (Box 5–5). Because FCTC negotiations are ongoing, whether the United States will support or oppose the WHO's effort to create new international law on tobacco control remains to be seen. The January 2001 proposed FCTC text includes a provision requiring states parties to regulate and prohibit the export of tobacco products that do not conform to the exporting country's own domestic standards.[22] This proposed provision would require the United States to change federal law on cigarette exports, which currently does not require that exported cigarettes comply with U.S. domestic standards (15 U.S.C. § 1340).

The United States has opposed international public health efforts to regulate commerce in pharmaceutical products, breast-milk substitutes, and genetically modified organisms. In the late 1960s and early 1970s, the United States opposed proposals to establish international monitoring of the quality of pharmaceuticals moving in international commerce. As a result of U.S. opposition, nonbinding guidelines on manufacturing, labeling, and quality control were adopted rather than internationally binding regulations. Public health experts argued that the marketing of breast-milk substitutes by Western multinational corporations in developing countries was detrimental to public health because such marketing reduced levels of breast feeding. The World Health Assembly adopted a nonbinding code on the marketing of breast-milk substitutes in 1981, with the United States casting the only negative vote. The United States also has opposed international regulations on trade in genetically modified organisms, as evidenced during the Cartagena Protocol negotiations, in part because the United States does not believe that scientific evidence supports the health threat ostensibly posed by genetically modified organisms.

Box 5–5. Proposed Framework Convention on Tobacco Control

In 1995, the World Health Assembly (WHA) asked the World Health Organization (WHO) Director-General to report to it in 1996 on the feasibility of developing an international instrument on tobacco control. In 1996, the WHA called on the WHO Director-General to begin the development of a framework convention on tobacco control (FCTC). In 1999, the WHA established a working group to prepare for intergovernmental negotiations on the FCTC; and the working group completed its work in May 2000. Three intergovernmental negotiating sessions on the FCTC have been held in Geneva. The objective is to present the final treaty for WHA adoption in May 2003.

U.S. positions on other areas of international law have also been part of global controversies. The United States is currently embroiled in a global dispute that pits international legal protection of patent rights in pharmaceuticals against needs in many developing countries for affordable access to drugs and vaccines. The United States challenged South Africa and several developing countries that legislation designed to use compulsory licensing and parallel importing to increase access to HIV/AIDS drugs violated the WTO Agreement on Trade-Related Aspects of Intellectual Property Rights (TRIPS). Major U.S. and European multinational pharmaceutical companies also began litigation against the Government of South Africa, claiming that such legislation violated their constitutional and legal rights in South Africa.

The actions of the U.S. government and the major pharmaceutical multinationals helped spark a global campaign to increase access to essential drugs and medicines and to balance TRIPS' protection of patent rights with emphasis on access to drugs and vaccines as a human right. In the face of global criticism, the U.S. government and the major pharmaceutical multinationals retreated from their positions with respect to South Africa. The "TRIPS v. access to drugs and vaccines" controversy continues, however, as evidenced by the special discussions held by the TRIPS Council on intellectual property and access to medicines.[23]

CONCLUSION

Public health and public health law in the United States are intertwined with U.S. participation in international politics and economics and have been since the Republic's founding. The traditional neglect of international considerations in analysis of U.S. public health law leaves out an aspect that is important for not only historical understanding but also an accurate picture of the global public health environment in which the United States is embedded. The federal exercise of the powers to regulate foreign commerce and to enter into treaties have been and remain key legal instruments for the U.S. government's responsibility for the health of the U.S. population. The United States is a leading power in the "anarchical society" of sovereign states; international law also has been and continues to be central to U.S. international activities that affect public health in the United States and beyond its shores.

Much of the federal and international law mentioned in this chapter is currently in flux, which makes future attention to the international considerations of U.S. public health law even more important. The CDC is revising federal quarantine regulations. The WHO is revising the IHR to strengthen this regime in the face of global infectious disease problems. The place of public health in international legal regimes involving trade and the environment has not been definitively determined, as illustrated by WTO treaties and cases and controversies over international environmental treaties. The WHO's effort to develop new international law on public health through FCTC also bears close observation. The perceived clash in international law between international protection of intellectual property rights and access to drugs and vaccines will not disappear anytime soon. All these federal and international legal issues directly affect U.S. public health law now and for the foreseeable future.

This chapter has focused on international considerations that arise in the exercise of U.S. public health sovereignty and to assist in correcting the traditional neglect of these issues and encouraging public health practitioners, experts, and scholars to view U.S. public health and public health law in their proper global context.

Notes

[a] U.S. public health officials believe this list is outdated, but it has not been updated by Executive Order or legislation since 1983.

[b] The SPS Agreement essentially replaces GATT Article XX(b) for purposes of trade-restricting food-safety measures imposed by WTO member states.

[c] Certain adulterated drugs or devices cannot be exported (21 U.S.C. § 382[f][2]).

References

1. Yach D, Bettcher D. The globalization of public health, I: threats and opportunities. *Am J Public Health* 1998;88:735–8.
2. Yach D, Bettcher D. The globalization of public health, II: the convergence of self-interest and altruism. *Am J Public Health* 1998;88:738–41.
3. Tobey JA. *Public Health Law*, 2nd ed. New York: The Commonwealth Fund, 1939.
4. Wing KR. *The Law and the Public's Health*, 5th ed. Ann Arbor, MI: Health Administration Press, 1999.
5. Grad FP. *The Public Health Law Manual*, 2nd ed. Washington, DC: American Public Health Association, 1996.
6. Gostin LO. *Public Health Law: Power, Restraint, Duty*. Berkeley: University of California Press, 2000.
7. Fidler DP. Challenging the classical concept of custom: perspectives on the future of customary international law. *German Yearbook Int Law* 1996;39:198–248.
8. Birnie PW, Boyle AE. *International Law and the Environment*, 2nd ed. Oxford: Clarendon Press, 1992.
9. Maloney SA, Cetron MS. Investigation and management of infectious diseases on international conveyances (airplanes and cruise ships). In: DuPont HL, Steffen R, eds. *Textbook of Travel Medicine and Health*, 2nd ed. London: BC Decker Inc, 2001: pp. 519–30.
10. Howard-Jones N. *The Scientific Background of the International Sanitary Conferences 1851–1938*. Geneva: World Health Organization, 1975.
11. Pan American Health Organization. *Pro Salute Novi Mundi: A History of the Pan American Health Organization*. Washington, DC: Pan American Health Organization, 1992.

12. Gordenker L. The World Health Organization: sectoral leader or occasional bene-factor? In: Coate RA, ed. *U.S. Policy and the Future of the United Nations.* Washington, DC: The Twentieth Century Fund, 1994: pp. 167–91.

13. CDC, National Center for Infectious Diseases, Division of Global Migration and Quarantine. Technical Instructions for Medical Examination of Aliens in the United States, March 1998. Available at http://www.cdc.gov/ncidod/dq/pdf/ti-civil.pdf. Accessed September 21, 2001.

14. CDC, National Center for Infectious Diseases, Division of Global Migration and Quarantine. Medical examinations. Available at http://www.cdc.gov/ncidod/dq/health.htm. Accessed September 21, 2001.

15. Miller JM, Boyd HA, Ostrowski SR, et al. Malaria, intestinal parasites, and schistosomiasis among Barawan Somali refugees resettling to the United States: a strategy to reduce morbidity and decrease the risk of imported infections. *Am J Trop Med Hyg* 2000;62:115–21.

16. WHO. Global Health Security—Epidemic Alert and Response: Report by the Secretariat. Geneva: WHO, April 2, 2001 (Doc. A54/9).

17. Gostin LO, Lazzarini Z. *Human Rights and Public Health in the AIDS Pandemic.* Oxford: Oxford University Press, 1997.

18. European Community—Affecting Asbestos and Asbestos-Containing Products, Appellate Body Report, issued March 12, 2001. Geneva: World Trade Organization, 2001 (WTO Doc. WT/DS135/AB/R).

19. European Community—Measures Concerning Meat and Meat Products (Hormones), Appellate Body Report, adopted February 13, 1998. Geneva: World Trade Organization, 1998 (WTO Doc. WT/DS26/AB/R).

20. Public Citizen. *NAFTA's Broken Promises: Fast Track to Unsafe Food.* Washington, DC: Public Citizen, 1997.

21. Thailand—Restrictions on Importation of and Internal Taxes on Cigarettes, adopted November 7, 1990, GATT Doc. DS10/R.

22. World Health Organization. Chair's Text of a Framework Convention on Tobacco Control, Intergovernmental Negotiating Body on the WHO Framework Convention on Tobacco Control, Second Session. WHO Doc. A/FCTC/INB2/2, January 9, 2001.

23. World Trade Organization. TRIPS Council's Discussion on "Intellectual Property and Access to Medicines." Available at http://www.wto.org/english/tratop_e/trips_e/counciljun01_e.htm. Accessed September 21, 2001.

II

THE LAW AND
CORE PUBLIC HEALTH
FUNCTIONS

6

Interaction Between Public Health Practitioners and Legal Counsel

WILFREDO LOPEZ AND BENJAMIN MOJICA

Public health practitioners within a government agency constitute a broad array of titles and functions—positions ranging, for example, from the Secretary of the U.S. Department of Health and Human Services, the Surgeon General of the United States, and the Director of the Centers for Disease Control and Prevention to the commissioner of a state or local health department, deputy and assistant commissioners, bureau directors, epidemiologists, public health advisors, and inspectors. All are integral to the practice of public health. Legal advisors to these practitioners can be internal or external to the agency and may comprise one or more lawyers with limited or broad roles.

Medical schools, and even schools of public health, limit the amount of curriculum addressing the roles and activities of government public health agencies. Similarly, law schools rarely provide insight into the field of public health law. Therefore, many public health practitioners and their attorneys, even those with considerable experience in the fields of health-care delivery or health-care financing, find themselves in need of on-the-job training regarding the relation between the practitioner and legal counsel. The purpose of this chapter, therefore, is to provide a practical framework for understanding and guiding the relationship between public health practitioners and legal counsel. We first suggest issues to be reviewed when a public health practitioner and his or her legal counsel initially meet or when the legal counsel writes the practitioner an introductory memo; we then describe in detail the different roles and responsibilities of the legal counsel in relation to the practitioner-client.

For simplicity in illustration, this chapter focuses primarily on the relationship between the head of a state or local health agency and its chief legal officer who supervises an internal Counsel's Office comprising several attorneys. Legal citations will focus on New York City and State to accommodate the authors' areas of expertise and to emphasize that the heart of public health law and practice is at the local and state level.[a] However, the concepts addressed here most likely apply to any practitioner and can, or should be made to, apply to any level of legal advisor, whether internal or external. Because law is so fundamental to public health—and because public health is so grounded in law— we believe that the optimum arrangement is for a public health practitioner to have an internal lawyer to provide readily available legal services.

INITIAL ENCOUNTER BETWEEN PUBLIC HEALTH PRACTITIONER AND LEGAL COUNSEL

The Statutory Framework

As administrative agencies, state and local health departments are creatures of statute. The state laws and the city charters that create state and local health departments usually will have particular sections that set forth the powers, functions, and duties of the health commissioner, sometimes called the "health officer," or of the health department.[1-4] Generally, the health officer can exercise all of the powers of the health department so that both terms can be read interchangeably.[3,5] These jurisdictional statutes and the court decisions that have interpreted them are a good place for counsel to start elucidating what the practitioner can do and why.

A memorandum from counsel should be provided to a new health commissioner as part of an introductory or transition document. The memorandum should point out where the law states that the prime directive is to protect the health of the public.[1,2,4] or what might be thought of as the "Three-M" theory of public health: to mitigate morbidity and mortality.[6] The document should explain that these jurisdictional statutes set forth the agency's core activities of "assessment, policy development, and assurance." Assessment mandates for the department to supervise the reporting of vital events, such as births and deaths, or to supervise the reporting and control of communicable and chronic diseases. Policy development mandates for the health officer to regulate many activities through the issuance of permits to safely operate hospitals, clinical and environmental laboratories, food-service establishments, radiation facilities, and others. Assurance mandates to safeguard the food and drinking water supply and generally to develop programs and interventions that will reduce morbidity and mortality. These statutes also will provide the authority, if not the mandate, for the health agency's other activities related to personal health issues such as health-care access, maternal and child health, school health, or correctional health.

The Police Power

Health departments, along with police, fire, and sanitation departments, are fundamental to the exercise of the state's police power. Indeed, most constitutions will declare that the reason for government's existence is to provide for the *health*, safety, and welfare of the people.[7] The introductory memorandum should clearly indicate to the health *officer* that he or she is constitutionally and legislatively charged with the exercise of the police power. Simply put, it is the power to issue orders. In New York City, this extraordinary authority includes the powers to

- Regulate commercial and noncommercial activities as the Permit Issuing Official
- Issue Commissioner's Orders to abate nuisances and, when those orders are not obeyed, to actually abate the nuisance and impose a lien on the offending premises
- Compel the attendance of witnesses and the production of records through the issuance of subpoenas in any matter before the health officer, including to subpoena records necessary to the conduct of an epidemiologic investigation;
- Isolate individuals, quarantine premises, and even detain persons who present a danger of transmitting disease to others.

The breadth and depth of this authority usually surprises a new public health practitioner.

The Rule-Making Power of Boards of Health and Health Officers

An initial memorandum from counsel should also explain to the public health practitioner the parameters of the authority vested in the particular jurisdiction's board of health and how that authority differs from the practitioner's inherent authority to promulgate rules. Commissioner's regulations generally fill in the details necessary to implement a state or local law. However, a board of health enactment, depending on the nature of the board's underlying authority, may have a vastly different force and effect, sometimes even the force of a state law. Extensively elaborating in the memorandum on the role of a board and giving a few illustrations of its value to the practitioner may be worthwhile. Boards, like legal advisors, may follow different models and have varying roles and functions. Some may act as a governing body of a health department, much like a board of directors of a corporation. Others may act in a quasijudicial capacity to hear appeals from certain commissioner of health decisions such as permit denials or revocations. The traditional role for most boards, however, is to promulgate a health code. We focus here on this latter function.

In New York City, the board of health has been accorded the ability to legislate in the area of health through the promulgation of the health code, which to some extent has the force and effect of state law and otherwise may be viewed as equivalent to a local law.[8] The force and effect of state law may result from either the state legislature enacting or amending the City Charter directly or from the fact that a state law may exempt the city from its application. The parallel to local law stems from several provisions of the Charter and is discussed in more detail below. The courts long ago found this extraordinary delegation of legislative authority to be constitutional as a time-honored exception to the principle that the power to legislate cannot be delegated.[9] The rationale for the delegation is that public health requires the exercise of professional and expert judgment and that it often needs to be exercised more quickly than what a typical city council or state legislative process would permit. The result is that similar boards of health can, if used properly, swiftly enact provisions that have greater force and effect than mere regulations. Counsel should impress on the practitioner the opportunity that such a board presents as a tool to protect the health of the public.

The possibility also exists that health officers will choose to accomplish their goals by administrative regulations, which most agency heads have the authority to promulgate, rather than by working through their board of health. However, this approach carries several risks. First, an administrative regulation generally needs specific enabling legislation. A commissioner's regulation that cannot demonstrate its enabling source runs the risk of being easily challenged. In contrast, when a board has broad legislative power, no specific enabling legislation is necessary in a particular case before taking action. In effect, the above-cited New York City Charter's legislative delegation is the enabling authority for all of the board's health code enactments. This principle is not as arcane as it may appear. For example, in the 1990s, New York City wanted to codify the ability of domestic partners, legally registered as such, to have the same rights as spouses. The concept applied to many aspects of life, requiring the local legislature, known as the City Council, to amend many local laws and other affected agencies to change regulations. However, because it needed no enabling legislation, the New York City Board of Health was quickly able to change the health code to put domestic partners on the same priority footing as spouses with regard to claiming the bodies of deceased loved ones and the issuance of burial permits.[10]

A second risk associated with the use of a commissioner's regulation, rather than board of health enactments, is that the courts generally grant greater deference and weight to the provisions of the health code than to commissioner's regulations.[11] Some proposals need to be enacted by a board, rather than by a commissioner, because they need the greater authority and deference to survive legal challenge. For example, if a board of health has the authority to enact laws requiring reporting of individualized medical information to the health officer for surveillance purposes, then the law should be at a level sufficient to establish the confidentiality of that information. In our view, such a confidentiality provision should be at least a board of health enactment, if not a statute. However, it should not be the subject of a mere administrative regulation, for such a rule will most likely not be sufficient to, for example, form the basis for a motion to quash a judge-signed subpoena seeking the inappropriate disclosure of confidential information.

Furthermore, the confidentiality of public health information should be the province of at least a board of health, not of a commissioner's regulation, to better protect such information from the incursions of "data snoopers" using freedom of information laws (FOIL). A somewhat subliminal principle that underlies much of public health is that individualized health information, once reported to the health officer, should be accorded a higher level of confidentiality than that accorded the same information in the hospital or physician's office. If a physician believes that public health reporting may result in his or her patient's confidentiality being compromised (or, to use FOIL terminology, the patient's personal privacy being invaded), then the physician may be less willing to make a complete and prompt report.

The centralized, populationwide nature of public health information makes health agencies an increasingly attractive target of data manipulators using the vehicle of these laws. Parenthetically, by obtaining supposedly de-identified information (i.e., apparently redacted of personal identifiers), it is also possible, through the use of other easily available data bases, to link "de-identified" information to an individual.[12] Therefore, a reporting requirement established by a board of health should be associated with a provision that addresses the confidentiality of that information—such as a provision that specifies that the information will not be disclosed even with the consent of the subject of the report, that it will not be subject to disclosure under FOIL, or that disclosures under FOIL will be limited to aggregated data. However, depending on the language of a particular state's information laws, even a board of health enactment might not be sufficient to adequately protect individualized medical information, and a state law might be required.[13]

The Line Between a Board of Health and a Local Legislature

Counsel should also advise the health officer about the limits of a board of health's jurisdiction. Although no bright line separates the authority of a city council from that of a board of health with regard to public health regulations,

the following analysis as it relates to New York City may be a useful model
for other jurisdictions.

The government of New York City, like that of many other municipalities,
is modeled on the tripartite distribution of powers among the three branches of
government: executive, legislative, and judicial.[14] Despite this functional separation, the Court of Appeals has recognized that "the duties and powers of the
legislative and executive branches cannot be neatly divided into isolated pock-
ets."[15] Many public health-related matters may be common to the powers and
authority of both the City Council and the Board of Health.[16] "Public health" is
not a term that is easily defined; the scope of what may be viewed as "public
health" is constantly evolving. The difficulty in reconciling the jurisdictions of
the Board of Health and the City Council regarding authorities to enact health
regulations is reflected in the New York City Charter Revision Commission
Report (dated August 17, 1936), which provides that "the charter, effective January 1, 1938, is intended to confer 'extraordinary' and 'plenary' powers of
legislators for the protection of health upon the Board of Health." The report
further states that "The Board of Health exercises extraordinary police powers
affecting the health of the City. By its power to adopt a Sanitary Code the Board
has plenary powers of legislation."[17] However, as referenced in an earlier case,
the report stated: "The Council is the legislative body and is vested with the
entire legislative power of the City."[18]

It is reasonable to postulate that certain areas of public health regulation are
exclusively within the domain of the New York City Board of Health and for
which only the Board would be authorized to enact health regulations. Although
an all-inclusive listing of these areas is not possible, examples of such areas are
the control of communicable diseases and requirements concerning the detention
of noncompliant tuberculosis (TB) patients. These areas of public health regulation link to the essence of the Department of Health's role.[19,b]

In assessing the appropriateness of a law enacted by the City Council rather
than by the Board of Health, we should note that in vesting the City Council
with legislative authority the City Charter stipulates that the Council may only
enact local laws that are not inconsistent with the Charter.[20] Legislative action
taken by the City Council in certain areas (e.g., those identified above) would
be inconsistent with the Charter by usurping the authority vested in the Board
of Health. For example, the Council could pass a law limiting the number of
swimming pools or restaurants within a geographic area, but could not specify
the temperature at which hot foods must be maintained in a restaurant because
that probably would be the prerogative of the Board of Health.

For other areas, both the Board and the City Council may have jurisdiction,
including domestic violence. The Board of Health clearly would have authority
to issue regulations in this area. If the City Council wished to enact a local law
addressing domestic violence, such legislation also would seem to be appropri-

ate. If, however, the Board of Health amended the Health Code with regard to domestic violence, the City Council could not enact a local law that would be inconsistent with a requirement imposed by the Board. If the City Council proposed legislation regarding a public health matter not exclusively vested in the Board of Health, then the Board would continue to be authorized to impose more stringent requirements at its discretion. To hold otherwise would be inconsistent with and impede the required and statutory mission of the New York City Department of Health.[19] Furthermore, a decision to the contrary would be inconsistent with the Charter, which specifically grants the Board of Health the authority to "publish additional provisions for security of life and health in the City. . . ."[8]

However, the delegation of legislative authority to a board of health should not be taken for granted. Current legislators seem less inclined to cede such authority to a nonelected body like a board of health. The line between public health policy, which should be the province of a board of health, and social engineering, which should be a legislative prerogative, has never been clear. Examples of such issues are whether requirements for window guards in multiple dwellings where children reside should be set forth in a health code; whether the board should determine the degree of abatement necessary to render a lead paint hazard safe; and whether prohibiting smoking in restaurants of a certain seating capacity is more appropriate for the legislature because it considers economic impact. Myriad issues exist about which counsel can only provide advice on the basis of applicable statutes and case law.[21] Even though public health practitioners must understand the principles underlying such questions, the legislature and the board of health also must be attuned to these matters so that they both can act effectively without interfering with one another.

Overlapping Jurisdictions: The Example of Lead

One example of the difficulty of sorting out the overlapping jurisdictions of a local legislature, like the New York City Council, and a board of health is the class action suit involving lead abatements in multiple dwellings. Although this case involved many issues, the key point regarding counsel's advice to the public health practitioner concerns a direct inconsistency between the city's Administrative Code, enacted by the City Council, and the Health Code. For many years, the Health Code had defined lead-based paint as interior paint containing 0.5% metallic lead or more and that a reading on an X-ray fluorometer of 0.7 micrograms of lead per square centimeter ($\mu g/cm^2$) would be deemed the equivalent of 0.5%. In 1981, the City Council amended that part of the city's Administrative Code known as the Housing Maintenance Code to create a lead-abatement mechanism in multiple dwellings where children aged 6 years or less resided. The Council defined lead-based paint in a similar manner to the Board by using the 0.5% lead *or* 0.7 μg/cm^2 standard. Although the Administrative Code did not mention whether intact, rather than peeling, paint was a hazard, a court in the course of the litigation had required the abatement of intact lead-based paint (0.7 μg/cm^2). In 1996, the Board of Health focused on two points that were particularly within its field of expertise: first, the X-ray fluorometer machine was found not to be reliable at readings of less than 1.0 μg/cm^2; and, second, the Board found that disturbing intact lead-based paint in the course of abatement was more hazardous for children than abating the peeling or damaged paint only. Therefore, the Board amended the Health Code by changing the definition of lead-based paint to reflect the 1.0 μg/cm^2 threshold and by requiring abatement only when the Health Department finds lead-based paint that is peeling; on a window friction surface; or on any surface where a hazard exists because of the paint's condition, location, or accessibility to children.

The Board's determination created a direct contradiction between the Health and Administrative Codes. The court, in an unpublished order, struck down the Health Code amendment on the ground that it violated the Administrative Code provisions. The City appealed this ruling, vigorously defending the Board's authority. By then, however, the 15-year-old class action suit was so mired in other issues that the appeal was denied with no mention of the relative authority of the two legislative bodies.[22] Subsequently, the City Council passed Local Law 38 of 1999, amending the Administrative Code in a manner that adopted the Board of Health's position relative to not disturbing intact lead-based paint and as to the 1.0 μg/cm^2 threshold.

In an area as unique and sensitive as this, another important function of a legal advisor to a health department is to educate the litigating attorney—whether it be a corporation counsel or an attorney general—for whom delegated legislative authority is counterintuitive, with regard to the extraordinary authority of a board of health. Such effort will assist in providing a vigorous defense in upholding this fundamental legislative power.

Due Restraint: The Example of Tuberculosis

Counsel should help the health officer understand that fundamental public health laws that constitute a public health agency's statutory framework are usually among the oldest in the annals of state and local laws and must be interpreted carefully. In some respects, such laws require updating to strengthen the public health infrastructure. For example, a state statute to clarify that reported information is not to be disclosed at the line item level (i.e., in a nonaggregated manner, even if redacted of identifiers) would be useful.

The ability to order an individual or an entity to cease and desist from committing or maintaining a nuisance and to order the abatement and correction of the nuisance is crucial. However, establishing an all-encompassing list of specific public health nuisances is not possible. Efforts to attempt to define a health nuisance more specifically than "anything that is dangerous to life or detrimental to health" most likely would limit the health officer's ability to protect the public from some unforeseen risks.

Nevertheless, the broad authority conferred by these statutes must be exercised with restraint and with due consideration, particularly when individual civil liberties need to be limited for the public's health and safety. This principle is illustrated through review of the following problem involving TB in New York City during the early 1990s. Review of this problem demonstrates how law can assist the public health practitioner's efforts to protect the public in a manner that safeguards it against the arbitrary and capricious use of the police power. It is also illustrates how both the practitioner and counsel can fully engage the communities affected by a proposed public health intervention.

For many years, the City's Health Commissioner has had the authority—on determining that the health of others is endangered by a case, contact, or carrier of a communicable disease—to order such an individual to be removed and detained in a hospital.[23] This authority had been exercised almost exclusively in the context of TB. In a typical scenario, an infectious disease nurse or physician from a local hospital would phone the health department on a Friday afternoon to report that a patient with infectious TB was threatening to leave the hospital against medical advice. A public health advisor would be quickly dispatched to the hospital to review the chart and interview the patient. If a detention order was deemed necessary, one would be issued to both the hospital, ordering it to hold the patient, and the patient, ordering him or her to remain in the hospital. However, no mechanism was in place to effectuate these orders: No locked medical wards existed for such patients; Medicaid did not pay for the cost of posting a guard around the clock at the patient's door; and, although the patient could, in theory, petition the Commissioner for release and a writ of habeas corpus, a detained patient had no meaningful way to access an attorney. In short, full compliance with detention orders was difficult to achieve and maintain.

Even when the patients stayed in the hospital, once they were no longer infectious, they would be released with some medication and a referral. In 1991, the Health Department realized that a significant number of patients were developing antibiotic resistance to multiple antimicrobial drugs used for treating TB. Drug resistance resulted from the failure of many of these patients to continue their medications beyond their period of infectiousness to completion, followed by relapse and the resumption of treatment. Infectious, drug-resistant TB patients who left the hospital, or noninfectious TB patients who stopped taking medication and then had recurrences of infection, would in turn transmit the drug-resistant strain to others. The risk was compounded by the co-morbidities of acquired immunodeficiency syndrome (AIDS) and TB so that a patient with infectious, drug-resistant TB who was living in an AIDS residence, for example, presented an even greater danger to others.

Completion of treatment became an imperative that led to the innovative program of directly observed therapy (DOT). Making detention orders enforceable also became a priority. New locked isolation wards with negative air pressure and air exchanges had to be built to detain recalcitrant patients with infectious TB. However, options were unclear for those with noninfectious TB and a history of noncompliance. Modern concepts of due process held that, to sustain civil detention, an individual had to constitute a clear and present danger to others. At first blush, it might have appeared that patients with noninfectious TB presented no immediate danger to others. Discussions catalyzed by the Counsel's office at the City Health Department ensued and included representatives of the New York Civil Liberties Union, the City's Corporation Counsel, and others.

The process was one of mutual education not without points of serious contention. One area of initial disagreement involved the ability of a Health Commissioner (rather than a judge) to order someone detained. Ultimately, the practicalities of the situation prevailed; it simply was not practical to let an individual leave a hospital and then seek a court order, then try to find and seize the person. Another area of contention involved the government's right to civilly detain a noninfectious person until completion of therapy. This option seemed counterintuitive to many who were grounded in the due process principles of least-restrictive alternatives and the need for clear and convincing evidence of imminent danger.

However, dialogue led to recognition that public health is preventive. This idea was illustrated by the well-recognized, although still occasionally challenged, right to exclude unvaccinated children from school. Such children do not present a danger to others until they become infected by and are contagious with a vaccine preventable disease. Yet, because the prevailing belief is that the majority of children must be vaccinated if the community is to be protected, the proposition that the unvaccinated present a risk to the public is accepted. Similarly, because a patient with noninfectious active TB who does not complete therapy can, at any time, relapse into infectiousness and possibly transmit a drug-resistant strain, the argument held that such a person constitutes a current and significant threat to the public health.

The result was a Health Code enactment by the New York City Board of Health that allowed for Commissioner-ordered detention of patients with either infectious or noninfectious TB. The provision (Section 11.47 of the City Health Code) also incorporates many due process protections, such as requiring the department to seek a court order within 72 hours of a request for release by the detained person. The patient cannot be held for more than 60 days without a court order, regardless of whether he or she has requested release. The detained person has a right to be represented by counsel and, on request of the person, the City must provide and pay for counsel. In a related resolution, the Board of Health found that individuals who fail to adhere to their prescribed course of TB treatment constitute a public health nuisance.[c] The provision has survived legal challenge and has been upheld at the appellate level.[24] It also provides a recent example of how a fundamental public health police power such as detention can still be exercised in a practical manner, with due restraint and safeguards, and of how a law can be updated to strengthen the public health infrastructure.

The public health authority must also be exercised with restraint in relation to the possible primacy of other units of government. Potential exists for overlap between health departments and other agencies, at both the state and local levels, such as departments of environmental protection with regard to environmental and chemical hazards, departments of sanitation relative to rodent or vector control, and housing agencies concerned with lead paint. Therefore, the fundamental, jurisdiction-setting public health statutes cannot be read as a simple list of absolute mandates but rather should be viewed as an aggregation of the areas where the health officer can act. For example, a health officer will always have the authority to control and abate public health nuisances, generally accepted to be anything that is dangerous to life or detrimental to health. However, even the simplest act or condition can be converted into a public health issue by, for example, asking whether it is safe. If other agencies have greater primacy, then the health officer may not need to act. However, if other agencies do not have the authority or the resources to implement the appropriate remedy, then the health department's participation may be brought in to ensure the public's health.

THE ROLE OF COUNSEL TO A PUBLIC HEALTH AGENCY

An attorney to a health department needs to be experienced in the distinct field of public health law. Some lawyers, particularly academicians, may know about the concepts of public health law, but it is not a field of law that is practiced outside of government. Furthermore, as demonstrated in the preceding discussions, it is broad and complicated. Therefore, expertise in the practice comes only from years of work in the field itself—meaning that the health commissioner or the chief counsel (hereinafter "counsel") would be well advised to hire attorneys at entry level positions to develop their exposure to the breadth and depth of the practice over time. Such development and expertise will enhance the ability of an attorney to render accurate legal advice spontaneously at a meeting. As any public health practitioner knows, many crucial decisions are made quickly in response to an emergent situation. Whether that situation is an outbreak of communicable disease or an immediately dangerous environmental health risk, rarely does sufficient time exist to ask for a legal opinion if a question arises about the legality of a particular public health intervention. In times of crisis—which are invariably frequent—access to a knowledgeable public health lawyer is necessary. To ensure immediate access to such, an attorney should be available in-house.

The role of in-house counsel should not be confused with that of a private lawyer to the public health practitioner. As a governmental lawyer, counsel's duty as a matter of legal professionalism is to report wrongdoing. Therefore, the limits of attorney–client privilege should not be crossed or compromised. For example, if a practitioner finds himself or herself the target of an Inspector General investigation, the practitioner should not ask counsel to represent him or her at a sworn interview before the investigators. Fortunately, such complications rarely, if ever, intrude into the relationship.

The day-to-day operational interactions between counsel and the various public health practitioners within a health department are numerous and varied. They involve many kinds of legal skills, activities, and areas for which legal counsel is required.

Legal Advisor

The core function of counsel is to provide legal advice and to render legal opinions. Typically, this function involves two kinds of activities: (*1*) participating in policy planning discussions and (*2*) researching and writing legal opinions. In a narrow, but important, sense, the role of a lawyer at a policy meeting is to advise on matters such as the agency's legal authority to undertake a particular course of action, the exposure to liability inherent in the action or intervention, and the procedural requisites involved.

However, policy meetings can be challenging in that focusing on the line between legal advice and programmatic direction is sometimes difficult. In addition to the role of advising on whether something can be done, the risks associated therewith, and the legal requirements for doing it, lawyers often are asked for advice on which course of action to take. This can be a slippery and perhaps dangerous road. Ideally the practitioner with decision-making responsibility will know and be sufficiently confident to set forth what needs to be done. Certainly a practitioner can ask a high-ranking attorney for a policy recommendation from among possibilities. However, asking an open-ended question about what can be done in a particular situation is another matter entirely and can too easily result in inappropriate transfer of decision-making authority. For example, a public health practitioner might ask about dealing with mold that is a potential health risk in an apartment, and the lawyer might reply that the practitioner can issue a vacate order. The practitioner should then weigh in with his or her own professional judgment about whether the health risk warrants that kind of intervention or whether a more appropriate remedy (e.g., bleaching the walls) exists that would adequately mitigate an immediate danger. It is possible, however, especially if the query to the lawyer is by a lower echelon practitioner, for the lawyer's advice to be accepted without benefit of the practitioner's independent technical assessment. Thus, counsel should be cognizant of situations where appropriate legal advice becomes inappropriate programmatic direction and decision making.

Of course, many legal questions cannot be answered on the spot. Many issues—such as a physician's duty to warn the contacts of his or her patients or the health officer's emergency powers—are complex and evolving. Researching the applicable law and writing a legal opinion are often necessary to render legal advice adequately. However, counsel should not entertain internal requests for opinions unless they are made by an individual with policy discretion, such as the commissioner, deputy or assistant commissioners, or program directors. Often, legal questions have been asked and answered previously, and a program director should be aware of previous advice so that he or she can provide direction without checking with counsel on every issue.

For several reasons, opinions should be requested in writing. First, a written request assists inquirers in determining whether they are asking a legal question or a programmatic one. Second, it creates a record that connects the question to the answer, thereby minimizing dangerous extrapolations of legal answers to fact patterns that were not contemplated when the answer was developed. Such unwarranted extrapolations can lead to mistakes and subsequent recriminations such as "Legal said it was okay." Maintaining a database of legal questions and answers is also advisable to facilitate future research. Of course, past opinions in the database should be used only as a starting point and not as the absolute answer in every instance because statutory, regulatory, or common law changes might produce a different legal answer at a later time.

Protector of Confidentiality

The public health practitioner needs to have broad and easy access to individualized medical and demographic information to protect the population at large. For example, statutes and regulations that authorize such access must, of necessity, be open ended to allow the practitioner conducting an epidemiologic investigation to demand more information than is initially required to be reported. The corollary to such broad authority is, however, an increased obligation to protect such information. Of course, different levels of confidentiality apply to different kinds of information in the custody of a health department. In addition to the FOIL forays discussed above, counsel must be vigilant to subpoenas that seek protected information.

For example, the results of a lead hazard inspection of an apartment obviously would be readily available to the landlord of the dwelling, the tenant of the unit, or their attorneys. The blood lead level of a child residing therein would not be available to the landlord except with the consent of the tenant-parent or on the issuance of an appropriate subpoena. In New York State, the disclosure of confidential human immunodeficiency virus (HIV) information requires a specialized court order,[25] and HIV-related information reported to the practitioner is accorded an even higher level of protection.[26,27] Sexually transmitted disease information in the custody of the health department, whether obtained through surveillance or through the provision of clinical services by the department, is similarly protected and not subject to disclosure by regular subpoena.[28] Obviously, the disclosure of information by a health agency is a complicated matter that requires the review, and often the intervention, of an attorney. Relevant, common activities for counsel include discussions with lawyers seeking information and with judges signing subpoenas and the development and arguing of motions to quash or motions for protective orders.

Compliance with the requirements of confidentiality is not a matter just for lawyers. Program staff and their supervising practitioners need to be trained in and familiar with the nuances of confidentiality to appropriately use and maintain the protected information. Because the laws that apply to public health information differ from those that govern clinical information in a hospital or physician's office, the training of personnel needs to be specialized and can be provided only by attorneys familiar with these principles and experienced in their application. This need underscores the importance of developing expertise in the distinct field of public health law within a health agency.

Contracts

Increasingly, health departments are forming partnerships with medical and academic institutions for the delivery of clinical or research services, community-based organizations for outreach and education, technology companies for specialized software, or other vendors for myriad activities and services, such as pesticide spraying to control mosquitoes to prevent arthropod-borne diseases. Although the process-related functions associated with contracting (e.g., ensuring competition through bids or requests for proposals) may be the province of nonlegal procurement specialists, the drafting of contract language remains largely a legal function that is best met by attorneys within the health agency.

Historically, health-related services have not been easy to quantify, resulting in contracts that reimburse contractors for actual expenses. However, in recent years the philosophy of government contracting has shifted toward presumably more accountable approaches, such as performance-based contracting or outcome funding. Vendors, particularly community-based organizations with few resources and little familiarity with such approaches, need to be given a clear and early understanding of the contractual expectations. Negotiating and drafting such contracts in the "human services" arena require close collaboration between the attorney drafting the agreement and the departmental programs that need outside services.

As governmental downsizing continues, the need for outsourcing will increase. However, because a health department is a police power agency, it should be careful not to contractually vest a nongovernment entity with the police power. Sometimes keeping this bright line in focus is not easy. For example, in this era of electronic reporting, a health department might be tempted to contract with a company to electronically receive and sort mandated surveillance reports. Aside from issues of confidentiality, the line can become blurred if the contractor is assigned the responsibility to call a physician to advise him or her that the report was not complete and to *demand* that additional information. Such a contract can be viewed as an unconstitutional delegation of the police power. In 1996, the U.S. Department of Defense gave considerable thought to the inappropriateness of contracting out "inherently governmental functions."[29]

Legislative and Regulatory Counsel

A significant role for counsel is to ensure that health code changes or agency head rules are within the statutory authority of the health board or commissioner to adopt and that they are enacted in compliance with laws that dictate the procedures to be followed in the promulgation process. The following typical process illustrates an appropriate interaction between counsel and practitioner.

The practitioner (e.g., a program director or a deputy commissioner) prepares a Certificate of Necessity that describes the problem that needs to be addressed by rule making and the proposed solution and suggests the language of a proposed rule. The Certificate is then transmitted to counsel's office for analysis of the statutory basis and legal viability of the proposal. Counsel then prepares a document setting forth the basis and purpose of the rule and the actual resolution language to be promulgated. After preliminary approval by the board or commissioner, the information is published, and notice of the proposal is provided to known interested parties (e.g., licensees or trade associations) to give them an opportunity to comment. Also, a public hearing may be held during which testimony may be taken. The proposal may be amended to reflect comments and submitted to the board or commissioner for adoption. The final rule is then published. In addition, board of health meetings are subject to the Open Meetings laws. Counsel must ensure compliance with all of these procedural requisites.

Another function of counsel relative to legislation and regulations is to coordinate the agency's comments on legislation or regulations proposed at the federal or state level or by sister agencies. Such coordination may involve tracking and distribution of proposals within the agency, synthesizing various internal comments, and drafting the agency's position.

Enforcement

As previously mentioned, one of the basic ways that a health agency exercises its police power is through the issuance of valid and enforceable orders. These can take the form of a commissioner's order issued to recalcitrant TB patients compelling them to complete their medical regimen, or they can be subpoenas issued to a physician refusing to disclose information necessary to an epidemiologic investigation. More typically, however, commissioners' orders are issued to landlords (or others in control of property or premises) requiring abatement of a health nuisance that presents a danger. Such orders can be standardized, as in the case of orders to abate peeling lead paint in an apartment in which a lead-poisoned child resides, orders to install window guards where a child aged 10 years or younger lives, or orders to clean a vacant lot strewn with garbage that provides harbor for rats. Individualized commissioner's orders also can be issued to others, such as a dry cleaning establishment releasing dangerous fumes to adjoining residential units, to require cessation of operations until the activity can be safely conducted.

Drafting orders, whether standardized or individualized, requires close working relationships between the practitioner and the attorney. The issuance of an order should be taken seriously. Program experts should be clear on the existence of a danger. The practitioner should provide the attorney drafting an order with direction as to the appropriate remedy to be required. For example, whether a lead hazard should be abated by wet-scraping and repainting, by encapsulation, or by complete removal are scientific or technical, not legal, decisions necessitating professional public health judgement combined with environmental and engineering input. Once the practitioner articulates the nature of the danger and the means of abatement, the attorney can draft an order that provides adequate notice to the subject of the order.

Due process usually requires an opportunity to be heard, although the opportunity need not be a full-scale hearing. Such a requirement can be met by affording the subject of an order the ability to call or appear before a supervising practitioner, such as an assistant commissioner, to challenge the scientific underpinnings of the order or to dispute ownership or control of the offending premises. Training by, and consultation with, an attorney is useful to make the opportunity to be heard fair and meaningful.

The issuance of an order is many times the beginning of an arduous process to achieve compliance. Follow-up inspections to ascertain compliance are necessary. If no action has been taken, a notice of violation may be issued that charges the responsible party with disobeying a commissioner's order and with maintaining a nuisance and requiring a return to an administrative tribunal. Some nuisances, however, are too dangerous to leave at that, for a fine is not abatement and does not by itself render a dangerous situation safe. Therefore, an order may need to be executed by the health agency directly or through another government agency. For example, a lot providing a rat harborage or containing water accumulations conducive to mosquito breeding can be cleaned by the health department or, if heavy equipment is necessary, by the sanitation department. Lead hazards are corrected and window guards are installed by the housing agency. These other units of government act as agents of the health officer in the execution of proper orders. The cost of the abatement work performed by the health agency and its agents is calculated and, pursuant to provisions of several local laws (enacted by the city council) that are specific to the authority of the health department, a tax lien is imposed on the premises.[30]

Sometimes access to offending premises is not possible without breaking down an obstruction such as a fence. Realizing that a rat harborage or a water accumulation, while constituting significant risks that require quick action, do not rise to the level of a boiler about to explode and destroy an occupied building, New York City seeks access warrants from the courts to forcibly gain entry for inspecting or abating these types of conditions. All of these activities attendant to the issuance and enforcement of orders require close interaction between the program and legal staffs of a health agency.

Conflicts of Interest

Among government agencies, health departments in particular have a high percentage of professional staff with a concomitant high degree of outside interests. For example, some may be medical doctors with positions at area hospitals or doctors of public health teaching at universities; others may sit on boards of directors of health-related organizations, and some may collaborate with outside entities in the conduct of research. All of these raise conflicts with regard to potential misuse of "city time" or, of greater concern, relative to relationships with entities that do business with the city or department. To help staff avoid difficulties after unknowingly entering into questionable activities, counsel can act as an advisor and a liaison to a central authority such as a conflicts of interest board. Employees can request approval from the agency head and, if necessary, from the central board. Counsel will provide advice to the agency head about the propriety of the activity.

Disciplinary Matters

Counsel also may be responsible for investigating and prosecuting wrongdoing by agency employees, other than criminal or corrupt behavior that usually is within the jurisdiction of an inspector general. Such allegations may relate to time and leave abuse, incompetent performance, insubordination, fights, arguments, or harassment. If the allegations are borne out, charges are brought against an employee who, by virtue of civil service status or contractual rights, is entitled to be served with charges and afforded a hearing to determine whether he or she should be terminated, suspended, or fined. Legal staff will work closely with the inspector general in situations of overlapping jurisdiction, with the employee's supervisory chain of authority, and with the human resources department and will represent the agency in the prosecution of the charges before administrative bodies authorized to hear and determine such cases.

Human Rights Cases

Counsel's office, as representative of the agency, will investigate the matter when employees or other parties bring formal charges before the local, state, or federal human rights agencies accusing the department of unlawful discrimination, usually in the context of employment practices or of condoning sexual harassment. If the charges are substantiated, the agency may settle the matter with the aggrieved party and may bring disciplinary charges against an employee who committed the wrongful act. If, after investigation, the charges are deemed to be inaccurate, agency legal staff will defend the department before the administrative human rights bodies. If these bodies find probable cause to believe that the allegations are true, or if the aggrieved party takes his or her claim to court, then the matter is turned over to the city's law department to represent the department in court.

Litigation Liaison

Except for motions to quash subpoenas, as discussed above, counsel's office does not engage in litigation. However, it is integrally involved as liaison to the litigating attorneys at the law department. Whether the litigation is against the health agency—for example, as in the case of a coalition of plaintiffs suing to stop the city's spraying of pesticides to prevent West Nile virus infection—or the city is suing lead paint or tobacco manufacturers affirmatively, the legal staff at the health department serves various functions. In such cases, legal staff may facilitate the gathering of information from the agency that may be necessary to defend or prosecute the case or respond to discovery demands. In addition, staff may explain the nuances of public health law to the litigating attorneys, often conducting legal research, for example, as discussed above in relation to lead litigation, explaining the authority of a board of health to the litigating and appellate lawyers. Counsel also explains the nuances of legal theories and strategies to the public health practitioner so that the client can be an active and informed participant in the litigation.

CONCLUSION

The interaction between the public health practitioner and legal counsel is as broad and deep as the field of public health. The practice of public health is inextricably tied to law because so much of the health officer's powers, functions, and duties are founded in law. The requirements of law in public health practice represent a distinct specialty that is practiced only within a health agency, and expertise in the field can only be developed from within. The day-to-day role of counsel to a health agency touches every aspect of the practice of public health. Understanding and appreciating the role of law in the practice of public health will help a practitioner better achieve the agency's mission of protecting the public's health.

ACKNOWLEDGMENTS

Roslyn Windholz, the Deputy General Counsel, New York City Department of Health, over the years has conducted much research into the history of the New York City Board of Health's authority. We acknowledge and thank her for her tireless attention to detail, appreciation of public health history, and love of public health law.

Notes

[a] The views expressed in this chapter are those of the authors and do not necessarily express the views of the New York City Department of Health or the City of New York.
[b] "The protection from a disease which actually exists (e.g., rabies) and kills a number of persons each year is a *function of the Board of Health*" (emphasis added).
[c] See notes to 24 RCNY Section 11.47.

References

1. New York State Public Health Law, Section 201.
2. New York State Public Health Law, Section 206.
3. New York City Charter, Section 555.
4. New York City Charter, Section 556.
5. New York State Public Health Law, Section 204.
6. New York State Sanitary Code, 10 NYCRR, Section 2.6.
7. New York State Constitution, Article XVII, Section 3.
8. New York City Charter, Section 558.
9. *People v. Blanchard*, 288 NY 145, 42 N.E.2d 7 (1942).

10. New York City Health Code, 24 RCNY, Section 205.01(d).
11. *Grossman v. Baumgartner*, 17 N.Y.2d 345, 218 N.E.S.2d 259 (1966).
12. Lane E. A question of identity—computer-based pinpointing of "anonymous" health records prompts calls for tighter security. *Newsday* November 21, 2000, C8.
13. New York State Public Officers Law, Article 6.
14. *Kelly v. Dinkins*, 155 Misc.2d 787, 590 NY S.2d 166 (1992).
15. *Bourquin v. Cuomo*, 85 N.Y.2d 781, 652 N.E.2d 171 (1995).
16. *Knoblauch v. Warden of the Prison*, 216 NY 154, 110 NE 451 (1915) (which addressed the authority of the Board of Health and the Board of Aldermen—the body replaced by the City Council).
17. *Paduano v. City of New York*, 45 Misc.2d 718, 257 N.Y.S.2d 531, 535 (1965), affirmed 17 N.Y.2d 875, 218 N.E.2d 339, 271 N.Y.S.2d 305 (1966).
18. *LaGuardia v. Smith*, 176 Misc. 482, 27 N.Y.S.2d 321, 325 (1941), affirmed 288 NY 1 (1942).
19. *Knoblauch*, 89 Misc. 243, 245, 153 NYS 463 (1915).
20. New York City Charter, Section 28.
21. *Boreali v. Axelrod*, 71 N.Y.2d 1, 523 N.Y.S.2d 464 (1987).
22. *New York City Coalition to End Lead Poisoning, et al. v. Giuliani*, 248 A.D.2d 120 (1st Dept. 1998).
23. New York City Health Code, 24 RCNY, Section 11.55.
24. *City of New York v. Mary Doe*, 205 A.D.2d 469, 614 N.Y.S.2d 8 (1st Dept. 1994).
25. New York Public Health Law, Section 2785.
26. New York Public Health Law, Section 2135.
27. New York State Health Department regulations, 10 NYCRR Section 63.4(c).
28. New York Public Health Law, Section 2306.
29. 48 C.F.R. Subpart 7.5.
30. New York City Administrative Code, Sections 17–145, *et seq.*

7

Frontline Public Health: Surveillance and Outbreak Investigations

VERLA S. NESLUND, RICHARD A. GOODMAN, AND DAVID W. FLEMING

Public health surveillance and the investigation of disease outbreaks and clusters are critical, basic functions carried out by public health agencies at local, state, and federal levels. Each of the 50 states operates and maintains public health surveillance systems to monitor not only notifiable disease conditions—which primarily are caused by infectious pathogens—but also noninfectious disease conditions and public health indicators such as behaviors that are risk factors for injuries and chronic conditions.[1,2] Along with the traditional collection and analysis of vital records, state-level surveillance forms the foundation for national-level surveillance systems, which may be coordinated by federal agencies such as the Centers for Disease Control and Prevention (CDC) and the National Institutes of Health.[1-3]

In addition to conducting surveillance, local, state, and federal public health agencies must be able to respond to disease threats by investigating the hundreds of outbreaks and disease clusters that occur in the United States each year. Outbreak response relies not only on the legal authorities necessary for public health agencies to conduct surveillance and, therefore, to detect such problems, but also on the authorities and assurances required for carrying out the steps of an investigation and implementing appropriate control measures. Specifically, these legal authorities enable public health officials to obtain clinical specimens and data from persons affected by an outbreak, collect environmental samples,

143

protect the confidentiality of information, conduct analytic studies (e.g., case–control or cohort studies) to test hypotheses about sources for pathogens and modes of spread, and implement and enforce control measures, such as vaccination, chemoprophylaxis, quarantine, or even seizure or destruction of property.

This chapter reviews legal issues related to public health surveillance and outbreak investigations. It discusses the general legal authorities for surveillance and public health investigations provided by the U.S. Constitution and by state laws; legal milestones in the evolution of public health surveillance, outbreak investigations, and disease control in the United States; and legal issues related to the collection, analysis, and dissemination of surveillance data. In addition, the chapter presents information about new surveillance challenges that go beyond traditional infectious disease models, including how bioterrorism preparedness is influencing surveillance activities. Related aspects of legal authorities and issues bearing on surveillance and public health investigations also are addressed in other chapters in this book, including and especially those covering foodborne diseases and sexually transmitted and bloodborne infections (see Chapters 14 and 15).

GENERAL LEGAL AUTHORITIES FOR SURVEILLANCE AND PUBLIC HEALTH INVESTIGATIONS

Both federal and state governments have inherent powers to protect the public's health. Article 1, Section 8, of the U.S. Constitution gives Congress the authority to impose taxes to "provide for the general [w]elfare of the United States" and to regulate interstate and foreign commerce. The Public Health Service (PHS) and the CDC are both examples of federal agencies established under the authority of the Welfare Clause. Under the authority of the Commerce Clause of the Constitution, the federal government oversees such health-related activities as the licensing and regulation of drugs, biologic products, and medical devices. Although the provisions in the federal Constitution are broad, the activities of the federal government relating to health and welfare, nonetheless, must fit within the enumerated powers.

In contrast, the public health powers of a state are extensive, rooted in its inherent powers to protect the peace, safety, health, and general welfare of its citizens. The Tenth Amendment to the U.S. Constitution specifically reserves all powers not expressly granted to the federal government or otherwise prohibited by the Constitution to the states. Unlike the federal government, the states have vast, sovereign authority, including public health powers that are not limited to specific constitutional provisions. The states' police powers include the intrinsic right to pass laws and to take such other measures necessary to protect the citizenry. In many instances, states have delegated their public health responsibilities to county or municipal governments, which likewise exercise the state's broad authority to examine, treat, and, in the case of certain contagious diseases, to quarantine citizens to protect the public health. The state's public health laws include not only the established statutes of the state but also regulations, executive orders, and other directives from health authorities that may have the force of law.

The exercise of the state's police powers with respect to public health matters has limitations. The U.S. Constitution provides procedural safeguards to ensure that the exercise of these powers is not excessive or unrestrained. The Fifth Amendment prohibits the federal government from depriving any persons of life, liberty, or property without due process of law. The Fourteenth Amendment imposes similar due process obligations on states. Due process demands that the government use even-handed and impartial procedures in exercising its police power. The basic elements of such due process include notice to the person involved, opportunity for a hearing or similar proceeding, and the right to representation by counsel. In addition, the exercise of the state's police power necessitates the principle of using the least restrictive alternative that would achieve the state's interest, particularly when the exercise involves limitations of the individual's personal liberty.

Public health surveillance systems in the United States are established as an exercise of the states' police powers. These state-based systems are designed for reporting of diseases and conditions of public health interest by health-care professionals and laboratories. State laws and regulations mandate the reporting of a list of diseases and conditions, as well as timing and nature of information to be reported, and may prescribe penalties for noncompliance with the reporting laws. Required disease reporting varies greatly among states and territories. In some states, disease reporting is mandated by statutes that have not been reviewed by legislatures in decades. Other states have general statutes that empower the health commissioner or state boards of health to create, monitor, and revise the list of reportable diseases and conditions. Some states require reports under both statutes and health department regulations.

As in the public health activities discussed above, the inherent powers to protect the public's health provide the general authority for laws and regulations that empower health officials to conduct epidemiologic investigations. Although cooperation of institutions and individuals in epidemiologic investigations is usually voluntary, the intervention of state or local officials is within the scope of governmental legal authority. Furthermore, either specific legislation and/or the police power of the state provides the necessary authority to compel cooperation in such investigations in instances in which individuals or institutions are reluctant to grant access to certain properties, records, or individuals associated with information essential to the investigation.

Outbreak and *epidemic* are terms well known to the public and constitute problems for which the public expects aggressive responses. Regardless of the dimensions of any given outbreak, most health authorities employ a standard approach for investigating the problem. The goals of investigation are to provide a scientifically rational basis for identifying the source of and for implementing measures to terminate the outbreak and to prevent recurrences in as timely a manner as possible.[4] The elements of a typical outbreak investigation highlight many of the basic functional activities used more generally for the control and prevention of reportable conditions. In addition, both outbreak investigations as overall exercises in disease control and their component parts invoke a multitude of legal issues.

The basic steps of an investigation are detecting and confirming the occurrence of an outbreak; identifying and characterizing cases; developing and testing hypotheses regarding potential explanations for the outbreak; and implementing control measures.[4,5] These steps are carried out under legal authorities, which both compel and enable health agencies to undertake such investigations; these legal authorities are grounded in constitutional principles and in federal and state statutes, which are discussed in this and other chapters. In addition, however, myriad related considerations exist regarding responsibilities and authorities for the individual elements of an investigation. Such considerations include the authorities necessary to obtain microbiologic cultures and other laboratory specimens from hospitals and private laboratories; to review patients' medical records kept in the offices of physicians, dentists, and other health-care providers; to administer questionnaires to and collect specimens from persons affected in the outbreak, as well as persons who were not affected but who may be important sources of information for solving the outbreak; to retain information about medical histories and laboratory results; to protect confidentiality; and to enact measures to control the immediate problem and prevent recurrences. Such measures may include the ongoing collection of additional data, recall of an implicated product, closing of a business or restricting its activities related to the source of an outbreak, isolation or restriction of activities of affected persons, vaccination of or administration of antibiotics to exposed groups, and even compulsory treatment of some individuals or groups with antibiotics and other medications.

Certain statutory provisions may be absolutely necessary for epidemiologists to complete critical steps of outbreak investigations. Accordingly, epidemiologists need to be aware of any state laws—including statutes or regulations—that may affect their ability to conduct an outbreak investigation. For example, in one of the largest food-borne infectious disease outbreaks in U.S. history, the manufacturers of the implicated product (ice cream) agreed to disclose manufacturing and product distribution information only after the Minnesota's public health legal counsel provided written confirmation of state statutory provisions protecting corporate trade secrets.[6] Similarly, in an investigation of an infectious disease outbreak involving meals served to passengers of an international airline, the airline disclosed flight manifests only after learning of the state health commissioner's subpoena power to obtain such data.

THE ROLE OF SURVEILLANCE IN PUBLIC HEALTH

Public health surveillance is a cornerstone activity of virtually all public health programs. Although the nature of public health surveillance has changed during the past century, the definition applicable to this discussion is the one first discussed by Alexander Langmuir in the 1960s.[7] Langmuir redefined surveillance as the ongoing, systematic collection of public health data with analysis and dissemination of results and interpretation of these data to those who contributed them and to all others who "need to know."[8] Accordingly, an effective surveillance system includes both the capacity for data collection and the ability to disseminate the data to persons who can undertake prevention and control activities.[9] The public health surveillance definition employed by the CDC includes the concept of using the data for "planning, implementation, and evaluation of public health practice."[10]

Surveillance has played an especially vital role in the control and prevention of infectious diseases. For example, surveillance can be instrumental in detecting outbreaks of infectious diseases, then triggering the elements of an investigation, as described in the preceding section, and finally monitoring the long-term effectiveness of control measures put in place as a result of the investigation. In addition to the detection of epidemics, other examples of roles for surveillance systems in controlling infectious diseases include monitoring the natural history of certain diseases, assessing more slowly occurring changes in the interactions between organisms and populations over time, evaluating the impact of control and prevention programs, and monitoring changes in the biology of infectious agents.

The collection of vital records and other data for public health surveillance and during epidemic investigations may involve a variety of legal issues and considerations, which also are relevant to information gathering necessary for other basic disease-control activities (e.g., surveys, special studies, and categorical disease-control programs). Increasingly, surveillance is used for investigating the range of conditions affecting health, including injuries, chronic diseases, environmental exposures, and maternal and child health activities.[7] The underlying issues attendant to data collection in these situations are balancing the need for access to medical and other records against individuals' interests in privacy through the imposition of strict limits on access. These legal considerations, most of which are addressed by statutes or regulations, include protection available during and after investigations for records developed in relation to the investigation; special confidentiality provisions for medical and other information; and mandated reporting of specific infectious conditions, as noted above.

LEGAL MILESTONES IN THE EVOLUTION OF PUBLIC HEALTH SURVEILLANCE, OUTBREAK INVESTIGATIONS, AND DISEASE CONTROL

Legal Milestones in Public Health Surveillance

Surveillance was employed in colonial America as early as 1741, when the colony of Rhode Island passed an act requiring tavern keepers to report contagious diseases among their patrons.[10] Two years later, the colony enacted a law requiring reporting of smallpox, yellow fever, and cholera. In 1874, systematic reporting of disease in the United States began when the Massachusetts State Board of Health initiated voluntary weekly reporting of common diseases by physicians, who used a postcard reporting format.[11] The collection of morbidity data to be used by the U.S. Marine Hospital Service, the forerunner to the PHS, for quarantine measures against selected diseases (e.g., cholera, smallpox, plague, and yellow fever) was authorized by Congress in the Quarantine Act of 1878.[1] Fifteen years later, Michigan became the first jurisdiction in the United States to require reporting of specific infectious diseases.[10]

The federal Quarantine Act of 1893 authorized the weekly collection of data from all states.[11] By 1901, all states required that selected infectious diseases be reported to local health authorities. As the result of the intervening epidemic of polio in 1916 and the pandemic of influenza in 1918, all states were participating in national morbidity reporting by 1925.[11] In 1961, the CDC—at that time bearing the name "Communicable Disease Center"—became responsible for receipt of reports of notifiable conditions and for weekly dissemination of such data through the *Morbidity and Mortality Weekly Report*, a publication that by 1994 had begun to make these data available online. The Public Health Service Act authorizes the CDC to collect, collate, and analyze notifiable disease data at the national level; in fact, however, state health agencies provide these data to the federal government on a voluntary, cooperative basis. Moreover, each state promulgates its own set of reportable diseases by legislative enactment or regulation.[11,12]

Special Influence of Smallpox on Public Health Laws

Smallpox, the only disease to have been eradicated from the world, played an especially profound role in influencing the evolution of the legal basis for the control of infectious diseases in the United States; many of the key developments were reported by Hopkins.[13] An early example of the use of the functional strategies of local quarantine and isolation to prevent the spread of smallpox during the colonial era was an order issued in East Hampton, Long Island, in 1662.[13] In 1676, the colony of Virginia legislated mandatory home isolation of persons with smallpox. During a protracted outbreak in 1702, the Massachusetts Bay Colony enacted a law authorizing selectmen of local towns to carry out isolation and quarantine; this act superseded vaguer authority the Governor previously had delegated to selectmen.[13] Additional measures were authorized by the Bay Colony in 1731 with enactment of "An Act to Prevent Persons from Concealing the Small Pox," which required household heads to report cases to selectmen and to display a red flag on the home to warn others.[13]

As part of a more concerted effort to control smallpox, in 1813 the U.S. Congress established a National Vaccine Agency as part of the "Act to Encourage Vaccination"; however, the agency was closed and the act was repealed in 1822.[13] As the nineteenth century progressed, legislators were faced with the challenge of balancing the need for control measures such as vaccination to protect communities against evolving beliefs regarding personal freedom of choice. However, in the setting of an epidemic in Boston during 1855, the state legislature enacted "the first mandatory school vaccination law in the United States," although this law was not enforced until an epidemic occurred in the early 1880s.[13] Similarly, in Atlanta, regulations mandating vaccination of school children were enforced only months before an outbreak occurred in that city in 1882. Improvement in the smallpox situation led to public resistance to vaccination and vaccination laws in the early 1900s, and California went so far as to repeal its law mandating vaccination for school children. However, following a resurgence of smallpox beginning in 1920, in 1922 the U.S. Supreme Court held that school authorities could mandate vaccination for school entry regardless of whether an immediate local smallpox threat existed.[13]

As a historical footnote, in addition to prompting laws and other control measures, smallpox affected the legislative and judicial processes in colonial America in other ways. For example, in 1636 and 1659, the General Court of the Massachusetts Bay Colony was forced to convene in locations outside of Boston, where it usually met.[13] Similarly, in 1696, an outbreak in Jamestown, Virginia, caused the colony's assembly to recess, and in 1702, smallpox in Manhattan caused both the assembly and the supreme court to adjourn to Long Island.[13]

Impact of other infectious disease influences on current laws

Although smallpox is one of the earliest of the infectious diseases to prompt legislative responses in the United States, many others also fundamentally influenced current laws related to such diseases.[14] For example, yellow fever and cholera epidemics during the 1800s led to the enactment of state and local disease-control laws providing for sanitation, quarantine, and isolation. Recognition of the impact of TB led to changes in disease reporting and surveillance, including the establishment of case reporting in New York in the 1890s; and syphilis control initiatives in the early 1900s prompted enactment of laws for premarital screening, reporting, contact tracing, and involuntary treatment.[14] The federal government had only limited early involvement in public health, including the control and prevention of infectious diseases; however, one example of such involvement was a law enacted by Congress in 1813 requiring the federal government to both ensure the effectiveness of cowpox vaccine and distribute the vaccine free.[15]

Some of the earliest sanitary legislation in the American colonies was an enactment in 1647 or 1648 by the General Court of the Massachusetts Bay Colony that provided for maritime quarantine against ships from the yellow fever-affected West Indies.[16] In 1678, local regulations against smallpox were adopted in Boston, Salem, and Plymouth, and in 1742 a law to prevent smallpox and other infectious sicknesses was passed by the Massachusetts Bay Colony.[16] The first local boards of health in the United States were created during 1793–1794 in Baltimore and Philadelphia as a consequence of a yellow fever epidemic.[16]

MANDATORY REPORTING OF DISEASES AND CONDITIONS

All states have legislated requirements for reporting specific conditions.[11] These requirements may be enumerated directly by statute, through authorities delegated to state boards of health, and under health department regulations. Reporting may be required of a variety of professionals and organizational entities, including physicians and other health-care providers, diagnostic laboratories, and clinical facilities[9,11,17] Although state disease reporting is generally mandated by law or regulation, reporting of disease and death information by the state or territorial health department to the CDC is voluntary.

The scope and nature of reporting requirements vary considerably by state, differing, for example, by the number of conditions required for reporting, time periods within which conditions must be reported, agencies to which reports must be submitted, and persons or sources required to report. Moreover, despite the legal requirements for reporting, the adherence to and completeness of reporting also vary substantially by infectious disease agent, ranging from 6% to 90% different common infectious conditions.[18] The deficiencies in reporting by physicians are accounted for, in part, by limitations in physicians' knowledge of reporting requirements and procedures, as well as the assumption that laboratories have reported cases of infectious diseases.[11,19].

Since the early 1900s, the PHS has attempted to collect disease information from all states about the occurrence of certain infectious diseases.[1,10]. In 1951, the Council of State and Territorial Epidemiologists (CSTE) was authorized by its parent body, the Association of State and Territorial Health Officials, to decide what diseases states should be reported to the PHS and to recommend reporting procedures. The CSTE meets annually and, in consultation with the CDC, recommends additions and deletions to the list of diseases and conditions.

An assessment of state laws and regulations in 1989 highlighted an important impediment to the surveillance and control of infectious diseases—namely, the variations in case definitions the states used for identifying and acting on reports of cases and the effect this lack of uniformity had on limiting the ability to compare patterns of infectious disease occurrence between states.[11] For example, some states required reporting any person with a positive culture for *Salmonella*, while others required reporting only culture-positive persons who were symptomatic. To address these differences and to facilitate comparison of surveillance between states, the CSTE and the CDC developed standardized case definitions for nationally notifiable infectious diseases.[20] Implementation of uniform case definitions and related procedures was expected to provide for interstate reciprocal notification for cases of infectious disease when onset was in one state but the patient was hospitalized in or transferred to another state and cases for which public health action (e.g., contact tracing) might be involved in different states. However, reporting requirements by states have continued to differ: As of January 1999, of the 52 infectious conditions agreed on for national surveillance, only 19 were reportable in all states.[9]

In 1995 and 1996, the CDC and CSTE expanded the list beyond the traditional list of infectious diseases, recommending that elevated blood lead levels, silicosis, tobacco use, and acute pesticide poisoning be added.[9] The number of diseases and conditions on the list varies from year to year but is usually 65 to 75. The list of diseases and conditions under national surveillance is published each year in the annual summary of notifiable diseases published in the *Morbidity and Mortality Weekly Report*. The CSTE also keeps information on state disease and condition reporting requirements on its Internet website, http://www.cste.org.

Even though few states choose to penalize physicians for not reporting notifiable conditions, disciplinary measures may be invoked in instances when failure to report has serious untoward effects. For example, the California Board of Medical Quality Assurance (BMQA) took action against a physician in that state for "gross negligence and incompetence, failure to report to local health authorities a suspected case of an infectious disease in a known food handler."[21] At that time, California law set forth legal responsibility of physicians, dentists, nurses, and others to notify local health authorities of persons ill with specified infectious diseases. In this instance, the physician had examined a patient he knew to be a food handler. Although the physician recognized that the patient was jaundiced and possibly had hepatitis, he failed to report the patient's condition to local public health authorities. An outbreak of foodborne hepatitis followed in which at least 62 cases of hepatitis were associated with the food handler; one patient died. In suspending the physician's license for 1 year (the suspension was stayed, and the physician was placed on 5 years probation), the BMQA declared that the "failure to report a suspected if not a known case of an infectious disease in a food handler was an extreme departure from the standard practice of medicine."[21] More recently, in Minnesota, a small proportion of physicians initially refused to report the identity of human immunodeficiency virus (HIV)–positive persons to the state health department as required, even though violation of any health department rule was a misdemeanor.[22]

INTERPLAY OF FEDERAL AND STATE LAWS IN PUBLIC HEALTH PRACTICE

When an outbreak of disease or other event threatens public health, state or local public health authorities are responsible for investigating it because of their inherent police powers. In practice, institutions and individuals generally cooperate voluntarily in epidemiologic and outbreak investigations. However, if investigators meet with resistance, local or state public health officials can take legal actions, such as applying to a court with jurisdiction over the agency (or individual) for a subpoena or court order to compel the agency (or individual) to grant investigators access to the premises or records at issue. An individual can be compelled by court order to provide the information necessary to the public health investigation.

In contrast to the broad state public health authorities, federal public health officials have limited statutory authorities to initiate independent epidemiologic investigations. For epidemiologists and public health officials employed by the federal government, the laws relating to the general powers and duties of the PHS for research and investigation are found in Title III of the Public Health Service Act. The general statutory authority that applies to federal epidemiologic investigations is Section 301(a) of the Public Health Service Act, 42 U.S.C. Section 241(a):

The Secretary shall conduct in the Service, and encourage, cooperate with, and render assistance to the other appropriate public authorities, scientific institutions, and scientists in the conduct of, and promote the coordination of, research, investigations, experiments, demonstrations, and studies relating to the causes, diagnosis, treatment, control, and prevention of physical and mental diseases and impairments of man. . . .

In addition, subsection 6 of Section 301(a) indicates that the Secretary is authorized to "make available to health officials, scientists, and appropriate public health and other nonprofit institutions and organizations, technical advice and assistance on the application of statistical methods to experiments, studies, and surveys in health and medical fields." Although these provisions are broadly worded and are permissive rather than compulsory, they nonetheless give legal authority for intervention by federal epidemiologists in disease outbreaks and other instances in which such assistance is requested. In practice, local and state public health officials may request federal assistance in the epidemiologic or outbreak investigation. Federal public health employees who collaborate with state and local public health authorities in such investigations generally are not exercising specific federal authority but rather are assisting the state or overall investigation.

LEGAL ISSUES RELATED TO DATA COLLECTION, ANALYSIS, AND DISSEMINATION

The processes of collecting data for public health surveillance activities or as part of an outbreak investigation involve numerous legal considerations, including (1) protection available under state or federal law during and after the investigation for the records collected and generated in relation to the investigation; (2) confidentiality provisions for medical and other information; (3) required reporting of particular diseases or conditions; (4) status of information in investigative files on the federal Freedom of Information Act (FOIA), 5 U.S.C. Section 552, or state FOIA counterparts; and (5) the possible applicability of federal or state human subjects research regulations, including the need for review of study protocols by institutional review boards and the need for informed consent for participation in the investigation or for procedures related to the investigation.

To determine what records will be kept or generated and where and how such records will be stored, federal, state, and local public health officials need to be familiar with legal protections applicable to documents and other records that will be examined, extracted, and compiled in association with the surveillance activity or outbreak investigation. Most states provide specific statutory and regulatory confidentiality protections over medical and public health records. In general, the confidentiality protection prevents the disclosure of a name-identified record without the consent of the person on whom the record is maintained. Accordingly, such medical records in the hands of an investigator generally are protected by state law. Furthermore, such state laws frequently require that only certain authorized personnel have access to such confidential records and that such records be maintained in a secure manner. Public health investigators would usually be authorized access to such records for surveillance and related public health activities but would be bound to maintain the records in a manner that would protect the confidentiality of the identifiable information from unauthorized or inadvertent disclosure.

In the course of an outbreak investigation or surveillance activities, investigators may create or compile a variety of documents, including questionnaires, forms, investigative notes, copies or extractions of patient or other records, letters, reports, memoranda, drafts, manuscripts, and final reports. Depending on the nature of the records and the status of the investigation, these documents may not be protected from disclosure to the public by state or federal laws. Except for records afforded specific protection by state or federal laws (such as state laws protecting medical records), public health investigators should assume that all records collected may at some point be open to public scrutiny. This may include personal notes by the public health investigator, drafts of documents retained in the files, and other related information that is within the scope of the request.

Freedom of Information Act

Federal investigators need to be cognizant of the provisions of FOIA. As noted above, most states have similar laws that give citizens access to certain records that are not otherwise privileged or specifically protected by statute. In general, the federal FOIA provides that all documents in the hands of federal employees, on federal premises, or within the control of federal employees are available to the public unless specifically exempted by FOIA. FOIA contains nine exemptions. In general, four of these exemptions may affect epidemiologic investigations:

- *Interagency and intra-agency communications.* Exemption (b)(5) permits the federal government to withhold from disclosure interagency and intra-agency memorandums or letters that would not be available "to a party other than an agency in litigation with the agency." An example of the use of this exemption would be to protect from disclosure a draft memorandum written by the investigator to his supervisor describing the early findings of the investigation.
- *Personnel and medical records.* Exemption (b)(6) permits the federal government to withhold from mandatory disclosure "personnel and medical files and similar files the disclosure of which would constitute a clearly unwarranted invasion of personal privacy." The federal government may invoke this exemption to protect confidential medical information about an individual contained in a record collected by the federal investigator.
- *Information otherwise exempt from disclosure by statute.* Exemption (b)(3) provides that a federal agency may withhold from disclosure information "specifically exempted from disclosure by statute." If an epidemiologic investigation is conducted under an assurance of confidentiality authorized by a federal statute (such as Section 301[d] or Section 308[d] of the Public Health Service Act), the information collected pursuant to the confidentiality assurance is protected from disclosure under FOIA in a manner that would contravene the statutory provision. Assurances of confidentiality are not commonly used. Instead, with legal counsel and on a case-by-case basis, such assurances generally are limited to exceptional circumstances in which the sensitivity of

the information demands additional confidentiality measures or when the co-operation of the study participants would be impeded in the absence of such an assurance.

• *Trade secret and commercial or financial information.* Exemption (b)(4) permits the federal government "to withhold from disclosure commercial or financial information obtained from a person and privileged and confidential." Although this exemption may be less commonly applicable than the other three outlined above, it would be relevant to an epidemiologic investigation that involved, for example, a commercial product on which the investigator has records containing trade secrets or confidential information about the components of the product. Likewise, confidential financial information may be contained in investigative records, even records that might otherwise be disclosed under FOIA.

Privacy Laws

Federal and state laws provide protection for name-identified records that contain medical and other confidential information. The federal Privacy Act, 5 U.S.C. Section 552a, applies to any investigation conducted by a federal employee and to the retention of personally identifiable records retained within a federal system of records. The Privacy Act generally allows an individual to have access to his or her records held by a federal agency. Certain national security and criminal law enforcement records are exempt from the Privacy Act. Although the level of privacy protection varies among state laws, all states accord protection of medical, public health, and certain vital statistics records.[24]

EMERGING DEVELOPMENTS IN PUBLIC HEALTH SURVEILLANCE, INVESTIGATION, AND RESPONSE

Reporting of Bioterrorism-Related Diseases

The CDC recently examined the disease reporting laws of 54 jurisdictions (50 states and Chicago, Los Angeles County, New York City, and Washington, DC) to determine how many jurisdictions had laws mandating the reporting of diseases caused by "critical biological agents."[24] Critical biologic agents were those designated by the CDC to have the potential for use in a bioterrorist weapon. The study looked at which of 24 of the most critical biologic agents are explicitly reportable by law, as well as the required time frame for reporting. The 24 critical biologic agents or disease conditions chosen for the study included anthrax, botulism, brucellosis, cholera, cryptosporidium, *Escherichia coli*, glanders, hantavirus, hemorrhagic fevers (viral), meliodosis, mycotoxins, plague, psittacosis, Q fever, ricin poisoning, salmonella, shigella, smallpox, staphylococcal enterotoxin B, toxic syndromes, tularemia, typhus fever, *Vibrio cholerae*, and viral encephalitis.

The study showed that particular deficiencies existed in the immediate reporting of diseases associated with Category A agents (anthrax, botulism, viral hemorrhagic fevers, plague, smallpox, and tularemia). Although anthrax, botulism, and plague were immediately reportable in most jurisdictions, tularemia was immediately reportable in less than half of the jurisdictions. The study also identified deficiencies in reporting requirements related to Category B and C agents, although these may be of less concern because of their less critical nature. The findings underscore the need for states and other jurisdictions to review existing disease reporting laws to determine whether they include the most critical biologic agents associated with bioterrorism.[24]

New Surveillance Concepts

New surveillance concepts have been introduced in the past decade to public health practice. Through changes in state public health reporting statutes, regulations, or executive orders, conditions and syndromes that fall outside more traditional infectious diseases have been added to reporting requirements. These include chronic diseases, environmental and occupational health conditions, emerging infectious diseases, and injury-control data. For example, in 1996, the CSTE, by an unanimous vote, added prevalence of cigarette smoking to the list of conditions designated as reportable by states to the CDC.[25] The addition of prevalence of cigarette smoking marks the first time a behavior, rather than a disease or an illness, has been considered nationally reportable. Moreover, the CSTE maintains information on its website identifying indicators for chronic disease surveillance, including access to current data to assist public health practitioners to assess indicators for their locales. In addition, publication of data regarding firearm-related injuries has significantly increased awareness of these public health issues, as well as the importance of surveillance to the consideration of law and policy interventions.

In recent years, the CSTE and CDC have cooperated in publishing numerous surveillance summaries, including hazardous substances and emergency events, infant mortality, childhood lead poisoning, low birth weight, neural tube defects, occupational asthma, occupational hazards, and smoking. Perhaps even more than traditional reportable disease surveillance reports, the analysis of these surveillance summaries has provided essential information at both the state and national levels for developing policy and evaluating programs.

State and Federal Cooperation in Emergency Responses

Beginning in 1999, federal government initiatives designed to improve national public health capabilities to respond to acts of chemical and biologic terrorism raised questions about the adequacy of state quarantine, isolation, and other compulsory public health powers. A preliminary review of state quarantine, isolation, and other critical agent laws conducted informally by the CDC in 2000 showed that most of these laws had not been revised since the 1940s. This is most likely true because voluntary cooperation of the public and advances in medical interventions have made use of compulsory actions less frequent. However, in the context of public health threats related to potential bioterrorism events, the infrequent use of such actions also presented the possibility that public health officials were inexperienced or unfamiliar with the proper procedures for invoking the compulsory powers. Accordingly, the CDC and other federal officials involved in bioterrorism preparedness have suggested that states examine public health laws—including quarantine and isolations powers—that affect their abilities to effectively respond to potential chemical and biologic threats. Such assessments can help ensure that the laws enable public health officials to act promptly while still providing adequate due process protections for individuals who may have been detained as part of a bioterrorism response. In addition, bioterrorism initiatives increasingly are focusing on the need for advance coordination, planning, pharmaceutical stockpiling, and training that involves public health officials and officials from various law-enforcement, emergency-response, and other civilian agencies, as well as military intelligence experts.

The events following the September 11, 2001, attacks in New York City and Washington, DC, illustrate both the strengths of and challenges to traditional concepts of primary state and local responsibility for public health investigations. The catastrophic nature of the events rapidly taxed the abilities of local and state public health officials to respond to the needs for surveillance of hospital and emergency department admissions, injuries, hospital-based syndromic surveillance, and various environmental monitoring activities. Resources from the CDC and other public health agencies had to be deployed to gather this important surveillance information. Yet, the legal authority and oversight of the overwhelming public health activities remained with local and state public health officials. The consistency in training, advance planning, and prior collaborative relationships between state, municipal, and local public health practitioners made possible an effective response during this emergency situation. In the aftermath of the events of September 11 and the anthrax attack in the United States, a draft model law (The Model State Emergency Health Powers Act) was created and made available for public review and use (see Chapter 10).

References

1. CDC. Summary of notifiable diseases, United States, 1999. *MMWR* 1999;48 (no. 53):v–vi.

2. Holtzman D, Powell-Griner E, Bolen JC, Rhodes L. State and sex-specific prevalence of selected characteristics—Behavioral Risk Factor Surveillance System, 1996 and 1997. *MMWR* 200;49(no. SS-6):1–12.
3. National Cancer Institute. About SEER. Available at http://search.nci.nih.gov/search97cgi/s97_cgi. Accessed December 1, 2001.
4. Goodman RA, Buehler JW, Koplan JP. The epidemiologic field investigation: science and judgment in public health practice. *Am J Epidemiol* 1990;132:9–16.
5. Gregg MB. Conducting a field investigation. In: Gregg MB, ed. *Field Epidemiology*. 2nd ed. New York: Oxford University Press, 2002:62–77.
6. Fidler DP, Heymann DL, Ostroff SM, O'Brien T. Emerging and reemerging infectious diseases: challenges for international, national, and state law. *Int Lawyer* 1997; 31:773–99.
7. Birkhead GS, Maylahn CM. State and local public health surveillance. In: Teutsch SM, Churchill RE, eds. *Principles and Practice of Public Health Surveillance*, 2nd ed. New York: Oxford University Press, 2000: pp. 253–86.
8. Langmuir AD. The surveillance of communicable diseases of national importance. *N Engl J Med* 1963;268:182–92.
9. Rousch S, Birkhead GS, Koo D, Cobb A, Fleming D. Mandatory reporting of diseases and conditions by health care professionals and laboratorians. *JAMA* 1999;282: 164–70.
10. Thacker SB. Historical development. In: Teutsch SM, Churchill RE, eds. *Principles and Practice of Public Health Surveillance*, 2nd ed. New York: Oxford University Press, 2000: pp. 1–16.
11. Chorba TL, Berkelman RL, Safford SK, Gibbs NP, Hull HF. The reportable diseases: I. Mandatory reporting of infectious diseases by clinicians. *JAMA* 1989;262:3018–26.
12. Koo D, Wetterhall SF. History and current status of the National Notifiable Diseases Surveillance System. *J Public Health Manage Pract* 1996;2:4–10.
13. Hopkins DR. *Princes and Peasants: Smallpox in History*. Chicago: University of Chicago Press, 1983.
14. Gostin LO, Burris S, Lazzarini Z. The law and the public's health: a study of infectious disease law in the United States. *Columbia Law Rev* 1999;99:59–128.
15. Christoffel T. *Health and the Law: A Handbook for Health Professionals*. New York: Free Press, 1985.
16. Tobey JA. *Public Health Law*, 3rd ed. New York: The Commonwealth Fund, 1947.
17. Thacker SB. Surveillance. In: Gregg MB, Dicker RC, Goodman RA, eds. *Field Epidemiology*. New York: Oxford University Press, 1996: pp. 16–32.
18. Thacker SB, Berkelman RL. Public health surveillance in the United States. *Epidemiol Rev* 1988;10:164–90.
19. Konowitz PM, Petrossian GA, Rose DN. The underreporting of disease and physicians' knowledge of reporting requirements. *Public Health Rep* 1984;99:31–5.
20. CDC. Case definitions for public health surveillance. *MMWR* 1990;39(RR-13):1–43.
21. California Department of Health Services. Disciplinary action by Board of Medical Quality Assurance for failure to report a reportable infectious disease. *Calif Morbid* 1978 (August 11).
22. Fidler DP, Heymann DL, Ostroff SM, O'Brien T. Emerging and reemerging infectious diseases: challenges for international, national, and state law. *Intl Lawyer* 1997; 31:773–99.
23. Gostin LO, Lazzarini Z, Neslund VS, Osterholm MT. The public health information

infrastructure: a national review of the law on health information privacy. *JAMA* 1996;275:1921–7.

24. Horton H, Misrahi JJ, Matthews GW, Kocher PL. Critical biological agents: disease reporting as a tool for bioterrorism preparedness. *J Law Med Ethics* 2002. In press.

25. CDC. Addition of prevalence of cigarette smoking as a nationally notifiable condition—June 1996. *MMWR* 1996;45:537.

8

Public Health Research and Health Information

NANETTE R. ELSTER, RICHARD E. HOFFMAN,
AND JOHN R. LIVENGOOD

Key roles of public health agencies are to support and to conduct research to quantify the presence and impact of diseases, conditions, or behaviors of public health importance; to identify risk factors that can be used to target appropriate diagnostic, therapeutic, or (more likely) preventive interventions; and to develop and evaluate innovative strategies to reduce the associated societal impact of these conditions. Although basic science research applies widely in public health settings (e.g., discovering an immunogenic protein common to various subtypes of human immunodeficiency virus [HIV] that could be developed as a candidate HIV vaccine), public health research is more often directed toward translating existing scientific findings into broad, population-based programs.

Public health research uses a variety of methods to achieve its goals. Examples include a clinical trial to evaluate new medications to treat tuberculosis (TB); a laboratory investigation to identify a new or previously unrecognized pathogen, such as hantavirus; a survey of physicians to assess the barriers to implementing a new vaccine recommendation; a survey of laboratories to determine what tests the laboratory is performing to detect antibiotic resistance; telephone surveys to estimate the prevalence of a particular condition; or a behavioral intervention to reduce tobacco use in a particular population. These illustrate the diverse activities designed to improve the health of the community rather than one methodology or research design to accomplish its goal.

160

The goals of public health research often address issues associated with identifying groups at risk, defining the effectiveness and monitoring the impact of intervention projects to develop and evaluate intervention strategies, and improving access to effective services and proven interventions to bring the benefits of these findings to the community. Public health research frequently is designed to complement the practice of public health in terms of identifying problems in the community; intervening to reduce or prevent their impact; and searching for ways to accomplish these tasks in an efficient, equitable, ethical, and comprehensive manner. These characteristics can lead to difficulties in distinguishing public health research from practice.

The goal of research in public health is primarily to benefit populations, but the involvement of individuals in the research process necessitates protection of participants or human subjects. Legal requirements for the minimal protections that must be provided to subjects of research funded in whole or in part by the U.S. Department of Health and Human Services (DHHS) are found within the Code of Federal Regulations (C.F.R.). This chapter discusses the applicability of these regulations to public health practice and research, including background and general information about institutional review of research, the difficulties in determining whether a particular activity is public health research or practice, the imperative and mechanisms for protecting privacy and confidentiality of data, and the interests that must be balanced in conducting public health research.

BACKGROUND AND GENERAL INFORMATION ABOUT INTERNAL REVIEW BOARDS

The "Federal Policy for the Protection of Human Subjects (Basic DHHS Policy for Protection of Human Research Subjects)," found at 45 C.F.R. 46, was adopted in its current form in 1991. In fact, the evolution of the regulations found at 45 C.F.R. 46 seems to indicate that the regulations were intended to apply to more than just biomedical research. According to a statement by the Surgeon General in 1966, the requirement of institutional review "applies to all investigations that involve human subjects, including investigations in the behavioral and social sciences."[1]

The regulations were developed and adopted largely in response to a history of research abuses culminating in the public disclosure of the events of the Tuskegee Syphilis Study. The study was conducted and supported by the U.S. Public Health Service from 1932 to 1972. The purpose of the study was to investigate the natural progression of syphilis. To do so, treatment for the disease was withheld from poor black men in a rural southern community. The men who participated in the study were not told that they had syphilis; they were simply told that they suffered from "bad blood."[2]

In 1972, a newspaper article brought the study to the public's attention. The public outrage and growing distrust of the research and public health enterprises[3] led to hearings on Capitol Hill about the inadequate protection of human research participants. The hearings were the impetus for the enactment of the National Research Act of 1974 and the subsequent adoption of regulations for the protection of human subjects. Additionally, the National Research Act led to the development of the Office of Protection from Research Risks (OPRR) and the National Commission for Protection of Human Subjects. The OPRR was renamed the Office of Human Research Protections (OHRP) in 2000 and relocated from the National Institutes of Health (NIH) to the Office of the Secretary of Health and Human Services.[4] The OHRP's responsibilities include "Developing and monitoring as well as exercising compliance oversight relative to HHS Regulations for the protection of human subjects in research conducted or supported by any component of the Department of Health and Human Services."[5]

The regulations were promulgated by the then Department of Health, Education, and Welfare (DHEW) pursuant to the DHEW's rule-making authority as delegated in its enabling statute. An agency's rule-making authority requires that certain steps be taken for an agency to promulgate and enact regulations. First, the agency must publish the proposed rule in the *Federal Register* for a time to allow individuals and interested groups or organizations to comment; the agency then reviews any comments and revises the proposed rule accordingly. The revised rule is then published in the *Federal Register* for a period before it becomes effective. Once it is effective, it will be codified in the annual publication of the C.F.R. In 1991, pursuant to this process, 45 C.F.R. 46 was adopted by 16 other governmental agencies and, hence, the term *Common Rule* was adopted.

The regulations set forth basic conditions that apply to research supported by the 17 federal agencies: (*1*) ethical review by an independent body in advance of initiation of research, (*2*) voluntary and informed consent of participants, (*3*) protection of privacy and confidentiality of participants, and (*4*) institutional assurance of compliance with the regulations. The DHHS also has defined supplemental regulations providing additional protections to pregnant women and fetuses, prisoners, and children.[6] This combined set of regulations governs public health research supported by DHHS agencies, such as the Centers for Disease Control and Prevention (CDC) and the NIH as well as research conducted at selected institutions with a DHHS Multiple Project Assurance (MPA)[a] that has been expanded to apply to all research conducted at that institution.

Obtaining an assurance of compliance for each site engaged in research has been particularly problematic in public health research. Most state and local health departments do not have an MPA and have had to rely on project-specific, single project assurances (SPAs), which are often time consuming to obtain, resulting in delays in the initiation of research projects. Recently, however, the

OHRP modified the assurance process to phase out MPAs and SPAs and instead began issuing federal-wide assurance (FWA) to each institution covering all research studies conducted at the institution. The FWA is renewable on an ongoing basis without additional paperwork as long as the institutional review board (IRB) roster and other information associated with the FWA is updated at least once every 3 years. This process will help streamline one facet of the often unwieldy regulations. Nonetheless, because each IRB is autonomous, and a given activity may involve IRB review by several agencies and institutions—each of which has different perspectives, understandings, and approaches to the informed consent process, definition of research, and review of protocols—difficulties in coordinating multiple IRB reviews are likely to remain.

The regulations, although detailed, do not preempt state or local laws governing basic public health functions, the ability to give informed consent to participate in research, or protection of privacy and confidentiality, but instead provide a baseline level of protection to human participants in research. (See, for example, Colorado law [Box 8–1], which is more specific and detailed than federal law.) For public health research, applicability of federal regulations is mostly related to support by the CDC or NIH. Support in this context means more than direct financial support through grant or contract mechanisms. Support for public health research also includes contributions of federal personnel

---

Box 8–1. Colorado Revised Statute 25-1-122 (2000)

(4) Reports and records resulting from the investigation of epidemic and communicable diseases, environmental and chronic diseases, reports of morbidity and mortality, reports of cancer in connection with the statewide cancer registry, and reports and records resulting from the investigation of venereal diseases, tuberculosis, and rabies and mammal bites held by the state department of public health and environment or local departments of health shall be strictly confidential. Such reports and records shall not be released, shared with any agency or institution, or made public, upon subpoena, search warrant, discovery proceedings, or otherwise, except under any of the following circumstances:
  (a) Release may be made of medical and epidemiological information in a manner such that no individual person can be identified.
  (b) Release may be made of medical and epidemiological information to the extent necessary for the treatment, control, investigation, and prevention of diseases and conditions dangerous to the public health; except that every effort shall be made to limit disclosure of personal identifying information to the minimal amount necessary to accomplish the public health purpose.

(3) Release may be made to the person who is the subject of a medical record or report with written authorization from such person.

resources through direct interaction with research participants or collaboration on laboratory testing, protocol design, or data analysis. This latter interpretation is particularly salient for public health research where a long history exists of partnership and collaboration in the conduct of public health practice and research between the CDC and state and local health departments, even in the absence of direct funding support.

The basic premise underlying the federal regulations is that participation of human subjects in research is a privilege for investigators and investigating institutions.[7] Therefore, appropriate protections must be afforded to these volunteers. In determining the applicability of the regulations, two essential questions must be answered: (1) Is it research? and (2) Does it involve human subjects? To answer these questions, the definition in section 46.102 must be reviewed. "Research means a systematic investigation including research development, testing and evaluation, designed to develop or contribute to generalizable knowledge."[8]

This definition of "research" articulated in the Common Rule does not apply to any one particular type of research. The regulations are intended to apply to all research involving human subjects, including biomedical, behavioral, and public health research; however, as with the difference between clinical research and the practice of medicine, the regulations governing public health research are not intended to be applied to public health practice.[8] Public health practice can be roughly defined as the set of activities undertaken by local, state, or federal organizations (usually health departments) that are designed to fulfill their legal mandate to protect the health of the community. Examples of public health activities that are generally considered to be practice include disease surveillance, outbreak investigation, program evaluation, and other efforts to monitor the health of the population.

The CDC has published guidelines to assist investigators in determining whether an activity is research or practice.[9] Determining that an activity is public health practice in no way diminishes the need to ensure that participants are treated ethically, with appropriate procedures for informed consent and safeguards to protect privacy and confidentiality where needed.

Once the proposed activity has been determined to meet the definition of research, the next question is to determine whether the research involves human subjects. The regulations read: "Human subject means a living individual about whom an investigator (whether professional or student) conducting research obtains (1) data through intervention or interaction with the individual, or (2) identifiable private information."[10]

On the basis of this definition, the regulations do not apply to generalizable data gathered by public health agencies about persons who have died. The agency may collect mortality data in the normal course of performing its duties to compile and tabulate vital statistics, although some public health investigations require gathering data in addition to what is contained on the death certificate. Additionally, the definition does not encompass research involving information about persons when no identifiable information is available, meaning that no link whatsoever exists between the information and the individual, even in the form of a code.

The regulations require research involving human subjects to be approved by an IRB[11] in advance of contact with human participants unless such research is specifically exempt by the regulations.[12] The regulations list six categories that are exempt from the requirements. The most common two exempt types of public health research are (1) research involving the use of educational tests, survey procedures, interview procedures (including focus groups), or observation of public behavior unless the participants can be identified and disclosure of the response could place them at risk for criminal or civil liability or be damaging to their employability or reputation[13] and (2) "research involving the collection or study of existing data, documents, records, pathological specimens, or diagnostic specimens, if these sources are publicly available or if the information is recorded by the investigator in such a manner that subjects cannot be identified, directly or through identifiers linked to the subjects."[14]

Institutional review boards comprise at least five members with diverse backgrounds, at least one of whom is a nonscientist and at least one of whom is not otherwise affiliated with the institution.[15] The IRB is charged with ensuring that appropriate information is provided to research subjects through the informed consent process[15] and that risks to subjects are minimized and reasonable in relation to the anticipated benefits of the proposed research.[16]

Institutional review boards conduct two levels of review of research: expedited and full board review. Expedited review does not require review and approval by the fully convened board, merely review by the chair or one or more experienced members of the IRB.[17] Such review is appropriate only when the research involves no more than minimal risk and falls within a category of review specifically articulated by the Secretary of Health and Human Services.[17] Nine categories are currently published in the *Federal Register*[18] and include such types of research as "prospective collection of biological specimens for research purposes by noninvasive means" and "research on individual or group characteristics or behavior . . . or research employing survey, interview, oral history, focus group, program evaluation, human factors evaluation, or quality assurance methodologies."[18] As these examples illustrate, the categories appropriate for expedited review pose no more than minimal risk to subjects, are not physically invasive, and commonly apply to types of behavioral and social science research.

Full board or convened review is required for all other research that is not exempt under 45 C.F.R. 46.101 or subject to expedited review under 45 C.F.R. 46.110. For this type of review, a majority of the IRB members must be present, including at least one member whose primary interests are not scientific.[19] The types of research that typically are subject to full board review include research involving invasive procedures, special populations (see Chapter 11), surveys of a sensitive nature (e.g., involving drug and alcohol use or criminal behavior), and research involving deception.

One of the most critical roles of IRBs is to review the appropriateness and adequacy of informed consent. Informed consent in this context refers to more than the written documentation; it refers to the entire process, including who is seeking the informed consent, where it is being sought, when it is being sought, and the method being used to convey the information. Consent must be both voluntary (i.e., free from coercion or undue influence) and informed. To optimize the readability and understandability of the document, IRBs will often spend a substantial amount of time reviewing it. The document must accurately and clearly state the risks and benefits of participation, as well as the alternatives without minimizing risks or overstating benefits. The language used in the document must be straightforward and comprehensible—typically at an eighth-grade reading level or less. Additionally, the federal regulations require eight specific elements to be included in all informed consents.[20] For example, all informed consents must contain "a statement describing the extent, if any, to which confidentiality of records identifying the subject will be maintained.[21] Each of these elements must be specifically included in the informed consent unless the IRB reviews and approves any alteration.[22] Additionally, an IRB may approve a waiver of informed consent or a waiver of documentation of informed consent if certain requirements are satisfied.[23]

The process of obtaining informed consent is often complex and can be influenced by such factors as the availability of alternative treatments for the disease or condition under study, the amount of remuneration offered as an incentive for participation, or the existing relationship between the researcher and the subject (e.g., an existing physician–patient relationship). Institutional review boards will consider these factors as part of the review process because they could seriously affect an eligible person's decision to participate in research. For example, a person who is terminally ill may be willing to accept a high-risk procedure or intervention, even if the direct benefits may be limited or nonexistent or a person of lower socioeconomic status may be unduly influenced to participate by the promise of monetary remuneration.

In addition, IRBs must conduct continuing review of ongoing research projects—meaning that IRBs must review active protocols at least annually.[24] In their review, IRBs have a range of authority, including the authority to approve research, require modifications to a particular research protocol, or disapprove the proposed research entirely.[25] This process for investigators may be time consuming and, at times, tedious, but the process is necessary to ensure that subjects are adequately protected.

PUBLIC HEALTH SURVEILLANCE: RESEARCH OR PRACTICE?

In public health, the distinction between research and practice is often unclear, and adherence to the federal regulations' requirement of IRB approval may interfere with or impede the goals of a particular public health initiative. Public health is "concerned primarily with prevention rather than treatment; populations rather than individuals, and collective goods rather than personal rights or interest."[26]

One of the essential functions of public health is the collection of data to assess the health of a community. Is this research or practice? According to one commentator, "The distinction between practice and research is unclear in public health because investigators do not undertake data collection and evaluation to primarily benefit the individual. Public health activities are intended for the benefit of populations."[27] This distinction is important because, according to some public health professionals, "routine public health practice activities—like routine clinical practice activities—cannot be effectively carried out in a timely manner if they are subjected to the considerable administrative burdens associated with an Institutional Review Board (IRB)."[28]

Surveillance illustrates the sometimes difficult distinction between research and practice. Surveillance is defined as "the ongoing, systematic collection, analysis, and interpretation of data (e.g., regarding agent/hazard, risk factor, exposure, health event) essential to the planning, implementation, and evaluation of public health practice, closely integrated with the timely dissemination of these data to those responsible for prevention and control."[29] In analyzing and interpreting surveillance data, the practitioner may find that the results are generalizable and publishable, and this is where some would argue that the practice of collecting population-based disease surveillance becomes research as defined in the Common Rule.

Surveillance data are used for a variety of purposes that serve both individual and public health needs. Individual needs often include assurance of treatment for diseases such as TB and provision of official birth and death certificates. The use of the data to meet public health needs, however, truly captures the essence of disease surveillance data: The data are used to prevent uninfected or unexposed persons from becoming infected or exposed to a disease-causing agent. To accomplish this, disease surveillance data to the greatest extent possible must be all inclusive, that is, population based. For example, an outbreak of *Escherichia coli* O157:H7 cannot be easily stopped without an epidemiologic and laboratory investigation of all, or a representative sample of, affected persons (i.e., the cases). Likewise, determining whether a cluster of brain tumors in persons living near a source of nonionizing radiation exceeds the expected number is subject to error unless all the cases are ascertained. In both instances, erroneous conclusions (i.e., the absence of a statistically significant association between illness and exposure or a falsely positive association) may be reached without complete case ascertainment.

Traditionally, the data collected by public health agencies have included birth and death records, selected communicable diseases such as TB and pertussis, and cancer cases. More recently, public health agencies have regularly collected data assessing risk behaviors, health attitudes and knowledge, selected types of injuries and heavy metal poisoning, and the prevalence of biomarkers. For example, in June 1996, the Council of State and Territorial Epidemiologists (CSTE) agreed to include the prevalence of cigarette smoking among the list of conditions reportable by the states to the CDC, making this the first risk behavior to be reportable.[30]

The selection of which diseases and conditions must be reported is most often a function of state, rather than of federal or local, health agencies. Additionally, the selection process varies from state to state. In some states, the legislature itself makes the selection; in others, the determination may be delegated to the board of health or the health commissioner. Despite this variability, reportable conditions among states are common. Such consensus permits coordination of disease-control efforts in the event of multistate outbreaks and facilitates monitoring of national trends by the CDC.

The list of reportable conditions changes as new problems emerge and priorities evolve. For example, antibiotic-resistant *Staphylococcus pneumoniae* infections, cryptosporidiosis, cyclosporiasis, Lyme disease, and invasive group A streptococcal infections all have been added to the National Notifiable Disease Surveillance System (NNDSS) since 1990. The NNDSS is a national surveillance system of more than 50 diseases designated reportable to the CDC by the CSTE.[31] The origins of this system date back more than a century, and, as early as 1928, all states were reporting nearly 30 infections diseases to, at that time, the Surgeon General.[30]

In general, public health officers propose to the legislature, the board of health, or the health commissioner the addition or deletion of specific conditions. The proposals are often stimulated by the availability of categorical federal funds that support the costs of disease surveillance and control; in turn, the availability of federal funds represents acknowledgment by Congress of new or changing priorities in public health. For example, in 1995 and 2000, additional federal funds were distributed for surveillance of infections caused by hantavirus[32] and West Nile virus, respectively.[33]

Legislative mandates of the data to be collected often include a range of information about individuals, including personally identifiable information. Additionally, the data are often collected without the specific consent of the individual. This is one component of the overall compact that is typically part of the statutory authority for public health surveillance: the collection of information without the patient's consent. The other component of the compact, discussed below and in Chapter 11, is that the information will be kept strictly confidential. Few persons would choose to have their name and diagnosis reported to a government agency. If consent for reporting were required, the resulting aggregate data, therefore, would be incomplete because many people would be unwilling to provide information. From a disease-control perspective, the information would then be of significantly diminished benefit. The statutory authority for collecting surveillance data typically limits the initial collection of data to the essential amount needed for the health department to assess the community's health status and take action, as necessary, to protect the public health. Collection of disease surveillance information without patient consent and analysis of such data provokes discussion of whether this type of public health activity should be subject to the Common Rule. Formally trained public health workers are knowledgeable about research methods, are directed to assess the health of the people living within their jurisdiction, and are encouraged to disseminate their findings. Under what circumstances are their data collection activities appropriately labeled research? When is the individual's consent necessary for data collection? These questions are perpetually debated in meetings of IRBs.

In general, the view of public health professionals is that if disease surveillance and analysis, case investigation, and outbreak control are performed by a public health agency with the intent of providing care to the community, rather than advancing scientific knowledge in general, then the authority for participant protection (e.g., whether it is the reported case or the uninfected, unexposed citizen) derives from the public health statutes, regulations, and administrative codes. The dilemma is that public health workers are not only directed to assess the health of the people living within their jurisdiction but also encouraged to disseminate their findings. For example, during an investigation of an outbreak of salmonellosis, a state public health agency may institute active surveillance for cases and test hypotheses regarding the cause of the outbreak by performing a case–control study. When the staff of the agency interview patients and controls, they must explain the purpose of the investigation, use of the findings, nature of the subjects' participation in the investigation, and protections afforded the subject; otherwise the subject will not participate. The agency is conducting its investigation to determine the cause of the outbreak and to use the information to control the disease. Once the outbreak is over, the agency may choose to publish its findings with the intent of preventing outbreaks in other jurisdictions. Under what circumstances are such activities considered research? When are IRB review and approval and patient consent necessary before individual health data are collected? The federal regulations do not answer these questions, and the OHRP has not issued an official policy distinguishing public health practice. Because federally approved IRBs are autonomous, whether a project or activity is subject to 45 C.F.R. 46 typically is decided by public health officers and the individual IRB that reviews and approves the work conducted by the participating federal, state, or local health agency. However, the federal regulations have enumerated categories of research that are subject to review as discussed above in "Background and General Information about Internal Review Boards."

PRIVACY AND CONFIDENTIALITY OF COLLECTED DATA

Whether considered research, and therefore subject to the federal regulations at 45 C.F.R. 46, or practice subject to state and local laws, protection of privacy of the individual and confidentiality of the data are paramount considerations. For example, at the federal level, one of the most significant laws addressing the privacy of medical information is the Health Insurance Portability and Accountability Act and its Standards for Privacy of Individually Identifiable Health Information. The privacy regulations are intended to "protect and enhance the rights of consumers by providing them access to their health information and controlling the inappropriate use of that information.[34] In general, the regulations require an individual's consent to disclosure of his or her health information; however, certain public health activities do not require this. The regulations provide that health information may be disclosed to "a public health authority that is authorized by law to collect or receive such information for the purpose of preventing or controlling disease, injury, vital events such as birth or death, and the conduct of public health surveillance, public health investigations, and public health interventions. . . ."[35] This does not mean that such information is not protected—because the state laws that authorize such collection provide for protection of privacy and confidentiality. More recently, the National Bioethics Advisory Commission (NBAC) released its report and recommendations, *Ethical and Policy Issues in Research Involving Human Participants.*[5] With regard to protection of privacy and confidentiality, the NBAC recommended that "Federal policy should be developed and mechanisms should be provided to enable investigators and institutions to reduce threats to privacy and breaches of confidentiality."[7] For a more detailed discussion of state and federal laws addressing privacy and confidentiality of health records, see Chapter 11.

Even professional codes of ethics acknowledge the importance of protecting privacy and confidentiality. For example, the American College of Epidemiology's Ethics Guidelines assert that "Epidemiologists should take appropriate measures to protect the privacy of individuals and to keep confidential all information about individual research participants during and after a study. This duty applies to personal information about individuals in public health practice areas."[36] Unlike laws and regulations, guidelines are strictly voluntary and have no enforcement mechanism, but they are valuable in setting out the standard of a particular profession and informing such professionals of what is expected of them.

Arguably, with both surveillance and research, data are collected to gain generalizable knowledge—even though the primary intent of surveillance is to monitor disease to prevent its spread, and the primary purpose of research is often more amorphous. Despite this distinction, surveillance activities do threaten the privacy of the individual whose data are collected. One public health law expert describes the tension this way: "Society faces a hard choice between the collective benefits achieved by public health data collection and protecting individual privacy."[26] Balancing the interests of the individual and the community is not uncommon in research where often the subject may gain little from his or her participation, yet society may benefit greatly from the knowledge gained. This is the case with public health surveillance as well.

With respect to public health, the law has a long tradition of supporting the state's interest in protecting the health and safety of the community, even when the rights of the individual might be encroached upon. The Tenth Amendment to the U.S. Constitution reserves to states the power (better known as "police power") to take action to protect the health and welfare of its citizenry.[37] According to the U.S. Supreme Court in the seminal public health case *Jacobson v. Massachusetts*, "the police power of a state must be held to embrace, at least, such reasonable regulations established directly by legislative enactment as will protect the public health and the public safety."[7] Exercise of this power may, at times, interfere with the rights of an individual for promoting the greater good of the community.

Jacobson addressed the constitutionality of a Massachusetts compulsory smallpox vaccination statute. In determining the permissibility of such a requirement, the U.S. Supreme Court found that, "it is . . . true that in every well-ordered society charged with the duty of conserving the safety of its members the rights of the individual in respect of his liberty may at times, under the pressure of great dangers, be subjected to such restraint, to be enforced by reasonable regulations as the safety of the general public may demand.[37]

This rationale holds today as well. In 2001, an Illinois appellate court addressing the specific issue of confidentiality of information collected through public health action held that "it is unrealistic to try to mold a public health information system that promises both the ready availability of information and absolute privacy. Public health data collection is a worthwhile cause in the name of reducing morbidity and mortality. Although strict confidentiality of health data is a noble cause and is worthy of statutory protections, ultimately a balance must be struck between public health concerns and privacy concerns."[38]

Through the exercise of police power, every state has some form of surveillance mechanism in place. Collection of vital statistics data such as birth and death records, information about communicable diseases, and information about cases of cancer by state and local health departments is specifically authorized by state statute. This statutory authority typically involves a compact, discussed above, that permits gathering of medical data, including personal identifiable information, only when strong protection of the confidentiality of identifiable information is provided. Colorado law exemplifies this trade-off (see Box 8–1).

Statutes such as this are an attempt to balance the public's interest in acquiring this information against the individual's interest in maintaining the confidentiality of his or her medical records. Without such guarantees, individuals may avoid seeking treatment for particular conditions, further increasing the risk of an epidemic.

CONCLUSION

The Institute of Medicine defines public health as "what we, as a society do collectively to assure the conditions for people to be healthy."[39] Accomplishing this goal requires delicately balancing the individual's interest in privacy and confidentiality with society's interest in a healthy and productive population. This balancing requires give and take—a minimal loss of privacy for the individual in exchange for a maximum gain in health for the larger population. To achieve the greatest good with the least amount of harm to individuals, state and federal laws and regulations have been enacted and professional societies have adopted guidelines to help their members act ethically. Without collection and analysis of data, designing and implementing mechanisms to protect and promote the public's health would be difficult—if not impossible—because public health research and practice are often inextricably intertwined.

This is the challenge that public health professionals must confront and with which they must continue to grapple. The values that public health professionals must strive to maintain are reflected in the balance between the protection of the individual and protection of the community at large. The applicability of the state laws and regulations and the federal Common Rule is a secondary concern to the protection of the participants.

Note

[a] A document asserting an institution's commitment to upholding human subjects protection regulations and stating the institutions policies and procedures for satisfying these regulations for all research conducted at the institution. See: Office of the Inspector General. "Protecting Human Research Subjects: Status of Recommendations." April 2000. Available at http://oig.hhs.gov/oei/reports/a447.pdf. Accessed April 3, 2002.

References

1. Gray B. Memorandum from the Surgeon General to heads of institutions receiving public health service grants, December 12, 1966. The regulatory context of social and behavioral research. In: Beauchamp TL, Faden, R. Wallace RJ, Walters R, eds. *Ethical Issues in Social Science Research.* Baltimore: Johns Hopkins University Press, 1982: pp. 329–55.
2. Jones JH. *Bad Blood: Tuskegee Syphilis Experiment.* 2nd ed. New York: Free Press, 1993.
3. Mariner WK. Public confidence in public health research. *Public Health Rep* 1997; 112:33–6.
4. 65*Federal Register* 37,136 (June 13, 2000).
5. 65*Federal Register* 37,137 (June 13, 2000).
6. 45C.F.R. 46 Subparts B–D.
7. National Bioethics Advisory Commission. *Ethical and Policy Issues in Research Involving Human Participants. Volume I: Report and Recommendations of the National Bioethics Advisory Commission, August 2001*—Full Report. Washington, DC: National Bioethics Advisory Commission, 2001: p. v.
8. 45 C.F.R. 46.102 (f) (2001).
9. Speers MA. *Guidelines for Defining Public Health Research and Public Health Non-Research.* Issued October 4, 1999. Available at http://www.cdc.gov/od/ads/op-spoll1.htm Accessed December 23, 2001.
10. 45 C.F.R. 46.109 (2001).
11. 45 C.F.R. 46.101 (b)(1)–(6) (2001).
12. 45 C.F.R. 46.101 (b)(2) (2001).
13. 45 C.F.R. 46.101 (b)(4) (2001).
14. 45 C.F.R. 46.107 (2001).
15. 45 C.F.R. 46.109(b) (2001).
16. 45 C.F.R. 46.111(a) (2001).
17. 45 C.F.R. 46.110 (2001).
18. 63 *Federal Register* 60364–7 (November 1998).
19. 45 C.F.R. 46.108(b) (2001).
20. 45 C.F.R. 46.116 (2001).
21. 45 C.F.R. 46.116(a)(5) (2001).
22. 45 C.F.R. 46.116(c) (2001).
23. 45 C.F.R. 46.116(d)(1–4) (2001).
24. 45 C.F.R. 46.108(e) (2001).
25. 45 C.F.R. 46.109(a) (2001).
26. Gostin LO. Surveillance and public health research: privacy and the "right to know." In: Gostin LO, ed. *Public Health Law and Ethics: A Reader.* Berkeley: University of California Press, 2001.
27. Wedeen RP. Consent in epidemiology: implications of history for public policy. *Arch Environ Health* 2000;55:231–9.
28. Snider DE Jr, Stroup DF. Defining research when it comes to public health. *Public Health Rep* 1997;112:29–32.
29. Koo D. Public Health Surveillance Slide Set. Available at http://www.cdc.gov/epo/dphsi/phs/overviews.htm. Accessed June 24, 2001.
30. CDC. Notifiable disease surveillance and notifiable disease statistics—United States, June 1946 and June 1996. *MMWR* 1996;45:9–15.

31. CDC. Ten leading nationally notifiable infectious diseases—United States, 1995. *MMWR* 1996;45:883–4.
32. 60(140) *Federal Register* 37648–50 (July 21, 1995).
33. 65(118) *Federal Register* 37982–4 (June 19, 2000).
34. 65 (250) *Federal Register* 82463 (December 28, 2000).
35. 45 C.F.R 164.512 (2000).
36. American College of Epidemiology. American College of Epidemiology Ethics Guidelines. Available at www.acepidemiology.org/policystmts/EthicsGuide.htm Accessed February 21, 2001.
37. *Jacobson v. Massachusetts*, 197 U.S. 11 (1905).
38. *The Southern Illinoisan v. Dept. of Public Health*, 2001 Ill. App. LEXIS 219 (2001).
39. Institute of Medicine. *The Future of Public Health*. Washington, DC: National Academy Press, 1988.

9

Implementation and Management of Public Health Programs in a Managed-Care Legal Framework

BRIAN KAMOIE, SARA ROSENBAUM, AND PAUL V. STANGE

This chapter reviews the structure and legal basis of managed care and its relation to public health policy and practice. Managed care constitutes the dominant means of organizing, financing, and delivering medical care to the nonelderly U.S. population, and its impact on the core functions of public health is considerable. As a result, adapting managed care to accommodate public health administration is one of the basic challenges faced by virtually all public health agencies.

The five sections of this chapter address the legal basis of managed care and public health practice. First, we present a general overview of managed care. Second, we place the core functions of public health in a managed-care context and illustrate the relation between these core functions and the legal foundations of public health policy and practice in the area of health-care regulation. Third, we explore in greater depth the relation between managed care and public health. Fourth, we present a typology of legal interventions available to public health agencies as they approach the task of building the structural and governmental environment in which managed-care systems will operate in the future. Finally, we discuss the long-term prospects for further strengthening the legal framework under which managed care and public health accommodate each other.

The issues and challenges that lie at the intersection of managed care and public health are no greater—and in fact may more readily lend themselves to solutions—than those that existed in what is frequently termed the "fee-for-service" era of U.S. medicine. Indeed, with its structural integration of care, accountability for quality, focus on populationwide health improvement, and emphasis on cost-effective investment,[1] managed care probably tracks public health principles in ways that were never present in the "old" U.S. health system, which was dominated by thousands of largely unregulated small medical-care businesses whose core principles tended to function as a mirror image of public health in their focus on individual patients rather than on a broader community.

OVERVIEW OF MANAGED CARE

During the past two decades, the U.S. health-care system has evolved dramatically.[a] A generation ago, nearly all insured persons received health care from health professionals who and institutions that operated autonomously and retained near virtual control over health-care decision making and the pricing of health-care services and products. Today, the vast majority of persons with employer-sponsored coverage, half of all Medicaid beneficiaries, and a significant percentage of all Medicare beneficiaries are members of what is commonly called "managed-care systems."[2] Even in the case of the State Children's Health Insurance Program (SCHIP), studies suggest that most states with separately administered SCHIP plans (i.e., programs that are separate from Medicaid) use their SCHIP allotments to purchase managed-care arrangements.[3,4]

Experts in managed care note that "there is no universally accepted managed care terminology."[5] Despite its various forms, managed care can be defined as any arrangement in which for a pre-set fee (i.e., a premium or a capitation payment), an entity sells a defined set of medical care and administrative services to a sponsor or purchaser and offers services to enrollees through a network of participating providers that operate under written contractual or employment agreements and whose selection and authority to furnish covered benefits is controlled by the entity. This definition captures the essence of managed care regardless of whether the plan is labeled as a health maintenance organization (HMO), an individual practice association, a preferred provider organization, an integrated service network, a disease-management company, a provider services organization, or some other name.

Despite certain basic commonalities, there are numerous variations on managed care, and no single regulatory scheme completely encompasses the managed-care structure.[b] A managed-care organization (MCO) might function as a "prime insuring contractor," operating as a licensed insurer and selling fully insured services to employer groups or public group sponsors (e.g., state Medicaid agencies). The same company might alternatively operate as a "plan administrator," operating managed-care services for a self-insured group sponsor such as a large multistate employer or union. Other types of MCOs might sell certain discrete components of the overall enterprise to a prime contractor. An example of this arrangement is an independent physician practice association that sells medical services to an HMO or a community clinic network that sells its members' services to a state Medicaid agency operating a primary care case management program (essentially a self-insured, self-administered Medicaid HMO and a major form of Medicaid managed care).

Contracts comprise the primary legal instrument for building the modern managed-care enterprise. Although managed care's roots can be found in the staff and exclusive group model prepaid practice plans that appeared in the first half of the twentieth century, the modern managed-care corporation exists through a "cascade"[6] of contracts that binds together the intermediary, its network, and the portions of the enterprise that carry out the functions of utilization review, quality assurance, and business management.[2] As noted, managed-care entities may assume financial risk by offering "fully insured" products; alternatively, they may enter into "administrative services" contracts with entities that elect to self insure and retain some or most financial risk.[2] Approximately half of all private employers self-insure, and partial assumption of risk is present in an unknown number of state employee benefit plans and Medicaid managed-care systems.

Structural and Operational Design Features of Managed Care

A managed-care product comprises various structural and operational design features, each of which plays a significant role in making the managed-care enterprise function. Following is an overview of these critical elements.

A managed-care coverage agreement between a group sponsor and an MCO flows from a prime contract between the parties. Unlike a conventional insurance agreement, however, the prime contract not only delineates the services and items that will be covered and the terms and limitations of coverage but also obligates the MCO to make its contractual services available through a network of participating providers.[7] An MCO's network can be tightly or loosely structured, but the contract itself combines the elements of insurance coverage with a contractual undertaking of care. Because the prime contract represents both a contract of coverage and a contractual health-care undertaking, it effectively establishes a provider–patient relationship with each member, thereby triggering a professional duty of care and the application of professional liability law.[7–9] This is true regardless of whether the contract is with an HMO, a preferred provider organization, or any other MCO[10]; indeed, an undertaking arguably exists in any contractual arrangement where the service sold is networked health care, not merely insurance.

Most states regulate managed-care contracts under their purview to at least some degree, just as they regulate insurance contracts written in the state. The

Employee Retirement Income Security Act (ERISA) prohibits states from regulating "employee benefit plans."[11] However, in recent years the Supreme Court has interpreted this ERISA preemption statute as not reaching the regulation of health-care quality.[12,13] Furthermore, ERISA saves state insurance laws from preemption, thereby permitting states to regulate fully insured employer-sponsored health plans (i.e., health plans that purchase insurance and insured managed-care products and that do not self-insure). State statutes regulating managed-care contracts may establish minimum standards regarding coverage, access to health care, provider network composition, and other matters related to health-care quality.

By 1995, more than 80% of the approximately 600,000 practicing physicians in the United States reported that they were either employed by or had entered into at least one contractual arrangement with a managed-care plan. This represents a one-third increase in 5 years in the proportion of practicing physicians who report participating in managed care.[14] Managed-care participation thus has become fundamental to the ability to practice medicine in the United States.

As health-care purchasers, MCOs have exceedingly broad power to select their provider networks and negotiate the terms of participation through contracts with providers. Network selection is among the most closely guarded types of information maintained by managed-care plans. Until recently, neither state or federal law nor managed-care accreditation organizations had attempted to regulate provider selection (or the "de-selection" of providers with whom plans no longer wish to affiliate).[c] Consistent with recent judicial decisions regarding the managed-care provider credentialing process, current accreditation standards established by the National Committee for Quality Assurance (NCQA) require companies to maintain certain due process elements within their provider selection systems.[15] Several states have enacted provider due process statutes that extend to the relation of MCOs with one or more classes of providers.[d]

The fixed price, risk-based nature of managed-care financing effectively necessitates the creation of payment rules that encourage cost containment and adherence to a budget. As a result, risk sharing between MCOs and their providers is a basic feature of managed care,[8] regardless of whether the prime contract includes financial risk for the prime contractor or, in the case of a self-insuring plan, is for third party administration only.

Managed-care companies have at their disposal two types of risk arrangements. The first is called "upside risk" and denotes arrangements in which providers are paid an additional amount if they realize savings from practicing in an efficient fashion (usually through lower levels of referrals to specialists and reduced inpatient care). The second, called "downside risk," involves compensation arrangements in which a portion of a provider's fee is withheld and is returned to the provider only if he or she keeps costs below a stated target.

Although most states regulate managed care to some degree, few regulate the financial relation between MCOs and their network providers. However, federal standards covering Medicare and Medicaid managed-care agreements prohibit compensation arrangements that create "substantial" financial risk.[16]

Because MCOs furnish and arrange for health care, they engage in extensive oversight of health-care practice and quality. Prospective utilization management is by no means unique to managed care; prospective utilization review was a feature of conventional health insurance plans by the 1970s. Managed care differs in its emphasis on changing the practice style of its provider network to improve health-care quality. For this reason, experts who write about the industry focus on practices such as accreditation, credentialing, the development and dissemination of practice guidelines, and overall attention to health-care quality, emphasizing the extent to which these industry practices differ from those of physicians and hospitals in the fee-for-service system. Some state managed-care laws address the structure and operation of utilization management and quality assurance, while more than 40 states have established external review systems to allow for impartial oversight of various classes of managed-care medical treatment decisions.[17] Federal standards governing Medicare and Medicaid managed-care products establish minimum operational standards and provide for external review of certain treatment decisions.[18,19]

Information and Data

As with all private corporations, managed-care entities maintain a proprietary interest in the data they generate and thus may impose strict controls over the extent to which they will release information and data related to patient care, health-care operations, and corporate administration. Although federal privacy standards developed pursuant to the Health Insurance Portability and Accountability Act of 1996 (HIPAA)[e] establish certain minimum safeguards for individually identifiable health information and permit the disclosure of such information under certain circumstances,[20] no uniform state or federal standards exist that establish minimum public health reporting requirements in the case of data owned by MCOs. Although most states have privacy statutes, the extent to which they permit public health data disclosure varies.[21]

Impact and Regulation of Managed Care

Managed care has significantly affected health-care access, generally showing improvements in access to primary care among the poorest populations. In the case of Medicaid managed care, the managed-care structure ensures that all patients have a primary-care access point. A number of evaluations suggest increased access to primary health care, such as well-child exams, vaccinations, and decreased use of emergency departments; others demonstrate that there has at least been no loss of access to these services under managed care.[22] At the same time, these studies tend not to track "out-of-plan" utilization (i.e., use of health services and health-care providers who are not part of a member's health care network). Consequently, evidence suggests that hospital emergency departments, community clinics, and other parts of the "health-care safety net" may be furnishing care to enrollees and simply going without compensation for it. Furthermore, a number of studies suggest that managed care has had a potentially adverse impact on health-care access among persons with chronic physical and mental health conditions.[5,23–26]

Managed care's impact on health quality is less well understood, and studies vary in their results.[27] What is indisputable is that managed care has the potential to radically shift health care access through the formation of networks, the imposition of utilization management techniques, and the methods of network compensation and incentives. In the case of Medicaid beneficiaries, who historically have faced widespread barriers to health care, the contractual health-care undertaking and the ensuing right to health care created by managed-care coverage represents a fundamental advance in the "no duty" principle. This principle, one of the most basic in U.S. common law, holds that health providers have complete autonomy to select their own patients.[2] This contractual right to health care in publicly funded managed-care plans also creates a nexus between health-care providers and U.S. civil rights laws prohibiting discrimination on the basis of race in the case of health programs receiving federal financial assistance.[28]

At the same time, it is not clear that managed-care systems actually open up networks of previously inaccessible providers to the poor. Managed-care organizations may maintain separate provider networks for their members as a means of appeasing physicians who suddenly find themselves contractually obligated to serve all plan members under otherwise applicable "all products" clauses. Consequently, Medicaid enrollees may find that their actual choice of providers is limited to the very clinics and practices that treated them under the fee-for-service system. Managed-care systems also may fail to include in their networks certain providers deemed essential to public health, such as local vaccination clinics, public health clinics offering services for sexually transmitted diseases, programs funded by public health agencies that specialize in tuberculosis management, and other interventions created in furtherance of the core public health function of "assurance."

What appears to be an unquestionable impact of managed care is its effect on costs for purchasers. Numerous studies show managed care's effects on the use of hospital and specialty care.[2,26] However, in their extensive review of plan performance, Miller and Luft noted that many of the studies may be affected by "favorable selection" (i.e., the over-enrollment of healthy persons), which makes their results suspect.[5] Most observers credit employers' near-universal conversion to managed care by the mid-1990s, along with extensive use by public agencies, with having dramatically reduced the rate of medical care cost increases. Beginning in 1999, however, the high price of prescribed drugs, along with pent-up demand for systemwide cost increases, appears to have caused dramatic increases in the price of insurance. Regardless of whether managed care's significant savings have run their course, little doubt exists that the transformation slowed the overall rate of increase in health spending.

At the macro level, managed care may result in overall savings to the economy. At a community level, however, managed care may in fact cause the costs of other parts of the health system to increase in ways that can be difficult to measure. Consider, for example, public schools, which must buy significant amounts of health care for children with physical and mental disabilities who need health care to be able to attend school. Many managed-care companies refuse to pay for otherwise covered health services furnished in schools, excluding them as "educational" (an exclusion that is prohibited under Medicaid). In turn, schools must then buy what can turn out to be costly services to comply with federal and state special education laws. A school system that employs a clinical psychologist for children with emotional disturbance may find that its rates go up because the discounts that the psychologist must give to managed-care companies as a condition of network participation requires that he or she raise charges to other purchasers.

Although managed care has existed for decades, only within the past 20 years has it come to dominate the U.S. health-care landscape. A shift in organizational and financial policy as dramatic as managed care would inevitably have roiled U.S. medicine because the rise of the health-care corporation has diminished the independence of physicians and health-care institutions.[10] Because managed care on a large scale is a relatively recent phenomenon, governmental efforts to regulate managed care are also relatively young. Furthermore, because U.S. health-care financing is so fragmented, government regulatory schemes themselves are developing in a patchwork fashion, with the extent and nature of regulation closely tied to the source of group sponsorship. As a result, even where the identical product is sold by a single managed-care corporation to multiple public and private group sponsors, different legal and regulatory frameworks exist for each sponsor, depending on whether the product has been purchased by a private employer, a public employer, the Medicare program, a state Medicaid or SCHIP program, or the federal employee health benefits system.

The growth of legal regulation of managed care as a matter of public health protection is consistent with the evolution of public health laws over the past century. As markets mature and the consequences of their operations on public health are felt, formal legislative efforts to regulate the business of health care increase. Examples of health care regulation to advance core public health functions can be found at both the federal and state levels. Federal health-care regulation is embodied in such laws as the Clinical Laboratory Improvement Act

(CLIA) (establishing quality and safety standards for clinical laboratories)[29] and the Emergency Medical Treatment and Active Labor Act (requiring as a condition of hospital participation in Medicare the provision of certain screening and stabilization services in the case of medical emergencies).[30] In addition, Congress has debated federal legislation to establish minimum patient protections for managed-care organizations.[f] State laws that impose duties on health-care providers as a protection of public health include state notifiable disease reporting statutes and state statutes establishing licensure standards for hospitals, nursing facilities, and MCOs.

PUBLIC HEALTH CORE FUNCTIONS AND THE LEGAL FOUNDATIONS OF PUBLIC HEALTH OPERATIONS AND MANAGEMENT

To understand the impact (both actual and potential) of managed care on public health, it is important to review the core functions of public health in the modern health-care enterprise.

In carrying out their responsibilities, public health agencies perform certain core functions of assessment, assurance, and policy development.[31] Furthermore, for public health agencies to achieve their goals, they must be able to develop and sustain a reasonably integrated relation with the medical care system because proper patient management is essential to public health promotion and protection. As a result, changes in the underlying medical care system affect public health decision making and public health practice.

The core functions of public health not only remain valid in a managed-care era but may in fact also increase in importance in the modern health-care environment because the ability to measure the health of a population over time and adjust resources to meet evidence-based needs—a basic goal of public health—also is essential to the success of the managed-care enterprise. Viewed in this context, the successful execution of the core functions of public health can be said to be consistent with the managed-care enterprise because managed care may best succeed when evidence on the health of a population is available and timely, thereby allowing, to the maximum extent possible, the calibration of health resources (in both amount and availability) to meet population needs.

At the same time, however, fundamental differences exist between the duties of public health agencies and those of managed-care companies. As is discussed at greater length below, these distinctions have consequences for the public health/managed-care relation.

In carrying out their core functions, public health agencies use several basic legal tools: legislation, regulation, and contracting. In the case of contracting, public health agency activities can take two forms. The first is the use of formal legal contracts that create enforceable promises. Contractual relations are a staple of public health administration, particularly for the development of legally enforceable agreements.

The second type of arrangement that closely resembles a contract but is less formal is the use of memoranda of understanding (MOU), which are written instruments of negotiation and agreement. The MOU do not create enforceable promises, nor do they specify legal remedies if one party violates the requirements of the contract. Instead, the MOU outline an agreement or consensus among the parties. In the context of public health practice, an MOU between a public health agency and an MCO typically codifies informal expectations regarding the roles of respective parties with regard to a particular activity, such as sharing of information, explanation of available services and benefits to patients (such as treatment of partners of managed-care plan members with sexually transmitted diseases), and collaboration on needs assessment and planning.[32]

The authority of public health agencies to carry out legal tasks derives from several distinct bodies of law, which together form the legal foundation of public health. This legal foundation consists of federal and state constitutions, the constitutionally sanctioned federal and state legislative processes and the administrative actions that flow from this process, and judicial law (both judicially derived "common law" and law consisting of the interpretation of constitutions, statutes, regulations, contracts, and other bodies of law).[33] Public health agencies' authority to carry out core functions derives from law, and all of their actions—whether regulation of insurance, surveillance for disease, conduct of health planning, or personal health-care intervention—must be based in cognizable legal authority. A survey of state public health agencies throughout the United States in 2000 confirms agencies' extensive involvement in legal matters of all types, including the regulation of managed care and health-care delivery.[34]

Table 9–1 presents a typology of the core functions of public health and the legal authorities and tools available to public health agencies at both the federal and state levels.

IMPACT OF MANAGED CARE ON PUBLIC HEALTH PRACTICE

The growth of legal oversight of managed care during the past decade underscores managed care's potential to affect the health of the public and thus public health policy and practice. Even a brief consideration of how managed care is structured and functions illustrates the tensions and challenges that can arise at the intersection of public health and the managed-care enterprise.

In recent years, the relationships between public health agencies and MCOs often have been the debated,[21] yet the complexity of the issues is rarely well understood. At first glance, public health and managed care share a comple-

TABLE 9–1. Legal Authorities and Tools in Relation to Core Public Health Functions

LEGAL AUTHORITIES AND TOOLS	CORE PUBLIC HEALTH FUNCTIONS IN PROGRAM IMPLEMENTATION AND ADMINISTRATION		
	ASSESSMENT	ASSURANCE	POLICY/PLANNING
Constitutions (federal and state)	Police power of states, through public health agencies, to demand certain data	Compulsory treatment	Power of public health agencies to establish conditions of operation on health-care providers
Judicial law (common law and interpretation of laws)	Cases involving access to personal health data	Cases involving the power of public health agencies to compel treatment of people with communicable diseases	Decisions regarding the decision to grant or deny certificates of need
Statutes and regulations	Notifiable disease laws of general applicability	Conditions of participation for managed-care contractors	State certificate of need programs
Contracts	Contract terms related to data access	Contract terms related to network composition selection and membership, access standards, and other conditions of covered care	Needs assessment by contractor in the service area
Informal instruments of negotiation	MOUs to establish needs assessment collaborations at the community public health level between MCOs and public health agencies	MOUs to promote collaboration between school health clinics and MCOs serving children in a school district	MOUs related to the development of and support for community planning groups

MOU, memoranda of understanding.

mentary perspective: Both appear to rest on the premise that the provision of both primary and secondary preventive clinical services can improve individual health and achieve cost savings. Moreover, both public health and managed-care practice tend to focus on the group rather than on individuals; the essence of each enterprise is collective thinking and uniform practice in relation to a population, with a de-emphasis on the medical care needs of any individual.[1] Both managed care and public health thus tend to emphasize principles of populationwide intervention and "macro-allocation" rather than individualized coverage decision making and "micro-allocation," the hallmark of traditional insurance.

However, these broad assertions of common interest often obscure fundamental differences between managed care and public health. These structural issues are shaped by legal/jurisdictional, financial, and traditional worldview considerations.

Legal and Jurisdictional Differences

A public health agency's jurisdiction extends to the entire community that the agency is authorized to serve. Public health agencies have a social compact with their communities as well as a legal duty to serve the community at large; however, no individual within the community has a legally enforceable entitlement to population-based public health services. For example, communicable disease control and surveillance must be accomplished without regard to a particular individual's eligibility for Medicaid or any other form of insurance. Every member of the community, insured or not, "belongs" to public health, and public health agencies attempt to maximize their resources on the community's behalf.

In contrast, MCOs possess very different duties. As fiduciaries, managed-care entities owe a duty to their sponsors to restrict expenditures on members and to hold expenditures to preset premiums or, in the case of self-insured plans, capitation payments. Investments for which payments extend beyond the period of the contract may place the enterprise at major risk for losses, a problem that is further magnified by the legally enforceable right to coverage for the defined benefits in MCO enrollees' contracts—unlike for residents of a public health agency's service area. This entitlement further complicates the power of MCOs to divert resources from expressly covered medical benefits and into broad public health clinical and administrative investments, regardless of their contractual status.

At some point, the obligation to serve members properly may require MCOs to engage in services and activities that may also benefit nonmembers. Managed-care organizations also can elect to engage in certain communitywide service activities, and anecdotal evidence suggests that, like other health providers, MCOs frequently are actively involved in numerous communitywide programs.

Nonetheless, the duty of an MCO is defined by members who have a legal entitlement to coverage and care, and the duty of public health agencies is defined by their community jurisdiction.

Financial Considerations

Managed-care organizations operate on a financial risk basis—they sign contracts that require them to provide defined contractual services to enrollees for a fixed fee (typically paid monthly). Thus, for example, an MCO that contracts to furnish certain services cannot arbitrarily discontinue coverage for certain services (e.g., childhood vaccinations or drugs) during the term of its contract. This of course does not mean that an MCO cannot institute rationing procedures to slow consumption or seek to interpret its contract to reduce the scope and extent of its legal obligations. However, regardless of their ability to control resource consumption, MCOs are bound to live up to their contracts of coverage during the term of coverage.

Public health agencies, on the other hand, typically manage costs within global budgets, as supported by local, state, and federal categorical grants, as well as third party payments generated by participation in state and private insurance programs, especially Medicaid. Because no individual is legally entitled to certain defined benefits offered by public health agencies, an agency typically has the legal power to reduce or eliminate services and activities if funds run out during a budget year. Some states may in fact define certain public health agency duties as legally enforceable rights, thereby obligating the state to fund budget deficits incurred by the entitled service, but such a commitment on the part of state government is rare and, at the county level, even rarer.

Because public health agencies do not have legally enforceable duties to individuals, they also have greater latitude to commingle funds and engage in cross-subsidization practices to keep their basic activities afloat. Thus, for example, a public health agency may pool revenues derived from grants, contracts, patient fees, and third party payments (most typically Medicaid) to support the provision of subsidized personal health-care activities for uninsured people. In this way, shortages in one area can be compensated for by budgetary reallocations of dollars where not prohibited by law. Because grant and contract funding for public health activities tends to be modest and because a large proportion of the patient population is poor, third party revenues, especially Medicaid, take on crucial importance.

Differences in World Views and Perspectives

Differences in the traditional worldview perspectives of public health and managed care present complex challenges for understanding and collaboration. Managed care combines health-care delivery with the financial and structural principles of insurance, and managed-care companies focus on their members rather than on the entire community population. Meeting the needs of members over the period of the contract and within the constraints of premiums or capitation payments while still achieving an adequate profit margin or return on investment causes MCOs to focus intensively on short-range time frames. Public health, in contrast, takes a longer view of achieving community health status improvement, which may take many months, or even years, to reach. Public health agencies must also be equipped to respond rapidly to disease outbreaks with short-term dedication of labor and resource-intensive efforts to contain the spread of a particular disease. Managed-care organizations are an outgrowth of the world of employment-based health insurance. They gear their operations and activities to relatively healthy, relatively easy-to-manage patients. Public health agencies frequently specialize in the care, management, and oversight of complex patients with public insurance or other sources of public financing who present management challenges that include the provision of social supports to ensure completion of treatment (e.g., transportation, translation, "cultural competency" capacity). A fundamental question to any discussion of the possibility of public health and managed-care collaboration, therefore, is the extent to which each domain is aware of the other's perspectives and traditions.

The realities of managed care can put MCOs into conflict with public health agencies in a number of respects. First, managed-care companies may alter existing health-care delivery systems through their contractual network arrangements in ways that interrupt previously established relationships between public health agencies and providers of health care; that is, MCOs may shift members away from clinical-care arrangements that are either part of or work in collaboration with public health agencies and into other systems that do not share public health traditions. The shift away from "health-care safety net" providers, such as publicly managed maternity clinics, in favor of private health providers represents an example of this trend. Not only is the provider eliminated from the network but the insurance funds that might have helped subsidize care for uninsured maternity patients are lost.

Second, in altering health-care delivery arrangements and in establishing ownership over certain purchased services, MCOs may disrupt access to certain health-care data on which public health agencies historically have depended. As health care is purchased, the information generated by the care falls within the scope of the purchasing agreement. Such information may become inaccessible in the absence of special laws regulating disclosure. An example of this phenomenon is the tendency of MCOs to use out-of-state clinical laboratories in lieu of in-state public health laboratories. Not only are the in-state laboratories cut out of the health-care (and health-care financing) loop, but their access to specimens for secondary public health and epidemiologic analysis may be lost.

Third, managed-care entities may establish standards of treatment that differ from those recommended by public health agencies. This may be particularly important in the case of communicable diseases. Historically, public health agencies have played a significant role in setting standards of treatment for communicable diseases. Anecdotal evidence suggests that insurers, particularly Medicaid agencies, tended to honor these guidelines. For example, a community hospital treating a Medicaid patient with tuberculosis might have followed public health guidelines in determining the length of inpatient treatment, and the Medicaid agency would have adhered to such guidelines. Unless contractually obligated to do so, managed-care entities may instead use industry guidelines that may impose stricter limits that have been developed, not with an eye to public exposure, but with a view toward minimizing expenditures that cannot be absolutely clinically justified from an individual treatment point of view.

Put another way, managed care's impact can be seen in adherence to standards. Public health agencies, particularly the Centers for Disease Control and Prevention (CDC), have fostered the development of evidence-based standards in the area of prevention and management of communicable and chronic diseases. These evidence-based standards may reflect not only what is essential to patient management but also what should be provided to protect the broader health of the public. Managed-care companies may opt to create their own practice guidelines that depart from these standards, particularly to the extent that public health guidelines are viewed as requiring treatment that goes beyond what can be justified for a particular patient. In one important study of managed-care plan adherence to public health standards, researchers surveyed Medicaid MCOs for their compliance with a series of established guidelines for the prevention, treatment, and management of sexually transmitted diseases issued by the CDC. They found that MCOs overwhelmingly failed to follow the CDC's practices or even recommend them for their primary-care physicians. The reasons given by MCOs for not using or recommending the CDC standards included cost, legal liability, conflicts with networks, and a desire to give network physicians autonomy (a striking finding in light of the growing emphasis on guidelines in managed care as a means of contractually limiting coverage itself). Most importantly, MCOs noted the low priority they placed on preventive health service upgrading given the high rate of turnover in Medicaid enrollees.[36]

RESPONDING TO MANAGED CARE: THE TOOLS OF PUBLIC HEALTH LEGAL POWERS APPLIED TO PUBLIC HEALTH IMPERATIVES IN MANAGED CARE

As discussed above, public health agencies operate under and have access to numerous types of legal authority and tools, ranging from the development of legislation and regulatory standards (as well as regulatory intervention to enforce standards) to contracting powers. How each type of legal power is used is a complex matter of policy and political assessment. An agency may deem broadly applicable regulatory intervention to be essential in the case of a public health challenge such as management of communicable diseases. In the case of public protection against the transmission of communicable disease, the nature of the managed-care sponsorship is irrelevant; whether affluent and privately insured or poor and publicly insured, managed-care members can be exposed to and transmit communicable disease. Thus, how MCOs respond to, manage, and report communicable disease constitutes a matter of basic public health protection.

Other issues lend themselves to more tailored interventions. For example, certain public health concerns and patient protections arise with particular force in the context of publicly sponsored managed care purchased by Medicaid and SCHIP agencies. In the case of Medicaid managed-care products, public health agencies may have more product-specific concerns related to the minimum standards, competencies, and capabilities of publicly sponsored managed-care networks. For example, these network concerns might constitute inclusion of the school health clinics in provider networks by MCOs operating in medically underserved areas or adherence to CDC human immunodeficiency virus (HIV) prophylaxis guidelines in the case of Medicaid managed-care products given the dominance of Medicaid in the area of HIV/AIDS prevention and treatment. When public health concerns are specific to a type of product, intervention in the product-specific managed-care contracting process may be a particularly appropriate legal approach. Such interventions include the setting of both substantive performance standards and the methods by which adherence to contractual standards will be measured, the data that will be furnished to permit measurement, and the reporting of outcomes.[g]

Table 9–2 illustrates for selected public health priorities the types of public health legal tools that may be applied to emerging public health issues in managed care. Table 9–2 is meant to be illustrative and therefore is not exhaustive. The applications of legal tools noted for selected public health programs are transferable to other types of programs.

The choice of legal tool to use in implementing and administering public health programs depends on a variety of often competing factors. Each factor suggests questions to consider in determining the appropriate legal tool. These factors include

- *Identification of public health objectives.* Which legal tools address public health objectives? Does one tool achieve the objectives more effectively or efficiently than the others?
- *Compatibility with market principles.* Which legal tools facilitate market competition and private agreement? Does one tool promote market principles more effectively or efficiently than the others?

TABLE 9–2. Application of Public Health Legal Tools in Managed Care: Selected Issues

| LEGAL TOOL | SELECTED PUBLIC HEALTH PROGRAM | | | |
	VACCINATIONS	PREVENTION OF PEDIATRIC LEAD POISONING	CONTROL OF STDS	TUBERCULOSIS CONTROL
Statutes and rules	State/federal requirement that state Medicaid managed-care programs meet pediatric immunization coverage at the ACIP standard of practice	Federal legislation and regulation that require screening of certain children for elevated BLLs	State-level disease-reporting requirements	State-level public health reporting requirements
Contracts	Medicaid managed-care contract provisions to incorporate pediatric vaccination coverage at the ACIP standard of practice	Contract provisions to require that the CDC's *Screening Young Children for Lead Poisoning: Guidance for State and Local Public Health Officials* define the standard of care for all providers	Contract provisions to ensure that all laboratories comply with state disease reporting requirements, even if the MCO uses an out-of-state laboratory that might not be subject to the state's regulations	Contract provisions to ensure that an MCO provides all treatment that the public health department determines to be medically necessary
Informal instruments of negotiation	MOUs between local health departments and MCOs regarding the selection of immunization registry	MOUs to define the roles and responsibilities of the MCO in furnishing and coordinating services for children with elevated BLLs (e.g., clinical management, medical treatment, environmental investigation)	MOUs to address coordination of partner notification services for partners of MCO plan members who are not in the plan	MOUs to coordinate notification of contacts of people with tuberculosis MOUs to ensure health department access to clinical records to ensure therapy complies with public health standards

ACIP, Advisory Committee on Immunization Practices; BLL, blood lead level; CDC, Centers for Disease Control and Prevention; MCO, managed-care organization; MOU, memoranda of understanding; STDs, sexually transmitted diseases.

- *Feasibility.* Will any of the legal tools accomplish the public health objectives or imperatives? Does one tool have a greater chance of accomplishing the objectives or imperatives than the others?
- *Cost.* Which of the legal tools can be used within existing budgetary constraints?
- *Strength of evidence.* Do any of the legal tools have evidence supporting its effectiveness? Which legal tool has the best evidence of success for the public health objectives or imperatives?
- *Public health imperative.* Which legal tool will best enable a public health practitioner to meet public health imperatives?

This list of factors and questions to consider is by no means exhaustive, but it provides key considerations for public health practitioners when choosing among available legal tools to implement and administer public health programs.

CONCLUSION: MAPPING THE FUTURE FOR INTEGRATING PUBLIC HEALTH AND MANAGED CARE

The legal tools and applications in public health practice (e.g., use of MOUs in the prevention and treatment of sexually transmitted diseases) demonstrate that widespread adoption of managed care creates major opportunities for public health interventions; at the same time, it raises new challenges. Public health agencies need to reconsider their basic orientation to managed care, which affects more than direct health-care service obligations that devolve from the master managed-care contract. Similarly, as public and private managed-care purchasers become aware of managed care's potential impact on public health, they may wish to consider making certain public health-related practices a basic contractual duty on the part of the companies with whom they conduct business. At the same time, the ultimate responsibility lies with public health agencies themselves to ensure that both public and private purchasers understand managed care's potential public health effects and to develop a comprehensive approach for the modernization of public health policy.

Certain activities may help promote and speed the heightened integration of managed care and public health policy and practice:

- Evaluation of the ongoing evolution of the contractual relationship between MCOs and public and private sponsors to measure the growth of public health practice standards and principles as a contractual element[h]
- Ongoing efforts to monitor collaborations between public health agencies and MCOs in the areas of patient management, network development, data sharing, and unified planning and ongoing research into the impact of public health laws and standards on the operation and organization of managed care

- The development of model laws for the regulation of the public health aspect of the managed-care enterprise, including laws establishing minimum standards of practice with respect to data management and disclosure, coverage and management of communicable disease treatments, and managed care participation in certain community enterprises (such as duties to undertake emergency immunization activities in the case of disease outbreaks).

ACKNOWLEDGMENTS

The authors thank Tony Moulton, PhD, of the CDC's Public Health Practice Program Office for his helpful assistance in preparing and reviewing this chapter.

Notes

[a] This overview is adapted from Rosenblatt et al.[2] For additional resources on managed care, see the Center for Health Services Research and Policy's website at http://www.gwhealthpolicy.org.

[b] For years, the National Association of Insurance Commissioners has struggled to develop model state regulatory standards for managed care. Developing a model in this area is difficult because of the wide variation in corporate arrangements, delivery systems, and risk assumption. See http://www.naic.org for general information.

[c] Limitations exist on provider de-selection. See *Harper v. Healthsource New Hampshire, Inc.,* 674 A.2d 962 (N.H., 1996) (physician entitled to review of termination to ensure that an HMO's decision to terminate comports with good faith and fair dealing and is not contrary to public policy); and *Delta Dental Plan of California v. Banasky,* 33 Cal. Rptr. 2d 381 (1994) (dental plan must use fair procedures in decisions regarding fees and continued participation in the provider network).

[d] See, for example, New York (44 Pub. Health § 4406-d) and California (Cal. Bus. & Prof. Code Cal. Bus. & Prof. § 809; Cal. Health and Safety Code. § 1367.02).

[e] HIPAA protects health insurance coverage for workers (and their families) when they change or lose their jobs. The statute also contains administrative simplification provisions intended to make the administration of health insurance more efficient and effective through standardized electronic data transfer. In addition, the statute directed the U.S. Department of Health and Human Services to develop privacy standards to protect individually identifiable health information. These regulations are in 65 *Federal Register* 82462 (Dec. 28, 2000).

[f] Such legislation has been debated in Congress since 1994. The legislation would establish certain minimum standards for health-care quality and safety to be met by MCOs and employee health plans, establish certain procedures for both internal and external review of patient treatment decisions, and establish certain individual causes of action for persons who allege an injury by an MCO. See, for example, HR 2563 and S 1082 (107th Congress, 1st Session).

[g] State public health interventions into managed-care contracts range from extensive to limited. For a comprehensive review of the various approaches taken to key issues in public health in Medicaid managed-care contracting, see Rosenbaum et al.[6]

[h] For sample Medicaid managed-care purchasing specifications, see the George Washington University CHSRP website at www.gwhealthpolicy.org.

References

1. Eddy DM. Rationing resources while improving quality: how to get more for less. *JAMA* 1994;272:817–24.
2. Rosenblatt RE, Law SA, Rosenbaum S. The financing and organization of health care. *Law and the American Health Care System*. Westbury, NY: Foundation Press, 1997: pp. 543–73.
3. Rosenbaum S, Markus A, Sonosky C, Repasch L. *Policy Brief #2: State Benefit Design Choices under SCHIP—Implications for Pediatric Health Care*. Washington, DC: George Washington University School of Public Health and Health Services, Center for Health Services Research and Policy, 2001. Available at http://www.gwhealthpolicy.org. Accessed December 20, 2001.
4. Pernice C, Wysen K, Riley T, Kaye N. *Charting SCHIP: Report of the Second National Survey of the State Children's Health Insurance Program*. Washington, DC: National Academy for State Health Policy, 2001.
5. Miller R, Luft HS, Managed care plan performance since 1980: a literature analysis. *JAMA* 1994;271:1512–9.
6. Rosenbaum S, Smith B, Shin P, et al. Overview: Medicaid managed care and pediatric health care. *Negotiating the New Health System: A Nationwide Study of Medicaid Managed Care Contracts*, 2nd ed. Washington, DC: The George Washington University Medical Center, Center for Health Policy Research, 1999:1–37.
7. *Boyd v. Albert Einstein Medical Center*, 547 A.2d 1229 (Pennsylvania Supreme Court, 1988).
8. *Pegram v. Herdrich*, 530 U.S. 11 (2000).
9. *Shannon v. McNulty*, 718 A.2d 828 (Pennsylvania Supreme Court, 1998).
10. Weiner JP, de Lissovoy G. Razing a tower of Babel: a taxonomy for managed care and health insurance plans. *J Health Politics Policy Law* 1993;18:75–103.
11. 29 U.S.C. § 514.
12. *De Buono v. NYSA-ILA Medical and Clinical Services Fund*, 520 U.S. 806 (1997)
13. *New York State Conf. of Blue Cross & Blue Shield Plans v. Travelers Ins. Co.*, 514 U.S. 645 (1995).
14. Segal D. Doctors who dodge A managed care stampede. *Washington Post*, May 20, 1996:F5.
15. National Committee for Quality Assurance, *Standards for the Accreditation of Managed Care Organizations (MCOs)*. Washington, DC: National Committee for Quality Assurance, 2001.
16. 61 *Federal Register* 13430 (Mar. 27, 1996).
17. Pollitz K, Dallek G, Tapay N. *External Review of Managed Care Treatment Decisions*. Washington, DC: Georgetown University Institute for Health Care Research and Policy. 1998. Available at http://www.kff.org/content/archive/1443/. Accessed October 5, 2001.
18. 62 *Federal Register* 25844 (May 12, 1997) (Medicare managed care appeals regulation).
19. 66 *Federal Register* 43614 (Aug. 20, 2001) (proposed Medicaid managed care external review regulation).
20. 65 *Federal Register* 82462 (Dec. 28, 2000).
21. Pritts J, Goldman J, Hudson Z, Berenson A, Hadley E. *The State of Health Privacy: An Uneven Terrain* (A Comprehensive Survey of State Health Privacy Statutes).

Washington, DC: Georgetown University Institute for Health Care Research and Policy, 1999.

22. Rowland D, Rosenbaum S, Simon L, Chait E. *Medicaid and Managed Care: Lessons from the Literature*. Washington, DC: Kaiser Commission on Medicaid and the Uninsured. 1995: pp. 13–22.

23. Ware JE Jr, Bayliss MS, Rogers WH, Kosinski M, Tarlov AR. Differences in 4-year health outcomes for elderly and poor, chronically ill patients treated in HMO and fee-for-service systems. Results from the Medical Outcomes Study. *JAMA* 1996;276: 1039–47.

24. Retchin SM, Brown RS, Yeh SC, Chu D, Moreno L. Outcomes of stroke patients in Medicare fee for service and managed care. *JAMA* 1997;278:119–24.

25. Miller R, Luft HS, Does managed care lead to better or worse quality of care? *Health Affairs* 1997;16:7–25.

26. Wagner EH, Bledsoe T. The Rand health insurance experiment and HMOs. *Med Care* 1990;28:191–200.

27. Rechovsky JD, Kemper P, Tu HT, Lake TK, Wong HL. *Do HMOs Make a Difference? Comparing Access, Service Use, and Satisfaction Between Consumers in HMOs and Non-HMOs. Issue Brief 28*. Washington, DC: Center for Studying Health System Change, 2000. Available at http://www.hschange.org/CONTENT/54/. Accessed October 9, 2001.

28. 45 C.F.R. Part 80 (Department of Health and Human Services, Office of Civil Rights, Policy Guidance on the Title VI Prohibition Against National Origin Discrimination As It Affects Persons With Limited English Proficiency).

29. 42 U.S.C. § 263a (2001).

30. 42 U.S.C. § 1395dd (2001).

31. Institute of Medicine. *The Future of Public Health*. Washington, DC: National Academy Press, 1988:1–18.

32. Rosenbaum S, Mauery D, Blake S, Wehr E. *Public Health in a Changing Health Care System: Linkages Between Public Health Agencies and Managed Care Organizations in the Treatment and Prevention of Sexually Transmitted Diseases*. Washington, DC: George Washington University School of Public Health and Health Services, Center for Health Services Research and Policy. 2000: pp. 1–24. Available at http://www.kff.org/content/2000/1575/. Accessed October 9, 2001.

33. Turnock B. Law, government, and public health. *Public Health: What It Is and How It Works*, 2nd ed. Gaithersburg, MD. Aspen Publishers, Inc., 2001: pp. 123–62.

34. Rosenbaum S, Stewart A. *The Law and State-Based Public Health Practice: A Survey*. Washington, DC: George Washington University School of Public Health and Health Services, Center for Health Services Research and Policy, 2000.

35. Halverson PK, Kaluzny AD, McLaughlin CP, Mays GP, eds. *Managed Care and Public Health*. Gaithersburg, MD: Aspen Publication, 1998.

36. Brown ER, Nakashima J, Pourat N, Razack N, Chiu S. *Delivery of Sexually Transmitted Disease Services in Medicaid Managed Care*. Los Angeles, CA: University of California, Los Angeles, Center for Health Policy Research, 2000.

10

Legal Authorities for Interventions During Public Health Emergencies

JAMES J. MISRAHI, GENE W. MATTHEWS,
AND RICHARD E. HOFFMAN

> Every imaginable threat from civil suits to cold-blooded murder
> when they got an opportunity to commit it, was made by the
> writhing, cursing, struggling tramps who where operated upon,
> and a lot of them had to be held down in their cots, one big
> policeman sitting on their legs, and another on their heads, while
> the third held the arms, bared for the doctors.
> Account of the 1901–1903 smallpox epidemic in Boston[1]

The public health measures used to control the 1901–1903 outbreak of smallpox in Boston, as reflected in the media account quoted above, no doubt appear draconian to a modern-day public health officer. Recently, however, public health officers, academics, and government policy makers, motivated by concerns about the threat of bioterrorism, have questioned whether the intentional release of a biologic agent such as smallpox would necessitate a return to such coercive public health measures as compulsory vaccinations. Such concerns have been highlighted by recent events surrounding the unprecedented terrorist attacks on the World Trade Center and Pentagon on September 11, 2001. These tragedies underscore the importance of public health officers understanding their legal authorities to ensure an effective, well-reasoned, and appropriate public health response that will safeguard civil liberties in a national emergency.

This chapter describes the legal authorities for interventions during public health emergencies. Although this chapter focuses almost exclusively on acute events, namely, bioterrorism, pandemic influenza, and emerging and infectious diseases, many of the principles covered may also apply to noninfectious or nonacute events. The second part of the chapter provides a brief historical background explaining how the power of the state has traditionally been used to control infectious disease and describes the legal structure and sources of public health law in the United States. The third section discusses evolving issues related to bioterrorism, focusing on the government's use of emergency public health powers with respect to records, property, persons, and communications. Finally, this chapter emphasizes the need for public health officers to understand the use of legal authorities as a tool in protecting the public's health.

HISTORICAL PERSPECTIVE: SOURCES OF LEGAL AUTHORITY IN PUBLIC HEALTH INTERVENTIONS

The concept of using the power of the state to control infectious disease is neither new nor novel. The Old Testament—specifically, Leviticus, Numbers, and the First Book of Samuel—gave specific instructions for the sequestration of lepers and detailed how the priests were to examine people for leprosy.[2] In Medieval Europe, lepers were required to wear special costumes and to limit their walks to certain roads, and they were forbidden from gathering in public places such as marketplaces, inns, and taverns. The term *quarantine* is derived from the Italian *quaranta* and the Latin *quadragina* and refers to the period of time, 40 days, during which health authorities thought a disease to be contagious.[2] Torture, exile, and death were among the penalties for violating a land or maritime quarantine.[2]

Although many governments have used coercive measures in the name of public health, not all public health interventions are necessarily coercive. In 1855, Dr. John Snow published an expanded version of his pamphlet, "On the Mode of Communication of Cholera," in which he argued that cholera was spread primarily through contaminated drinking water and not through casual contact with infected persons.[3] Dr. Snow's theory was based on his investigation of the "Broad Street" pump, in which he discovered that all of the suspected cholera-associated deaths in London were among persons who had drunk from that pump rather than from one of the other public water pumps in the area.[3] Dr. Snow's public health intervention was simply to remove the pump handle, thereby ending the epidemic.

In the United States, the major source of legal authority for public health interventions is the police power, defined as the inherent authority of all sovereign governments to enact laws and promote regulations that safeguard the health, welfare, and morals of its citizens.[2] Under the authority of the police power, for example, states have enacted laws for nuisance abatement, traffic safety, and firearms safety. In Colonial times, public health interventions were primarily exercised at the local level, with the earliest municipal ordinances enacted by Boston in 1647 and New York in 1663.[2] Local boards of health were eventually organized, leading to more extensive state public health laws and regulations in the late eighteenth and early nineteenth centuries. At the time of the framing of the Constitution, such public health powers as quarantine were well-established.[2] The Tenth Amendment reserves to the states all powers not expressly granted to the federal government nor otherwise prohibited by the Constitution, including the police power (Table 10–1).[a]

Even though the Constitution reserves the police power to the states, the federal government nonetheless has extensive authority over public health by virtue of the Commerce Clause, which grants it the exclusive power to regulate interstate and foreign commerce.[4,b] Under this authority, for example, the federal government has enacted such diverse laws as those prohibiting racial discrimination, mandating environmental clean-up, and criminalizing certain activities such as loan-sharking.[5] In the area of public health, the federal government has authority under the Commerce Clause to medically examine immigrants seeking entry into the United States and quarantine infectious persons with certain communicable diseases when they are about to move from one state to another.[6,7] Although courts have construed broadly the Commerce Clause, the federal government's authority under that clause is not without its limits. For example, the Supreme Court has struck down key provisions of laws, such as the Gun Free School Zones Act and the Violence Against Women Act, where it found the connection to interstate commerce to be unsupported or too tenuous.[8] Accordingly, the scope of the federal government's authority under the Commerce Clause remains the subject of much debate.

The federal government also may effect public health policy under its constitutional authority to tax and spend. Article I, Section 8, of the U.S. Constitution states that "Congress shall have the power to lay and collect taxes . . . and provide for the common defense and general welfare of the United States." The federal government, for example, has spent money on programs that raise awareness of human immunodeficiency virus (HIV) and acquired immunodeficiency syndrome (AIDS) and imposed taxes on cigarettes to discourage people from smoking. Furthermore, unlike recent Supreme Court cases limiting the scope of Congress' Commerce Clause power, courts have been deferential to Congress' use of the Tax and Spend power, as long as Congress does not use that power in a manner that violates other constitutional protections, such as the separation of church and state.

The Constitution acts as both a source of authority for public health interventions and a restraint on what actions government may take. The state's interest in imposing such personal-control measures as quarantine, civil confinement, and mandatory treatment must be balanced against an individual's constitutional rights to due process, freedom of movement, and bodily integrity. Similarly, state-initiated programs that, without an epidemiologic basis, single out high-risk populations for screening or treatment may raise concerns under the Equal Protection Clause. Furthermore, disease reporting and collection of contact information may have freedom of speech and privacy implications. In addition to constitutional restraints, federal statutes also limit the manner in which state and local governments may act. For example, in the wake of the

TABLE 10–1. State Emergency Public Health Powers

POWER	SOURCE	RESTRICTION
Disease reporting and medical surveillance	Police power reserved to states under Tenth Amendment	Constitutionally recognized right to privacy; state statutes covering medical privacy
Subpoena of business information, for example, customer lists, shipping information	Derived from state statute	Fourth Amendment right against "unreasonable" searches and seizures; trade secrets and other information may be viewed as "property" under the Fifth and Fourteenth Amendments
Commandeer private buildings and seize pharmaceuticals	Police power	Fifth and Fourteenth Amendments' requirements of due process and just compensation
Abate nuisances	Police power	No compensation required if deemed a "nuisance," otherwise a "taking" requiring compensation
Personal-control measures, for example, quarantine, compelled medical testing, mandatory vaccination	Police power	Considered a significant deprivation of "liberty" requiring due process; Equal Protection Clause implicated if applied in a discriminatory manner; possibly First Amendment Freedom of Religion Clause
Legal immunity	State statute may provide legal immunity from lawsuits under state law	42 U.S.C. §1983 authorizes damage awards for violation of rights under the Constitution subject to doctrine of "qualified immunity"
Dissemination of public health information	Unclear whether the police power authorizes control of media outlets	First Amendment doctrine of "prior restraint" generally prohibits government from censoring information in advance of publication

outbreak of West Nile virus in 1999, a group of concerned citizens filed suit challenging New York City's mosquito-abatement program, contending that the program violated provisions of the Clean Water Act and the Resource Conservation and Recovery Act.[9] Accordingly, public health measures that arguably touch on areas of civil liberties may be the subject of a court challenge.

THE CASE OF BIOTERRORISM

Although public health officers may find an understanding of legal authorities useful in their day-to-day practice, the threat of bioterrorism and emerging infectious diseases has made such an understanding essential. One reason an effective public health response is critical is the unique nature of biologic weapons; a biologic weapon has the same potential to cause mass casualties as a nuclear weapon.[10,c] In 1970, the World Health Organization released a report estimating that a 50 kilogram release of anthrax spores along a 2 km line upwind of a city of 500,000 would in 3 days cause 125,000 infections and 95,000 deaths.[11] Furthermore, even without a large number of casualties, the disruption and fear caused by a potential bioterrorism event would be significant. In 1994, for example, a naturally occurring outbreak of bubonic plague in Surat, India, caused an estimated 500,000 residents—including a large portion of the city's private physicians—to flee.[12] This occurred despite the availability of antibiotics such as tetracycline and doxycycline, which are usually 100% effective if administered in the first stages of the illness or simply after a suspected exposure.[12]

If a bioterrorist event occurs, an effective, well-considered, and lawful response will help ensure public safety and ward off the panic and dread that a terrorist may hope to cause. Many of the legal authorities for responding to an epidemic, whether natural or human made, may already exist. For example, it is not unusual for public health officers to deal with tuberculosis (TB) patients, participate in nuisance abatement, or close hotels, restaurants, and other facilities for public health reasons. Although public health officers may use all or some of the same legal authorities during a bioterrorism event or an epidemic, the scale and implementation may be completely different. For example, legal authority may exist that allows public health officers to close buildings or condemn articles that are potential sources of infection. Because a public health administrative order, however, may not be sufficient to facilitate the commandeering of hotel rooms that operate on separate ventilation systems (and thus aid in isolating patients), the state's governor may need to invoke an executive order to compel such actions. Accordingly, it is incumbent on health officers and their legal counsel to determine what public health or executive powers would be needed in an emergency and examine whether existing legal authorities are sufficient.

To assist in reviewing and revising state public health statutes, the Centers for Disease Control and Prevention commissioned Georgetown and Johns Hopkins Universities, through the Center for Law and the Public's Health, to draft model legislation. This legislation, known as the Model State Emergency Public Health Powers Act provides states with strong public health powers to rapidly detect and respond to bioterrorism and other emergency health threats.[13] The act, among other things, requires the reporting of suspect illnesses or conditions to detect a serious threat to the public's health, provides standards for a governor's declaration of a public health emergency, allows a public health authority to access and use private facilities during an emergency, and contains provisions for mandatory medical examinations, isolation and quarantine, and access to patient records. The act also immunizes from legal liability the governor, public health authority, and other state executive agencies or actors for actions taken during a public health emergency. The goal of the act is to provide a public health authority with powers needed to respond adequately to a public health emergency while protecting an individual's right to liberty, bodily integrity, and privacy to the fullest extent possible. State legislatures can adopt any or all of the provisions of the model law or tailor individual provisions to meet their needs.

In this regard, a review of the Boston smallpox epidemic of 1901–1903, which resulted in 1596 cases of smallpox and 270 deaths in a city population of approximately 500,000, is insightful.[1] The Boston Board of Health took steps to control the epidemic, including isolating patients with smallpox in special facilities, placing persons who had been in contact with or exposed to patients under surveillance, and establishing a program of mandatory house-to-house vaccinations.[1] Persons who refused vaccination were subject to a $5 fine or a 15-day jail sentence.[1] Although ultimately successful in controlling the epidemic, the Board of Health engaged in activities that would not be tolerated today. The Board of Health, for example, employed "virus squads" that resorted to physical violence to vaccinate the homeless, whom the public had blamed for spreading the epidemic.[1] The Board also engaged in medically and ethically questionable practices by challenging vaccination opponents to expose themselves to smallpox and, in one case, allowing such an opponent to tour a smallpox ward without the benefit of vaccination.[1] Although unimaginable today, such abuses nonetheless underscore the importance of public health officers operating within a legal and ethical framework.

Several emergency public health powers exist that the government may need to control or mitigate a bioterrorism event or serious outbreak of disease. Although not an exclusive list, these powers fall under the broad categories of (*1*) collection of records and data, (*2*) control of property, (*3*) management of persons, (*4*) dissemination of information, and (*5*) legal immunity or indemnification for public health officers responding to an emergency.[13] The remainder of this chapter analyzes the legal authorities and restrictions on the use of each of these public health powers.

Collection of Records and Data: Disease Reporting, Surveillance, and Privacy

One of the most well-known public health powers is that of surveillance, derived from a French word meaning "a close watch or guard kept over a person."[2] In this respect, the police power authorizes states to mandate reporting of infectious diseases and sometimes injuries and other health conditions. Which diseases are reportable, under what conditions they must be reported, and who has the duty of reporting vary from state to state. To detect and respond adequately to an act of bioterrorism, however, public health officers may need additional authorities beyond surveillance and disease reporting. For example, because a terrorist may not necessarily announce the release of a biologic agent, public health officers may learn of an event only through unusual mechanisms, such as a large increase in workplace absenteeism or in the sale of certain types of medications. Similarly, access to hospital records and the ability to share that information with other agencies may assist law enforcement and public health officers to either track down the perpetrators or discover which biologic agent has been used. In addition, many infectious agents that affect human health, such as West Nile virus and certain strains of influenza virus, may first manifest themselves in animals. Accordingly, public health officers should examine whether authorities exist that would allow them to access hospital and provider records; share data with law enforcement and other entities; and mandate reporting of veterinary illnesses, workplace absenteeism, and sales of medications from pharmacies.[14]

Notwithstanding the public health importance of disease reporting and surveillance, the disclosure of medical information raises legitimate public concerns about privacy, particularly regarding sensitive information that may lead to stigmatization and discrimination. Although courts have recognized state authority under the police power to mandate reporting of medical information, states must have adequate procedural protections in place to safeguard patient confidentiality. In *Whalen v. Roe*, the U.S. Supreme Court upheld a New York statute requiring physicians to report information about certain prescription drugs because, among other factors, the state had adequate procedures in place to protect against unauthorized access.[15] At the federal level, statutes such as the Privacy Act of 1974, subject to certain exceptions (e.g., those governing "routine uses"), generally require that federal agencies not disclose "any record" that exists within a "system of records" controlled by those agencies.[16] State laws, to varying degrees, may also govern the privacy of medical records and public health reports gathered through surveillance and follow-up investigation. In addition, while creating exemptions for public health, proposed federal regulations enacted pursuant to the Health Insurance Portability and Accountability Act of 1996 may potentially limit a health-care provider's ability to disclose confidential patient information without consent.[17]

In addition to medical records, public health departments may also need access to nonprivileged business records such as customer lists, shipping information, and other information about business practices. For example, if an outbreak occurs in a hotel, the local health department may have to know what other guests have stayed in the hotel. A constitutional limitation on a health department's ability to obtain such information may be the Fourth Amendment, which guards against unreasonable searches and seizures. Generally, a search or seizure is unreasonable unless accompanied by a warrant that describes with particularity the places to be searched and the articles to be seized. Although health departments can inspect premises on an emergency basis to avert an immediate threat to health or safety, whether this authority allows them to seize documents is unclear. Health departments, however, may possess subpoena power to access relevant information during a public health emergency.[18] Although not necessarily rising to the level of medically privileged information, business information obtained through subpoenas may nonetheless contain valuable trade secrets or proprietary information that health departments should treat as confidential. Given the usefulness of this authority, public health officers who lack subpoena power may wish to consider obtaining such authority from their state legislatures.

Control of Property: Seizures, Takings, and Nuisances

Public health officers also should be aware of legal authorities concerning the control of private property. In general, state laws authorize health departments to take, destroy, or restrict the use of private property to protect the health and safety of the community. This often includes the authority to enter suspicious premises, close facilities on an emergency basis, and seize and destroy contaminated articles. A bioterrorism event or a large-scale epidemic, however, can require greater government control of private property than that to which the public is accustomed. For example, public health officers may have to designate certain hospitals to receive infected patients and transfer noninfected patients to other facilities. In addition, health officers may have to confiscate medicines from local hospitals and pharmacies and ration limited stockpiles of pharmaceuticals among the population.[14] Furthermore, public health officers may have to commandeer additional private facilities, such as hotel rooms that generally operate on separate ventilation systems and fast-food–type drive-through facilities that can easily be used to dispense medication.[14] Given a large-scale event, the government could conceivably seize cell phones and other communication devices to simply maintain open lines of communication during an emergency.[14] Finally, the disposal of human corpses may be radically different in a large-scale epidemic, and public health officers may be required to issue orders directing how corpses should be treated.

The major legal constraints on a public health department's use of private property are the constitutional requirements of due process and just compensation. The Constitution states that the government may not take private property for public use without compensating the owner.[19] Similarly, the government must generally provide notice and an opportunity for a hearing before depriving a landowner of the use of private property.[20] Although the concept of compensation for public use appears simple, under what circumstances the government must compensate private landowners has been the subject of extensive litigation.

In general, courts have defined two types of "takings" that require compensation: "possessory" and "regulatory."[2] Possessory takings, also known as physical invasions or "per se" takings, are relatively easy for courts to identify because they involve the physical possession by the government of private property.[2] Therefore, if the health department were to seize a drive-through facility and use it to dispense medications to the public, it would in all likelihood have to compensate the owner. Regulatory takings, on the other hand, are more difficult for courts to identify because they involve the diminution in economic value through government regulation of an owner's property.[2] In general, the more the regulation diminishes the economic value associated with the private owner's property rights, the more likely courts are to examine whether the regulation amounts to an unconstitutional taking.

One reason regulatory takings are difficult for courts to identify is that government may legitimately abate nuisances without compensation to the owner. A public nuisance is an activity that unreasonably interferes with the public's use and enjoyment of a public place or that harms the health, safety, and welfare of the community.[2] Public nuisances typically have included explosives; garbage and offal; decaying animals; improper sewage; and, more recently, places that promote high-risk sexual activity.[2] For example, under the nuisance theory, public health authorities in New York City were able to order the closing of bathhouses to prevent the spread of AIDS.[21]

Even though government may legitimately abate nuisances, it may not avoid paying compensation to private property owners by simply declaring their activities to be nuisances. Rather, the U.S. Supreme Court has held that government must rely on "background principles of nuisance and property law" requiring that government find some precedent, either in common law or in the law pertaining to private nuisance suits, that allows it to declare an activity to be a nuisance.[22] Some legal commentators have argued that this approach unduly hampers public health departments because it forces health officers to rely on often vague and outdated concepts of what constitutes a public health threat.[2]

One example of where public health concerns have clashed with private property rights is tobacco regulation. In *Philip Morris v. Harshbarger*, for example, a federal court of appeals preliminarily enjoined a Massachusetts law that required cigarette manufacturers to report tobacco ingredients on the ground that it could amount to an uncompensated taking of property, specifically, the manufacturers' trade secrets.[23] Accordingly, given the courts' protection of private property rights and the public's evolving understanding of what constitutes a public heath hazard, such clashes are likely to continue.

Management of Persons: Quarantine, Detention, and Treatment

A highly controversial area of public health is management of people. In general, public health officers possess authorities, subject to statutory and constitutional restraints, that allow them to restrict the liberty of persons through such measures as cease-and-desist orders, compelled physical examination, compelled vaccination, and possibly detention. A bioterrorism event or a large-scale epidemic, however, may require additional powers, such as the ability to suspend state licensing requirements for medical personnel from outside jurisdictions, authorization of other doctors to perform the functions of medical examiners, ability to waive informed consent requirements for collection of clinical specimens for laboratory testing, and procedures to allow for the safe disposal of corpses.[14] In addition, public health departments may need procedures in place to allow for large-scale isolation of infected persons and quarantine of persons believed to be exposed to an infectious agent. Although some health departments may have experience with personal-control measures with problems such as TB or measles, the scale and implementation of a bioterrorism event may be completely different. A bioterrorism event probably will require public health officers to collaborate with other agencies and organizations with which they do not have regular working relationships (e.g., public safety, law enforcement, or the National Guard).

Most public health interventions are accomplished through voluntary compliance, but coercive measures, such as detention, are sometimes necessary. Few states have a modern public health statute that specifically addresses bioterrorism. Rather, laws authorizing compulsory public health measures were enacted at different times, with different disease-causing agents or diseases in mind, and may rely on different or inconsistent medical and legal approaches to disease control. Typically, disease-control laws fall into three categories: (*1*) laws relating to sexually transmitted diseases, such as syphilis and gonorrhea; (*2*) laws targeted at specific diseases, such as HIV infection and TB; and (*3*) laws applicable to "communicable" or "contagious" diseases, a broad category dealing with a range of diseases from malaria to measles.[24] In addition, some states may have within their public health statutes laws that address environmental diseases or conditions. The problem with most of these statutes is that they are old; for example, laws enacted 50 to 100 years ago to deal with polio may not be sufficient to deal with viral hemorrhagic fevers, foot and mouth disease, West Nile virus, or a bio-engineered weapon. Moreover, these laws may not necessarily reflect a modern understanding of infectious disease, biology, or epidemiology; current treatment methods; or present-day standards of due process. As a practical consideration, however, adding specific statutory authority with respect to bioterrorism may be more prudent or expeditious than overhauling broad public health disease-control laws that have stood the test of time. Public health agencies must therefore decide whether to engage in wholesale revision of public health statutes or to modify existing regulations to deal with bioterrorism concerns.

The legal precedents authorizing compulsory public health measures, like the public health statutes themselves, also are old and of questionable value. For example, *Jacobson v. Massachusetts*, the U.S. Supreme Court case decided in the wake of the 1901–1903 Boston smallpox outbreak, while acknowledging that the state could pass laws mandating compulsory vaccinations, simply emphasized the state could not do so in an arbitrary or unreasonable manner.[2] Similarly, most state court cases addressing compulsory public health powers simply emphasize the importance of preserving the public's health without addressing the rights of the individual.[18] Accordingly, how courts today would react to a quarantine on the scale of the Boston smallpox outbreak is unclear.

One measure of how courts may react to a modern-day quarantine, however, may be the law surrounding involuntary detention of the mentally ill or TB patients. As the need for large-scale personal-control measures diminished through the advent of antibiotics and improved public health in the 1950s, courts became increasingly concerned with individual rights and due process. As a result, courts generally scrutinize very closely government actions that result in the involuntary commitment of persons. For example, courts have held, in the context of civil commitment to mental hospitals, that involuntary commitment is a significant deprivation of liberty requiring that the state afford the individual with due process of law.[2] In the context of detaining infectious persons, due process requires that the state provide written notice of the behavior or conditions that allegedly pose a risk to the community, access to counsel, a full and impartial hearing, and an appeal.[2] Even though the state must ordinarily provide notice and a hearing before detaining someone, the law recognizes emergency exceptions in which the state may be able to afford the person a post-deprivation hearing. In such cases, the government generally has the burden of proving its case by "clear and convincing evidence," a legal standard somewhat greater than a "preponderance of the evidence" but less than "beyond a reasonable doubt."[2] In addition to adequate procedural protections, the state may also have to show that its interest in confinement outweighs the individual's liberty interest and that no less restrictive means exists for accomplishing the state's objective.[2] This may require, for example, that the state prove that the person is actually infectious and that no other less restrictive treatment options are available. Furthermore, because public health powers are civil, designed to safeguard the public's health rather than punish the individual, the state may have to prove that detention is being carried out in a medically appropriate environment such as a hospital or other treatment facility.[2]

If a bioterrorism event occurs, detention of infected persons may not be sufficient; the state may have to compel exposed persons to accept chemoprophylaxis or vaccinations, despite personal or religious objections, to ensure that they do not become contagious and infect others.[25] The U.S. Supreme Court, however, has recognized a constitutionally protected right of competent persons to refuse medical treatment, which is derived from the common-law concept of informed consent.[26] As a practical matter, a public health department may therefore have to provide an exposed person with the choice of either accepting preventive therapy or being isolated until the incubation period passes and he or she is no longer at risk of becoming contagious. Today, in determining whether to allow compulsory vaccination, courts also are likely to balance the state's interest in protecting the public's health against the individual's liberty interest in bodily integrity. In *Washington v. Harper*, for example, the U.S. Supreme Court held in the context of prisoners that the state's interest in preventing dangerously mentally ill prisoners from harming themselves or others outweighed the prisoner's interest in refusing antipsychotic medications.[27] In addition to balancing the government's interest against the rights of the individual, courts may also subject state public health measures that single out high-incidence groups for compelled treatment to "strict scrutiny," the most rigorous and least deferential form of review, if such measures are found to discriminate along racial or ethnic lines.

The legal analysis applied to the compelled isolation of an individual with contagious pulmonary TB and the quarantine of a large number of people because of a bioterrorist's release of smallpox may be conceptually similar. In contrast, these problems are readily distinguished by factors such as the magnitude of a bioterrorist event, the fear created by the event, and the parallel criminal investigation of the perpetrators. Assuming that legal authorities are sufficient to allow public health officers to use personal-control measures, many practical questions such as who enforces a quarantine or detains an infected person and what actions government may take if a person disobeys a quarantine order may still be unanswered. Many public health officers may assume that, in the event of bioterrorism or a large-scale epidemic, the federal government will impose personal-control measures. Federal law, however, may limit the government's ability to control the movement of citizens. Regulations provide that the

Surgeon General, on recommendation of an advisory committee, may apprehend and examine individuals only if they are reasonably believed to be infected with a communicable disease and are about to move from one state to another or are a probable source of infection to individuals who, while infected, will be moving from one state to another.[28] Therefore, without such an interstate connection, the federal government may have to rely on state quarantine statutes. Similarly, the Posse Comitatus Act, subject to exceptions for insurrections and civil disturbances, generally prohibits the use of the military in civilian matters.[25] These restrictions, however, do not apply to the National Guard when in state status, which may be called on by a state governor to assist in an emergency.[25] Accordingly, in addition to ensuring adequate legal authorities, public health departments should begin addressing such practical considerations as who implements and enforces a quarantine order.

Legal Immunity

Even with sufficient legal authority, public health officers may feel constrained to act because of fears concerning legal liability. In general, people who believe state officials have violated their constitutional rights can file suit for damages pursuant to Title 42 of United States Code (U.S.C.) § 1983. In the public health context, for example, prisoners whom the state has compelled to accept TB treatment or those who have been involuntarily committed to mental hospitals have used 42 U.S.C. § 1983 to pursue damage suits against state public health officers.[29] In addition, most states recognize tort actions for battery, false arrest, and false imprisonment.

Regardless of the availability of damage suits, state officials may be shielded from federal liability for constitutional violations under the legal doctrine of qualified immunity. Qualified immunity provides that government officials performing discretionary functions are immune from civil liability under federal law if their actions do not violate clearly established statutory or constitutional rights of which a reasonable person would be aware.[30] Therefore, in theory, even if a court were to find a public health officer's actions to be unconstitutional, the officer would be shielded from liability if the officer reasonably believed he or she was acting pursuant to legal authority and his or her actions were objectively reasonable. In *Doe v. Marsh*, for example, a federal court of appeals found that a public health officer who had included the names of two HIV-positive persons in a government manual published in connection with an HIV/AIDS conference was entitled to qualified immunity.[31] Specifically, the court found that, although in error, it was objectively reasonable for the health officer to believe that the two persons had waived their rights to privacy by publicly announcing their HIV status at the conference.[31]

However, qualified immunity immunizes officials only from damages and not from suit, meaning that a government official would still have to defend himself or herself in court and bear the burden of showing his or her actions were reasonable. Furthermore, the doctrine of qualified immunity applies only to individuals, not agencies, and provides immunity from federal, but not state, liability. Even without immunity from liability, some states may nonetheless indemnify government employees from money judgments provided that they act in good faith and within the scope of their employment. Accordingly, public health officers may feel more comfortable making difficult decisions if they are either immunized or indemnified for decisions made in good faith.

Access to Communications: First Amendment and Media Strategy

Compulsory public health powers require that public health departments obtain the public's trust. Although public health departments play a large role in educating the public about health, for example, by warning about the dangers of smoking or obesity, bioterrorism requires a unique response. Such an event will probably cause fear and confusion, which, if government officials fail to address in an appropriate (i.e., timely, if not emergent) manner, may potentially lead to civil unrest and flight. At a minimum, public health officers will have to maintain clear lines of communication, for example, through a command center, to provide expert advice to the elected officials who will be managing such a crisis.[14] To dispel rumors and provide accurate information, public health officers should also consider using communications systems such as the emergency-response system, Internet-based websites, and toll-free telephone numbers.[14] Furthermore, experts in human relations and post-traumatic stress disorder may assist health officers in coordinating a message that will alleviate public concern. Public health officers, moreover, must be aware of cultural differences among ethnic groups that may require dissemination of information in different languages.

In the event of bioterrorism or a large-scale epidemic, government may have an interest in curtailing certain media outlets that could be perceived as endangering the public through dissemination of incorrect information. The First Amendment, however, generally prohibits government from censoring information in advance of publication. Under the legal doctrine of prior restraint, such measures are treated by courts with a great deal of suspicion and are presumed unconstitutional.[25] Furthermore, although the First Amendment does not encompass the right to endanger the public (the common example of shouting "fire" in a crowded building), attempts by government to control the media might lead to greater public mistrust and, therefore, prove counterproductive. A more realistic solution might be for government to formulate a media strategy in advance of a crisis that facilitates how public health officers will communicate with the media and the public.

CONCLUSION

Both historically and in modern times, people have looked to government to protect them against infectious agents and the diseases and epidemics caused by such agents. Although this responsibility falls primarily to state and local governments under U.S. constitutional structures, the federal government nonetheless plays a significant role in safeguarding the public's health. The threat of bioterrorism and of new and emerging infectious diseases, however, has compelled state and local public health officers to understand the role of legal authorities in responding to such health threats. Although public health officers may be familiar with using emergency public health powers to collect data, close dangerous facilities, control infectious persons, and disseminate information to the public, the scale and magnitude of a bioterrorism event requires a particularly well-coordinated and thoughtful response. Legal authorities must exist to allow public health officers to respond in a crisis, but such powers are useless unless public health officers possess the knowledge and ability to carry them out. This may, for example, require greater education of public health officers about their legal authorities and the formation of partnerships with outside communities— such as law enforcement, emergency-response managers, the governor's office, and federal health and emergency counterparts—that may be useful in managing the crisis. In some areas, legal authorities may be inadequate, but in others current operating procedures or a lack of planning may hinder the public health response to an emergency. Accordingly, public health officers should begin reaching out to groups outside the public health field and conduct exercises to test how public health and other executive powers would work in a real-life emergency. Only through such efforts will the public's trust in the ability of government to control and mitigate the serious public health consequences of a potential bioterrorism event be justified.

Notes

[a] The Tenth Amendment states that "the powers not delegated to the United States by the Constitution, nor prohibited by it to the States, are reserved to the states respectively, or to the people."

[b] Commentators have noted that the federal government's control over public health significantly increased as a result of the U.S. Supreme Court's broad interpretation of Congress' Commerce Clause and Tax and Spend powers during the New Deal.

[c] A few kilograms of anthrax has the potential to kill as many people as a Hiroshima-sized nuclear weapon.

References

1. Albert MR, Ostheimer KG, Bremen JG. The last smallpox epidemic in Boston and the vaccination controversy, 1901–1903. *N Engl J Med* 2001;344:375–9.

2. Gostin LO. *Public Health Law: Power, Duty, Restraint.* Berkeley: University of California Press, 2000: pp. 26–7, 116, 132–3, 185–7, 204–18, 264.
3. Vollmar LC. The effect of epidemics on the development of English law from the Black Death through the Industrial Revolution. *J Legal Med* 1994;15:416–8.
4. Hodge J. The role of New Federalism and public health law. *Journal of Law and Health* 1998;12:311–12.
5. Harsch BA. *Brzonkala, Lopez,* and the commerce clause canard: A Synthesis of Commerce Clause Jurisprudence. *NM Law Rev.* 1999;28:322–3.
6. 8 U.S.C. § 1222.
7. 42 U.S.C. § 264.
8. Sungaila MC. *United States v. Morrison:* the United States Supreme Court, the Violence Against Women Act, and the "New Federalism." *S Cal Rev L Women's Stud* 2000;95:303–10.
9. *No Spray Coalition, Inc. v. City of New York,* N.Y.L.J. October 2, 2000;38.
10. Siegrist D. The threat of biological attack: why concern now? *Emerg Infect Dis* 1999; 5:505–8.
11. Cieslak TJ, Eitzen EM Jr. Clinical and epidemiologic principles of anthrax. *Emerg Infect Dis* 1999;5:552–5.
12. Garret L. *Betrayal of Trust: The Collapse of Global Public Health.* New York: Hyperion, 2000: pp. 18–21, 366–8.
13. Model State Emergency Public Health Powers Act. November 27, 2001. Available at http://www.publichealthlaw.net. Accessed March 12, 2002.
14. State Emergency Health Powers and the Bioterrorism Threat. Cantigny Conference Series Chicago: National Strategy Forum, 2001.
15. *Whalen v. Roe,* 429 U.S. 589 (1977).
16. Glenn CL. Protecting health information privacy: the case for self-regulation of electronically held medical records. *Vanderbilt Law Rev* 2000;53:1605–35.
17. U.S. Department of Health and Human Services. HHS fact sheet: protecting the privacy of patients' health information. May 9, 2001. Available at http://aspe.hhs.gov/admnsimp/final/pvcfact2.htm. Accessed October 18, 2001.
18. Fidler D. Emerging and reemerging infectious diseases: challenges for international, national, and state law. *Int Law* 1997;31:788.
19. U.S. Constitution, Amendment V.
20. U.S. Constitution, Amendments V and XIV.
21. *City of New York v. New St. Mark's Baths,* 497 N.Y.S.2d 979 (1986).
22. *Lucas v. South Carolina Coastal Council,* 505 U.S. 1003, 1031 (1992).
23. 159 F.3d 670, 675–78 (1st Cir. 1998).
24. Gostin L. The law and the public's health: a study of infectious disease law in the United States. *Columbia Law Rev* 1999;99:108.
25. Kayyem J. US preparations for biological terrorism: legal limitations and the need for planning. BCSIA Discussion Paper 2001–4, ESDP Discussion Paper ESDP-2001–02. Boston: John F Kennedy School of Government, Harvard University, 2001.
26. *Cruzan v. Director, Missouri Dept. of Health,* 497 U.S. 261, 278 (1990).
27. 494 U.S. 210, 227 (1990).
28. 42 U.S.C. § 264.
29. Rothstein M. *Legal analysis of the institute of medicine recommendations to expand testing for and treatment of latent tuberculosis.* Houston: Health Law & Policy Institute, University of Houston.
30. *Harlow v. Fitzgerald,* 457 U.S. 800, 818 (1982).
31. 105 F.3d 106, 110–11 (2nd Cir. 1997).

11

Considerations for Special Populations

T. HOWARD STONE, HEATHER H. HORTON,
AND ROBERT M. PESTRONK

This chapter focuses on laws that pertain to special populations and their public health needs. We consider as "special populations" persons with mental disabilities; persons who are involved with the criminal justice system; homeless persons; children; and undocumented immigrants. At first glance, persons who are similarly situated with regard to one or more characteristics that are relevant to public health—such as persons with sexually transmitted diseases, drug dependency, or diabetes—might at one time or another be considered a special population. These persons may share attributes that facilitate identification and public health intervention. Our concept of "special populations" however, includes the additional attribute of vulnerability and therefore comprises persons who are not only underserved with regard to public health intervention but who also may be disenfranchised with respect to the legal status or social regard that is generally accorded our citizens.

Public health concerns about special populations are not new. Undocumented immigrants and homeless persons are generally transient populations who have always been difficult to reach for public health surveillance and service. Many of these persons try to avoid contact with public authorities at all costs, including their own health. Services for children and persons with mental disabilities are critical because they are situated at the nexus of the heightened value of early public health intervention and the potential for diminished capacity. For these persons, cost and other nonfinancial barriers often prevent more timely and appropriate access to needed health services. In addition, the health needs of undocumented immigrants, persons with mental disabilities, and persons who are involved in the criminal justice system are confounded by histories of past abuse or neglect. To this history is the added matter of legal capacity because many of these persons have reduced civil liberties and diminished legal rights to shape or determine the course of their treatment. To more effectively intervene with the public health needs of all persons, public health professionals should familiarize themselves with special populations and laws relevant to them.

This is not an exhaustive list of special populations and related concerns; limitations of space permit only a brief review of the public health issues and relevant laws pertaining to these special populations. This chapter is divided into sections, each focused on a special population. Each section begins with a case study of a member of a special population and his or her public health needs. The case study is followed by analysis of the pertinent legal issues. Each section closes with practice pointers that incorporate the pertinent legal issues in the context of the case study.

PERSONS WITH MENTAL DISABILITIES

Case Study 1

At the other end of the phone is an attorney who tells you he represents the wife of John H. The attorney states that John's recent behavior has left his client's health and welfare at risk. The attorney asks you to provide him with copies of your public health agency's treatment records for John, who, the attorney asserts, has previously received mental health and substance-abuse treatment from one of your agency's facilities or programs. In fact, the attorney states that you should take action to prevent John from further harming himself or others, including his wife. You are not aware whether John has in fact received any treatment through your agency or any of its contracting health service providers. Should you ask staff to search the department's files to produce the documents? Should you request the files from the contract agency? If you find the files, should they be released to the attorney? Whose rights are paramount? Whose are subsidiary?

Legal Analysis

At first, this case appears largely concerned with the confidentiality of health information for patients undergoing mental health and substance-abuse treatment and whether you should or are required to disclose such information in these circumstances. However, it also raises the important issue of John's dereliction and its attendant risks to John, his wife or other persons, and the apparently conflicting responsibility of public health agencies or professionals to intervene.

Confidentiality of health records

Patient health information is protected by a mixed bag of state and federal laws, the predominant characteristics of which are lack of uniformity and questionable effectiveness. State laws about health information confidentiality are based on a state's "police powers," which are a form of expansive sovereign authority intended in part to secure and protect public safety and are reserved to the 50 states under the U.S. Constitution.[1] Many state laws pertaining to confidentiality are actually situated within laws, the main purpose of which is to accomplish something other than protecting patient health information and which happen to include some level of protection for patient health information. For example, most state licensing laws or "practice acts" require, in addition to training in approved professional programs or continuing education, that health professionals observe or adhere to certain practice standards, including maintaining the confidentiality of their patients' health information. Professional licensees may have their licenses or privileges to practice revoked or suspended for failing to protect their patients' confidences.[2,3,a] The "willful or negligent violation of the confidentiality between physician and patient, except as required by law," is one of the grounds for disciplinary action against physicians in North Dakota (North Dakota Century Code, 1999),[4] while "willfully or negligently violating the confidentiality between advanced practice nurse, collaborating physician, and patient, except as required by law," can be the basis for disciplinary action against nursing professionals in Illinois.[5] Other health professionals also are subject to sanctions for violating patient confidences.[6,b]

Health institutions and agencies also may be legally obligated to protect the confidentiality of patient health information. These obligations are often subsumed under a state's health facility licensing authority. Under this scheme, a health facility may be required as a condition of receiving an operating license to provide its patients with certain rights, including the right to "confidentiality of all information and records pertaining to the patient's treatment. . . ."[7] A health facility's failure to provide these rights to its patients or to adequately protect patient health information from being impermissibly divulged may cost the health facility its operating license or result in some other sanction.

In addition to state laws, a number of federal laws pertain to the confidentiality of patient health information. Among the most significant of these is the Privacy Rule under the Health Insurance Portability and Accountability Act, which, with some exceptions, restricts the disclosure of identifiable health information.[8] Under the Privacy Rule, health-care providers may not use or disclose patients' protected health information except where permitted, such as when authorized by the patient, or where the use or disclosure does not require a patient's authorization, such as when the protected health information will be used to carry out treatment or where the disclosure is required by law for public health purposes. Under the Privacy Rule, public health entities may be considered health-care providers and therefore prohibited from disclosing protected health information without specifically permissible conditions that provide otherwise. One of these permissible conditions is disclosure by a health-care provider to other public health authorities for preventing or controlling disease, injury, or disability or disclosure to persons who may have been exposed to or are at risk of contracting or spreading a communicable disease.[8]

Medicare regulations are another federal source of laws pertaining to confidentiality that apply to public health agencies. Medicare regulations require that all hospitals—which would include public health agency facilities—that participate in the Medicare program have procedures "for ensuring the confidentiality of patient records."[9] In addition, because most hospitals participate in the Medicare program, most hospitals have instituted the requisite confidentiality procedures. More pertinent to this care, however, are federal regulations pertaining to substance-abuse programs and to the confidentiality of records created or maintained therein. Under Title 42 of the United States Code, "[r]ecords of the identity, diagnosis, prognosis, or treatment of any patient which are maintained in connection with the performance of any program or activity relating to substance abuse education, prevention, training, treatment, rehabilitation, or research . . . shall . . . be confidential and disclosed only for the purposes and under the circumstances expressly authorized. . . ."[10] One of these circumstances is the prior written consent of the patient about whom the records are maintained. Others include disclosure to medical personnel to the extent necessary in a medical emergency; for research or program evaluation in which the records are nonidentifiable; or by order of a court after demonstration of good cause, such as the need to avert a substantial risk for death or serious bodily injury. The authority of the federal government to mandate these confidentiality requirements is based on federal government funding or regulating authority. Health facilities or professionals who are either "directly or indirectly assisted by any department or agency of the United States" government are subject to these confidentiality regulations, as is any program that is conducted or regulated by any department or agency of the U.S. government. Where state and federal laws overlap, specific provisions apply: where disclosure permitted under federal law is nonetheless prohibited by state law, then federal regulations may not "be construed to authorize any violation of that state law.[11] Conversely, the federal law provides that "no State law may either authorize or compel any disclosure prohibited by these regulations." In this regard, the law of the jurisdiction with the strictest safeguards for patient health information confidentiality will prevail over the law with lesser safeguards.

*Mitigating risks posed by persons with mental and
substance-abuse disorders*

In most states and for many people, the only meaningful mental health or substance-abuse programs are provided or coordinated through the state or local public health authority through such providers as community mental health clinics or chemical dependency programs, crisis intervention, the inpatient and outpatient services of a local public psychiatric hospital, or the psychiatric service of a local public hospital. In particular, for persons with severe mental disorders, mental health care often occurs pursuant to law enforcement arrest or referral. For persons with substance-abuse disorders, the first encounter with substance-abuse treatment often results from a drunk driving or drug-related arrest.

The power of state or local authorities, including public health authorities, to compel mental health or substance-abuse treatment has a long history. For many years, the typical public health response to persons with mental disabilities was institutionalization, which transformed during the past few decades into civil commitment in only the most egregious cases of mental disability and the need for treatment coupled with some indication of a mentally disordered person's dangerous behavior or the risk for harm or injury posed thereby. In some jurisdictions, the lack of mental health and substance-abuse programs has resulted in arrest and jailing in lieu of treatment. Spurred by increasing public alarm over substance abuse, especially the abuse of drugs other than alcohol, some jurisdictions have tailored civil commitment laws that provide for the legally authorized confinement of substance abusers, sometimes in lieu of criminal prosecution.[12–15]

Civil commitment is essentially a statutorily structured process by which persons with qualifying conditions are legally confined within a mental health or substance-abuse treatment milieu for their own good or for the safety of others. Civil commitment laws are usually subsumed under state mental health laws and generally include provisions for referral, evaluation, treatment, release, notice, hearing, right to counsel, and the right to be present at the commitment hearing.[16–18] In fact, some state court decisions have indicated that the criteria for commitment of drug-dependent persons are guided by the same concerns for safeguarding public safety, the individual's health, and the individual's liberty interest under mental health laws.[19]

Civil commitment is intended to prevent persons with qualifying conditions from harming themselves and others and to provide them with treatment. In particular, drug-dependency civil commitment laws require sufficient evidence to establish that the person to be committed has "lost the power of self-control" with respect to the use of a controlled substance or is "incapable of self-management or management of personal affairs" by reason of the habitual and excessive use of drugs.[20,21] Most civil commitment statutes also require that the person for which commitment is sought actually poses a danger or substantial likelihood of *physical harm* to himself or herself or others; furthermore, the likelihood of this harm must be shown by clear and convincing evidence.[c] Finally, some states require that proper treatment programs be available and that benefit from such treatment to the person being committed be shown before commitment will be effected, an especially interesting requirement because mental health and substance-abuse treatment programs are in notoriously short supply.[22,23] Generally, courts will strictly construe the statutory provisions pertaining to civil commitment before permitting states to use their legal authority to take the drastic action of legally confining persons into such treatment settings.

Practice Pointers

Confidentiality of health records

Under the facts presented in Case Study 1, federal law pertaining to the confidentiality of protected health information—including mental health and substance-abuse treatment records—apply. Providing John's mental health and substance-abuse records to his wife's attorney may fall outside the boundary of permissible disclosure. No indication exists that John has consented to such a disclosure, and, without that consent, John's treatment records can be released only for one of several enumerated exceptions, none of which appears to apply here on the basis of the facts provided. The attorney is not a medical professional, so the exception for disclosing health information to further John's treatment is not applicable. In addition, the circumstances do not suggest that a medical emergency exists or that John poses an imminent risk of serious harm to himself or to others, which are common exceptions to the rule against disclosure. Furthermore, the records sought are identifiable, so this forecloses their use for research or program evaluation. Finally, no court order has authorized disclosure of John's treatment records, even if, as the attorney alleges, a potential risk exists to the attorney's client, John's wife. Even if the attorney were to invoke a state law that allowed the release of John's health records, less protective state law gives way to the more protective federal law, and the disclosure of John's records is still impermissible.

An exception may exist if John exposed his wife to a communicable disease, such as human immunodeficiency virus (HIV) infection, hepatitis C infection, or tuberculosis (TB). In that case, federal law might permit the public health department, as long as the department is so authorized under state laws, to notify John's wife of his communicable disease status for public health information or investigation. Even so, federal law permits only the disclosure of health information that is the minimum necessary for the public health department to conduct its intervention or investigation, so disclosures in this case may be limited to John's communicable disease status and not his mental health and substance-abuse treatment records.

Mitigating risks posed by mental disorders and substance-abuse dependency

The attorney's statement that more should be done to prevent further harm from John's mental health status and substance abuse raises a number of concerns. First, the existence of a potential for harm, the nature of the harm, and the legal steps that can be taken to mitigate such harm need to be determined. This is a calculus that should take place independently of the attorney's request for copies of John's treatment records, although the attorney's request may actually be part of a legal action of which the purpose is to initiate civil commitment. John's records may need to be reviewed to ensure that the agency or contractor is discharging its treatment responsibilities. If past or current treatment is inadequate and John's potential for harm is evident, then the agency may be required to take additional steps to safeguard public safety and John's own welfare. These steps might include enlisting John's wife to help guide subsequent agency intervention, but this still does not necessarily permit disclosure to the attorney of John's confidential health information. Even without the assistance of John's wife, public health officers are authorized to petition a court for a hearing to effect John's civil commitment. Depending on the jurisdiction, other petitioners may include the director of a community mental health center, a peace officer, the court, or the physician of the person for whom commitment is sought. The law's intent is to ensure that all persons who may have police powers or first-hand knowledge, including knowledge arising from the course of treatment, be permitted to ask a court to determine whether persons in John's situation should be civilly committed for evaluation or treatment. Under these circumstances, the requisite "emergency" or other need for hospitalization may exist that would permit disclosure of confidential health information, and a reviewing court may even order that John's health records be provided to the court. Both the potential for risk and the need for a court hearing on the matter of civil commitment may suffice as an exception to the limits on disclosure of John's substance-abuse records.

PERSONS WHO ARE CRIMINAL-JUSTICE–INVOLVED

Case Study 2

Jack T. was recently released from state prison. Now unemployed and living temporarily on public assistance and the services of local charities, he has been searching for a job. He stops by the local health department requesting medical services for chronic hepatitis C and HIV infections, for which he received treatment while incarcerated. Services of this nature are not available at the health department, so he is referred to the local emergency department and from there to a free medical clinic that operates just once a week. The free medical clinic does not provide Jack with the full range of services he received while he was in prison. Why was Jack's care better when he was a prisoner than when he is a free citizen? What are his rights to care in both environments?

Legal Analysis

This case illustrates an irony that is often difficult to explain: Once incarcerated, prisoners have a federal constitutional right to health care that is not accorded to nonprisoners, but that health care need not necessarily measure up to the standard of medical care for nonprisoner patients who are similarly situated. In the landmark 1976 decision of *Estelle v. Gamble*, the U.S. Supreme Court declared that governments have an "obligation to provide medical care for those whom it is punishing by incarceration . . . ," the denial of which violates a prisoner's rights under the Eighth Amendment of the U.S. Constitution.[24] The Court's reasoning, which in part appears deceptively simple, is that prisoners are essentially wards of the state; prisoners rely on prison officials for the most basic of their needs, including medical care; and if prison officials do not provide this care, the health-related needs of prisoners will not be met. Nonprisoners, on the other hand, generally do not stand in the same position as prisoners as wards or subject to government constraint; their limited or lack of access to health care is irrelevant to this concept. More fundamentally, denying medical care to prisoners may be tantamount to inflicting pain and suffering, which is essentially punishment without any legitimate penologic purpose that the Court construes is "inconsistent with contemporary standards of decency."

The *Estelle* case is unquestionably the progenitor of most improvements in prison-based health-care services in the United States, and, understandably, prisoners rely on its pivotal place in modern Eighth Amendment jurisprudence to assert other claims regarding their medical care, such as the right to psychiatric services, care ordered by a physician, exercise and recreational opportunities, housing that is free of environmental tobacco smoke (i.e., secondhand smoke), and follow-up health visits. Included among these is the government's obligation to screen or test prisoners for certain infectious diseases, the failure of which may be construed by a court as a negligent and reckless disregard of a known and obvious risk of contagion. In *DeGidio v. Pung*, for example, the Circuit Court of Appeals for the Eighth Circuit found fault with prison officials who failed to implement TB testing and control procedures despite a TB outbreak among over 200 prisoners and concluded that prison officials had violated the Eighth Amendment right of prisoners who had acquired TB while they were incarcerated.[25,d]

The public health implications of decisions such as these are profound; they may be interpreted as imposing on state and local prison officials an obligation—a violation of which could be punishable—to undertake public health measures to identify and prevent communicable diseases within jail and prison populations. In fact, prison officials who have taken an aggressive public health approach toward screening and testing prisoners for certain health conditions have been accorded substantial discretion by courts that have addressed prisoners' claims that such screening and testing violate a number of their legal rights. Courts have generally found that imposing mandatory screening and testing of prisoners for conditions such as communicable diseases furthers a government's "compelling interest in protecting inmates and [correctional] staff . . ."[26,e] and is permissible under the government's public health authority to take reasonable measures to prevent the transmission of communicable diseases.[27] In fact, in cases where inmates have sued prison officials over mandatory screening and testing, the legality of the screening and testing is not itself at issue, but rather whether the means used by prison officials impermissibly burdened prisoners' other rights, such as loss of certain prison privileges, when prisoners refused such testing.

The case of *Funtanilla v. Campbell* illustrates how courts have approached the tension between the government's public health authority and the rights of prisoners.[28,f] In *Funtanilla*, a prisoner sued a number of prison officials, claiming that they violated his federal constitutional rights by placing him in segregation for 4 months, limiting his visitation privileges, and restricting exercise privileges because he refused to have a tuberculin test or chest radiograph. The Ninth Circuit Court observed that prisoners may be provided with visitation and exercise privileges, but the court stated that "preventing disease and protecting the health of visitors and inmates are unquestionably legitimate penological goals." The court found that restrictions imposed on the prisoner's privileges while prison officials assessed his TB status were reasonable in light of these penologic goals. The court concluded that prison officials did not violate the prisoner's federal constitutional rights.

Less clear cut than cases involving a government's abject failure to provide prisoners with medical care are cases in which prisoners allege that prison officials provide *inadequate* health care. The precise parameters of the government's federal constitutional obligation to provide prisoners with medical care has rarely been clearly spelled out, often leaving government officials ambivalent about the nature, frequency, and degree of medical care for any particular condition. Paradoxically, the *Estelle* case involved a prisoner's claim that prison officials had failed to provide the prisoner with adequate medical treatment after a back injury caused by a prison farm accident, a claim the Supreme Court ultimately rejected, even while the Court cloaked prisoners' right to health care within federal constitutional protection. In relevant part, the Court observed that the decision to order diagnostic tests or other forms of treatment is "a classic example of a matter for medical judgment" and that a decision based on such judgment does not represent an Eighth Amendment violation but, at most, medical malpractice.

The limits of prisoners' federal constitutional right to health care—and the considerable discretion accorded by courts to clinical decision making—is vividly demonstrated in a more recent case. In this case, a court decided that, for a prisoner's Eighth Amendment rights, the medical care due incarcerated patients does not need to mirror the standard of medical care for nonprisoner patients who are similarly clinically situated.

In *Perkins v. Kansas Department of Corrections*, an HIV-infected prisoner claimed that prison physicians should have provided him with protease inhibitor therapy instead of treatment only with zidovudine (AZT) and lamivudine (3TC), which the prisoner considered inadequate and would lead to drug resistance.[29] Despite mounting evidence at the time that established appropriate treatment for HIV infection and acquired immunodeficiency syndrome (AIDS) (which was what the prisoner had requested), the court rejected the prisoner's claim, observing that prison officials were aware of and treating the prisoner's condition and stating that "a prisoner who merely disagrees with a diagnosis or a prescribed course of treatment does not state a constitutional violation." The court, similar to the Supreme Court in *Estelle*, explicitly maintained that these types of claims are medical malpractice issues for which federal constitutional protection is unavailing. In sum, in situations where prisoners are provided with a modicum of health care, even if that care departs from what may be provided to nonprisoners with similar clinical indications, prison officials do not fail in their federal constitutional obligations unless the prison officials are found to be deliberately indifferent to prisoners' medical needs.[g]

Practice Pointers

Given the conceptual underpinnings of the government's obligation to provide prisoners with health care, the predicament arising in Case Study 2, involving Jack's diminished access to medical services for his chronic hepatitis C and HIV infections, becomes easier to understand, although no less easier to resolve. As a prisoner, Jack's condition could not have been ignored by prison officials, including prison health professionals. That he received regular and excellent primary and specialty medical care during his incarceration is commendable, especially because most prison health care is, at best, minimally adequate given the health condition of prisoners and the resources of prison officials. Even if Jack's care while incarcerated was less than regular or not up to the prevailing standard of care for persons who are similarly clinically situated, prison officials' federal constitutional obligations still might have been discharged. Once Jack was released from prison, however, the state or local government's federal constitutional obligation under the Eighth Amendment to provide Jack or any other nonprisoner with public health intervention or with primary or specialty services for their health condition abruptly ceased.

If Jack is to continue to receive services, or receive medical attention for his chronic hepatitis C or HIV infections, then he must find an alternative right or privilege unrelated to his status as an "ex-convict," such as eligibility for state or federal insurance related to his medical circumstances or other qualifying conditions (e.g., long-term disability, age, armed services), or seek care as an indigent patient. Without eligibility or qualifications for these programs, Jack may have almost no right that would obligate or compel a government or health professional to provide him with care, with the possible exception of the right, imposed by federal law only on institutions participating in the federal Medicare program, to receive emergency medical treatment, which he cannot be denied.[30] Long-term medical treatment for his conditions is clearly not available under this law.

HOMELESS PERSONS

> [H]omelessness and health care . . . interact in three ways: (1) health problems cause homelessness; (2) homelessness causes health problems; and (3) homelessness makes health problems harder to treat.
>
> P.E. Phillips[31]

Case Study 3

Marie R. has been abused repeatedly by her husband. She and her 3-year-old son, Sean, are now homeless. They live in and out of supervised charitable settings but have settled for a time in the local women's shelter. While in the shelter, Marie tests positive for TB. She is reluctant to sign a release-of-information-and-consent form, which would allow medical information about her and Sean to be shared with local health department staff. Marie fears that the loss of confidentiality and the intervention of agencies outside the shelter may bring her in contact with staff of the local social services agency with whom she has had difficult relationships over time. Marie also fears the loss of her son. The director of the shelter is an acquaintance of the director of the health department. During a meeting at the shelter, the shelter director mentions to the health department director that a shelter resident tested positive for TB. While at the meeting, the health director notices conditions at the shelter both in the kitchen and in the living areas that appear unsanitary. What legal damage has been done by the shelter director? What legal obligation does the health director have to intervene at the shelter and with the TB-positive resident or her family? What are Marie and Sean's rights? What about cleaning up the shelter?

Legal Analysis

Homeless persons—many of whom are alcohol or drug dependent (40%); have mental illnesses (25%–30%); or are elderly, runaway children, physically disabled, or female heads of household—are defined as persons who lack a permanent residence or who live in public shelters. Homeless persons are a special population from a public health standpoint. Because of their socioeconomic status, poor lifestyle choices, lack of adequate health care, transient living conditions, or a combination of these factors, homeless persons are characterized by poor health status. They therefore face an elevated risk of contracting some infectious diseases such as TB. Tuberculosis, a highly communicable disease once thought to have been largely eliminated from the United States, has returned with a vengeance, especially in its multidrug-resistant form; TB is now the world's leading cause of death.[32,33] The resurgence of TB is attributed in part to persons at high risk of both acquiring and spreading the disease, including persons who are homeless. Compared with nonhomeless persons, homeless persons suffer disproportionately from TB and account for approximately 6% of reported cases in the United States.[34] When homeless persons are placed in such congregate settings as shelters or temporary housing, their risk for TB and other communicable diseases increases.

In almost all states, public health officials are accorded broad powers under state law to act to protect the public from highly infectious diseases such as TB or to take measures to protect the public from unhealthy or unsanitary conditions. This expansive authority was recognized long ago in the U.S. Supreme Court case of *Jacobson v. Massachusetts*, in which the Court rejected a challenge to local city health officials' efforts to curtail the spread of smallpox by requiring that all city inhabitants undergo smallpox vaccination.[27] One inhabitant refused the vaccination, claiming that a prior vaccination had caused him injury and that compulsory vaccination violated his federal constitutional rights to due process under the Fourteenth Amendment. The *Jacobson* case has been invoked many times since then to vindicate similar public health measures that were undertaken to address serious risks to public health, such as the obligation of health professionals to report communicable disease cases or the right of state and local officials to inspect public accommodations, services, or venues (e.g., water service, sewage and waste treatment, restaurants, other retail establishments) for health and sanitation reasons. Such legal intervention is considered by many to be particularly appropriate in the case of homeless persons and public shelters because of their higher incidence rates for TB and the difficulty of reaching this population for screening and treatment.

Many states have laws specific to the control of TB because of its communicable nature. Although states differ in their approach to controlling TB, some consistency exists. For example, one important intervention provided for by all states is the requirement that suspected or confirmed cases of TB be reported to state or local public health officials by health professionals (e.g., physicians, laboratory directors, and public health nurses) or other persons who have knowledge of such cases. Additionally, some states require reporting of TB patients who refuse treatment, and a few states require notification of the state health department when a patient has completed treatment for TB. Most states consider the deliberate nonreporting of TB a criminal misdemeanor and impose fines. Almost all state laws require the reporting of TB within a specific time frame, ranging from immediately to within 1 week of diagnosis. Federal guidelines, however, recommend that states require reporting of TB within 2 working days of diagnosis.[35]

State laws also permit public health officials to place TB-infected persons in isolation or quarantine under certain conditions. For example, most states provide for quarantine of anyone refusing TB treatment. Although many persons with TB may be quarantined within their own homes, many states designate appropriate residence facilities, including homeless shelters, for the care of homeless persons infected with TB. State laws also may permit public health officials to forcibly treat TB-infected persons, such as requiring them to undergo directly observed therapy (DOT), in which public health workers observe the taking of TB medications.

However, state laws that permit public health officials to intervene in TB cases do not exist in a total legal vacuum. Cases such as *Jacobson* clearly establish public health officials' legal authority to compel compliance with public health measures, but these measures can neither be taken arbitrarily nor violate other rights that persons may have. In fact, public health measures must usually be balanced against a number of rights that have been accorded to persons over time to protect them from abuses of power by state officials. Even in the case of *Jacobson*, the Court was careful to note that local health officials were acting within authority delegated to them by the state legislature and that, even then, if the health officials had acted arbitrarily by, for example, requiring vaccination without regard to a person's individual health condition or irrespective of the presence of smallpox, then their action would have been impermissible. More importantly for this case, the Court observed that if local health officials had "picked out one class of persons arbitrarily for immediate vaccination, while indefinitely postponing action toward all others," their action might violate the U.S. Constitution.

Within the context of state intervention regarding persons who may test positive for TB, competing individual rights may include a person's right to privacy as well as to refuse medical treatment, both of which are well grounded in state and federal law. For example, state law may require that public health officials provide "proof of actual danger to the community" before a homeless person with TB can be involuntarily civilly committed for isolation or TB treatment.

Ultimately, whenever legal interventions such as detention, quarantine or isolation, forcible treatment, or DOT are imposed, public health officials walk a fine line between acting in the interest of the TB-infected person and the public's health and impermissibly burdening a person's fundamental rights of liberty and privacy.

Practice Pointers

The rapid and accurate reporting of TB cases is critical to managing TB patients. Thus, health professionals and health facilities, and sometimes human services professionals (such as social workers), may be obligated to report known or suspected TB cases to local or state public health officials, the disclosure of which is usually an exception to laws regarding the confidentiality of a person's health information. The reporting obligation is generally a condition of the privilege of licensing or certification that is accorded health professionals or health facilities by state authorities. Reporting these cases not only alerts local and state public health officials to a TB incident for statistical purposes but also may be used by local or state public health officials to effect an infected person's isolation, confirmatory testing in cases of suspected TB infection, and treatment and monitoring.

Shelters such as described in this case, which are often regulated by local and state authorities, also may be required to report TB cases, particularly given the homeless state of their residents, congregate setting, residents' poor health status, and consequent risk for contagion. Even if Marie is unwilling to sign a release-of-information-and-consent form, shelter staff may be required by law to report her case to the local health department. Any court would be unlikely to find that Marie's right *not* to sign any release or consent outweighs a state's public health interest in TB prevention and the means for accomplishing its objective through such devices as mandatory reporting, testing, and isolation.

Marie's fears about losing her son might be addressed by making Marie aware that further withholding of information about her infectiousness, and thus the opportunity for local health officials to provide treatment or other intervention for Marie or testing for Sean, may be considered evidence of child neglect, which would almost certainly jeopardize her custody of Sean. In fact, Marie's willingness to disclose her TB status and seek treatment would speak far more positively of her ability to care for Sean than would her reluctance to be so forthcoming with shelter or health department staff.

The shelter director's disclosure to the health department director that a shelter resident has tested positive for TB is unlikely to be construed as a violation of law. The disclosure did not divulge the resident's identity, was directed toward an official to whom such disclosures are usually required, and—even if disclosed unwisely or in passing—may actually be legally mandated and require the identity of the infected person. Not only may the disclosure be permitted or required, but, depending on state law, such a disclosure may compel action by the local health department, such as confirmatory testing (depending on when Marie was originally tested and who performed the testing), detention, isolation, follow-up treatment, and testing of other residents (including Marie's son, Sean) or shelter staff. However, the federal due process protections discussed above may require that a public health officer who wants to impose isolation or treatment on Marie pursuant to a state law must first establish, by clear and convincing evidence, that Marie actually poses a serious risk of transmitting TB to others. Moreover, the health officer may be required to use the least restrictive means possible to achieve the clearly confined public health goal of preventing the spread of TB. For example, the involuntary commitment of Marie to a hospital may be appropriate only if no question exists about the diagnosis and, because she is homeless, there is no other place she could stay that would be less restrictive than a hospital. In this case, confining Marie until her TB is no longer active may be permissible and necessary.

The health department director's observation about the shelter's unsanitary condition, while perhaps related to the issue of TB control, simply provides the health department with an independent basis for taking action to ensure that the shelter does not pose a risk to public health, particularly to the health of the shelter's residents. Similar to health facilities, the privilege of operating a shelter or other public accommodation is generally conditioned on conformity to state laws, particularly laws pertaining to public safety such as sanitation. Any report made to local or state officials about the sanitation of public accommodations, reasonable or not, may be used to take official action, such as a site visit to ascertain any public health risks. In this case, the health department director's observation alone may justify action by the local health department, such as inspecting the shelter kitchen and living areas and requiring corrective action if necessary.

CHILDREN

Case Study 4

Sharie W., a 3-year-old child, is one of many participants in county Supplemental Feeding Program for Women, Infants, and Children (WIC) program. Her mother, Martha, received coupons for healthy foods, referrals for medical visits, and nutrition information and counseling during her pregnancy with Sharie. Sharie now eats well and nutritiously each morning before she leaves for school. Additionally, Sharie has had access to pediatric services from the time of her birth.

As part of the WIC program, Sharie is weighed and measured weekly at the WIC clinic. Unlike Sharie's prior visits to a variety of other local medical clinics—which did not yield careful and sequential monitoring of Sharie's growth and development—her mother's now regular visits to pick up coupons at the WIC clinic have made that site an ideal setting at which to monitor Sharie's health. However, abuse of Sharie is now suspected. During a recent WIC visit, severe facial bruising and welts were visible on Sharie. When asked about the bruises and welts by WIC staff, Sharie's mother left the clinic nervously. Clinic staff called the local child protective services agency (CPS) immediately, and CPS workers responded by visiting Sharie's house and removing Sharie to foster care.

Legal Analysis

Children are a special population from a public health standpoint because of their status as some of the most vulnerable members of society. Children depend on their parents or legal guardians for virtually all of their health and human services needs. If parents or legal guardians fail to discharge their parental responsibilities, their children's needs will be unmet. In these circumstances, the government may be authorized or compelled to provide for these children's needs. This section focuses on two important roles of the law in promoting the health and welfare of U.S. children: (1) improving the nutritional status of children and (2) combating child maltreatment.

Child nutritional status

The nutritional status of children is measured in a number of ways, including one described as "food security" or the percentage of children under age 18 years who live in households that experience food insecurity, with moderate or severe hunger.[36] Nearly 4% of all children and almost 12% of children classified as poor experience moderate or severe hunger. Most children have a diet that is poor or needs improvement and, not unexpectedly, children in families below poverty are less likely than children in higher-income families to have a diet that is rated as "good" under the federal government's Healthy Eating Index.

One federal program that is intended to improve children's nutritional status is the WIC program. WIC is an excellent example of law as a tool to improve the health status of children. Established by Congress in 1972 as an amendment to the Child Nutrition Act of 1966, WIC provides federal grants to states for supplemental food, nutrition counseling, and access to health-care services for certain pregnant, breastfeeding, and nonbreastfeeding postpartum women and to infants and children. WIC is administered by the Food and Nutrition Service of the U.S. Department of Agriculture and is available in each state, the District of Columbia, 32 Indian Tribal Organizations, Puerto Rico, the Virgin Islands, American Samoa, and Guam.

As with many federally funded programs, WIC gives states and local agencies substantial discretion in the administration of the program. Federal law authorizes the Secretary of Agriculture to make grants to state public health agencies, and states in turn contract with local agencies to effectuate the delivery of WIC services. States may choose to provide WIC services at county health departments, hospitals, mobile clinics, community centers, schools, public housing sites, migrant health centers and camps, and Indian Health Service facilities.[37] State WIC agencies and their local WIC service providers may design programs appropriate for their particular WIC caseloads. WIC is normally administered through statewide community networks, and the program's success relies on the coordinated efforts of local programs, sites, and retail food stores. In fact, one of the most successful models for providing children with WIC benefits is by combining public health programs for mothers and their children with an on-site WIC program component and allowing WIC-eligible persons to obtain needed services in one visit.[38,39]

Child maltreatment

Child maltreatment (including physical, sexual, and emotional abuse, as well as physical and emotional neglect) has traditionally been in the province of social services or the criminal justice system. However, child maltreatment is also a substantial public health problem, as evidenced by the detrimental health and psychosocial effects faced by abused and neglected children. The grave public health consequences of child abuse and neglect include depression, suicidal ideation, violent behavior, physical injuries, substance abuse, and chronic low self-esteem. Sexually abused children may engage in premature sexual activity, increasing their risk for unintended pregnancies or sexually transmitted diseases.[40]

Each year, approximately 1 million children are the victims of maltreatment, and approximately 1000 children die as a result of abuse or neglect. In 1998, the most recent year for which data are available, there were 12.9 victims of maltreatment per 1000 children and 1.6 child maltreatment fatalities per 100,000 children. Specified goals of *Healthy People 2010*, health objectives for the United States to achieve over the first decade of the twenty-first century, are to reduce child maltreatment to 10.3 victims per 1000 children and to reduce child maltreatment fatalities to 1.4 per 100,000 children.[41] Improved understanding and use of public health law can help meet these important public health goals.

Federal public health laws, in the form of statutes and administrative regulations, serve as effective interventions to combat child abuse and neglect. The U.S. Congress and President Clinton recognized the seriousness of child maltreatment when they enacted and signed into law the Adoption and Safe Families Act of 1997 (ASFA), establishing explicitly for the first time in federal law that a child's health and safety is of paramount importance for the nation's health. This federal legislation prioritizes safety and permanence for children who have been removed from their homes because of abuse or neglect.

ASFA was enacted ostensibly to promote the adoption of children in foster care; however, ASFA goes beyond this narrow goal to address comprehensively the public health concern of child maltreatment. Specifically, ASFA helps public officials and CPS professionals combat child abuse and neglect by specifying the circumstances under which, before placing an abused or neglected child in temporary foster care or with a permanent adoptive family, reasonable efforts need *not* be made to preserve or reunify the family (i.e., if parents pose a serious risk to a child's health or safety); giving incentives to states for providing adoptive families for children whose parents' rights have been permanently terminated because of abuse or neglect; and requiring that states move to terminate the parental rights of parents whose children have been in foster care for 15 of the last 22 months.[42]

More recently, the Child Abuse Prevention and Enforcement Act was enacted in part to reduce the incidence of child abuse and neglect. Under this federal law, funds are appropriated to enforce exiting child abuse and neglect laws (including laws protecting against child sexual abuse) and to promote programs designed to prevent child abuse and neglect.[43] Also in 2000, the U.S. Department of Health and Human Services issued child welfare regulations establishing a federal review process where state outcomes for children are measured in terms of safety, permanency, and family well-being. Under these regulations, federal funds are withheld from and financial penalties are imposed on states failing to improve outcomes for abused and neglected children.[44]

Federal legislation and guidelines for combating child maltreatment notwithstanding, state and local public health officials must often rely on their own state laws to address this public health problem. For example, legislatively mandated surveillance of child maltreatment by state or local health departments may reduce morbidity and mortality associated with child abuse and neglect. For surveillance purposes, all states have laws requiring the reporting of suspected or confirmed child maltreatment to public health agencies. Public health practitioners who are mandated reporters generally include physicians, mental health workers, social workers, and nurses. State licensing requirements for these public health professionals may include training in identifying and appropriately reporting suspected child maltreatment. All states have statutes specifying procedures for mandated reporters to follow when reporting child maltreatment. Reports are typically made by telephone to CPS; and the reports include age and address of the child, name and address of the parent or guardian, information about the alleged perpetrator, and type of suspected maltreatment (e.g., physical abuse, sexual abuse, or neglect). Almost all states have laws and regulations providing for immunity from civil and criminal liability for individuals (including public health practitioners) making good faith reports of suspected instances of child maltreatment.

Unfortunately, many cases of child maltreatment are neither reported nor investigated, even when suspected by public health professionals. To help address this underreporting and lack of investigation, nearly every state imposes civil or criminal penalties for the knowing or intentional failure of health professionals to report suspected cases of child maltreatment. Some states (i.e., Alabama, California, Delaware, Michigan, Minnesota, New Jersey, Rhode Island, South Carolina, and Wisconsin) impose sentences of imprisonment for failure to report. Other states (i.e., Maine, Massachusetts, Oregon, Vermont, and Virginia) penalize nonreporters with a fine. Additionally, many states (e.g., Arkansas, Colorado, Iowa, Montana, and New York) mandate that nonreporters be civilly liable for damages caused by the failure to report.[45]

Early identification of child maltreatment is necessary to intervene and prevent further abuse. However, the highest goal of the public health community and of laws related to child maltreatment should be intervention *before* abuse or neglect occurs. State laws may set aside funds and establish programs to serve families with multiple risk factors (including poverty, unintended or teen pregnancy, substance abuse, child with disabilities, or parents who were abused as children) that may lead to the abuse or neglect of children. For example, as part of a system of services and supports for children and their families, Oregon's Senate Bill 555 provides for increased public health nurse home visits to at-risk families and development of outcome measures for these visits.[46] This bill and similar legislation in other states are powerful tools for combating the significant public health problem of child maltreatment.

Practice Pointers

Case Study 4 demonstrates what may appear to be an awkward dilemma for many public health professionals: incurring and discharging a legal obligation to report suspected child abuse or neglect that arose from a public health encounter. In this particular case, Sharie's mother Martha left the WIC clinic when questioned by clinic staff about Sharie's visible bruises and welts. Subsequently, the clinic staff reported their suspicions to a CPS, and Sharie was removed from her mother's custody. Unquestionably, clinic staff are responsible for contacting a CPS once they suspect child abuse or neglect. However, the facts of the case do not indicate whether, pursuant to an investigation, CPS workers suspect abuse by Martha or by someone else in Sharie's family or household. Alternatively, Sharie's bruises and welts may not be the result of child abuse or neglect at all, and Sharie might have been removed from her mother's custody on an entirely unrelated basis. Regardless of the basis for revoking Martha's custody of Sharie, clinic workers may feel that by reporting the suspected child abuse or neglect, they may have deterred Martha from ever again obtaining WIC benefits for Sharie. Such a belief might be reinforced in the event Martha and Sharie are never again seen at the clinic, and WIC clinic workers are not informed about whether their suspicions had a basis in fact.

These concerns, although understandable, should not diminish the vigilance with which public health professionals tend to cases in which they suspect child abuse or neglect among their clients or patients. On the contrary, under circumstances such as these, public health professionals should exercise their continuing responsibilities pursuant to their authority under programs such as WIC. In other words, suspected or actual child abuse or neglect, the failure of Martha or Sharie to return to the WIC clinic, or the removal of Sharie from Martha's custody does not necessarily terminate Sharie's need for the nutrition made possible through the WIC program. Rather, the WIC clinic staff should take steps to ensure (if appropriate) that Martha and Sharie continue to receive WIC benefits to which they may be entitled. This will require that the WIC clinic staff develop and maintain effective communication with CPS staff. Otherwise, malnutrition may be added to Sharie's already difficult situation.

UNDOCUMENTED IMMIGRANTS

> Germs do not check for green cards.
> S.B. Drake[47]

Case Study 5

Artel is a 25-year-old man who, as an 18 year old, legally entered the United States on a student visa. Artel has overstayed his visa and is no longer a student. Artel works in a local small business that does not provide him with any health benefits; he and his wife are raising two children, both of whom are foreign born and will soon enter a public school. On the basis of the local school district's recommendation, Artel's youngest child is taken to the local health department's well-child clinic, where the child is found to need vaccinations and other physical and mental health services. During the visit, the staff determine that, on the basis of Artel's salary, Artel and his children are qualified to receive publicly funded health services. However, the staff also find out that neither Artel nor his children are legal residents of the United States, and they bring these findings to the attention of the department's director. What services may the health department provide to Artel and his family? Who will pay for these services? Should other local, state, or federal agencies be notified about Artel's and his family's undocumented status?

Legal Analysis

Undocumented immigrants[h] are a special population from a public health perspective: This population is characterized by relatively poor health and high rates of untreated communicable disease. For example, compared with U.S. citizens, undocumented immigrants have slower rates of declining infant mortality;

lower rates of vaccination; and higher rates of dental disease, delayed growth and development, poor mental health, and infectious diseases such as TB.[i] Moreover, many undocumented immigrants have severely limited access to public and primary-care health services because of their lower socioeconomic status, lack of familiarity with public health services, and other nonfinancial barriers such as language and culture. Confounding their poor health status, undocumented immigrants are at all times at risk for detention and deportation because of their unresolved legal status,

These facts and the above case illustrate an increasingly common dilemma for many public health officials: balancing the seemingly conflicting obligations to promote the public's health and prevent the spread of disease by providing preventive and other health services without regard to immigration status or ability to pay; and reporting undocumented immigrants who request or receive department services, and risk of discouraging undocumented immigrants from seeking needed services. This section describes the legal considerations pertaining to public health and undocumented immigrants.

Federal law

The federal government, acting through Congress, has plenary authority over immigration matters. As the U.S. Supreme Court has stated, "[t]he Federal Government has broad constitutional powers in determining what aliens shall be admitted to the United States, the period they may remain, regulation of their conduct before naturalization, and the terms and conditions of their naturalization."[48] In the 1976 case of *Matthews v. Diaz*, the U.S. Supreme Court ruled that the federal government may discriminate against immigrants and among different groups of immigrants regarding eligibility for federal benefits.[49] Relying on its broad authority over immigrations, the federal government enacted the Personal Responsibility and Work Opportunity Reconciliation Act ("Welfare Reform Act") of 1996, significantly limiting the rights of illegal immigrants to receive public health services.[50] This law restricts undocumented immigrants' access to almost all federally funded health services and requires states to deny state and local benefits to undocumented immigrants. Specifically, the Welfare Reform Act eliminated the eligibility of undocumented immigrants (with certain exceptions, described below) for "any State or local public benefit," defined as including "any . . . health . . . benefit for which payments or assistance are provided . . . a State or local government or by appropriated funds of a State or local government."[51] Importantly, however, states may choose to reject the general federal provision barring state assistance to undocumented immigrants as long as they pass affirmative legislation to that effect.[52]

One of the most controversial restrictions of the Act may be the denial of federally funded prenatal care for undocumented immigrants. Prenatal care for a mother undisputedly increases the likelihood of a healthy life for the child, and there is no doubt that a "child suffers after birth from lack of prenatal care in the womb."[53,j] On the basis of these considerations, plaintiffs in *Lewis* argued that denying prenatal care for an undocumented pregnant immigrant violates a born child's right to equal protection of the laws under the Fourteenth Amendment to the Constitution. The court in the case disagreed and ruled that denying federal funding for prenatal care does not violate the Constitution. First, the court stated that deterring illegal immigration is a rational basis for denying federal funding for prenatal care because Congress explicitly intended as one purpose of the Welfare Reform Act to remove the incentive for illegal immigration that might be occasioned by federal assistance. The court also stated that a fetus is not a "person" for equal protection purposes and therefore lacks the "constitutional protection to assure it enhanced prospects of good health after birth."

Despite Welfare Reform Act restrictions, a range of *both* federally funded and state-funded health services are available to undocumented immigrants. For example, undocumented immigrants may be provided with public health services such as child vaccinations; HIV- and AIDS-related care and treatment; TB screening, diagnosis, and treatment; sexually transmitted disease screening, diagnosis, and treatment; and testing and treatment of symptoms of other communicable diseases (regardless of whether those diseases are actually present).[54] Federal law also designates community programs, services, and assistance for which all immigrants, regardless of legal status, are eligible; these include (*1*) ambulance, sanitation, and other widely available services; (*2*) crisis counseling and intervention programs, including services related to child protection, violence and abuse prevention, and treatment for mental illness or substance abuse; (*3*) shelter and housing assistance for the homeless, victims of domestic violence, and abused or abandoned children; (*4*) community nutritional services, including food banks and senior nutrition programs; and (*5*) public health services that protect life and safety by preventing disease and injury.

Federal law also ensures that emergency health care and short-term, noncash disaster relief (including food, clothing, and shelter) are available to all persons without regard to their immigration status.[55] Emergency Medicaid, which pays for treatment of emergency medical conditions,[56,k] is available to undocumented immigrants who otherwise qualify for Medicaid and meet state residency requirements.[57] Undocumented immigrants can also access emergency care under the Emergency Medical Treatment and Active Labor Act (EMTALA).[58] EMTALA requires Medicare-participating hospitals with an emergency room to triage incoming patients to determine whether they have an emergency medical condition or are in active labor and, if so, to provide stabilizing treatment. These hospitals are prohibited from transferring patients before stabilization unless the physician on duty certifies that the medical benefits of transfer outweigh the increased risks to the individual. These obligations exist without regard to a patient's immigration status.

Federal law may also make available to some undocumented immigrants certain nonemergency health services. The Hill-Burton Act requires hospitals and nursing homes, in return for federal construction and renovation grant funds, to undertake an uncompensated care obligation and a community service obligation.[59,1] The uncompensated care obligation requires that facilities that receive Hill-Burton financial assistance provide a "reasonable volume of services to persons unable to pay," including undocumented immigrants. The community service obligation prohibits Hill-Burton facilities from discriminating on any ground unrelated to an individual's need for services or the availability of the needed services in the facility. Hill-Burton facilities must accept all persons, including undocumented immigrants, who are able to pay for their care either directly or indirectly through insurance coverage or through state or local government programs.

State law

States have no authority over immigration. The U.S. Supreme Court has clearly indicated that "the regulation of aliens is so intimately blended and intertwined with responsibilities of the national government" that federal laws regarding immigration will always take precedence over state laws.[60] Despite the federal government's broad power over immigration, states are not prohibited from enacting public health laws specifically directed at immigrants as an exercise of their broad power to protect the health and welfare of their citizens. A state statute directed at *immigrants*, as long as it is not a regulation of *immigration* (i.e., a regulation determining who should or should not be admitted into the country or the conditions under which an immigrant may remain), will not be preempted.[61]

Some states have made generous choices in providing public health services to undocumented immigrants. At least two states, California and Massachusetts, have laws that make available to qualified undocumented immigrants Emergency Medicaid, which ensures payment to participating providers who provide eligible recipients with bona fide emergency medical care. Several states have enacted laws that specifically provide public funding for prenatal care for undocumented immigrants. Other states mandate that pregnant immigrants are presumptively eligible[m] for publicly funded prenatal services. Nebraska law, for example, provides that, although undocumented immigrants are eligible for emergency medical care only, pregnant immigrants have "presumptive eligibility" for prenatal services. A pregnant immigrant may apply for ambulatory prenatal services, and the provider makes a presumptive determination of eligibility on the basis of income only. The provider is not required to investigate other eligibility requirements, such as immigration status. The provider must notify the applicant that to continue receiving prenatal care, she must apply for the Nebraska Medical Assistance Program (NMAP) by the last day of the month after the month of presumptive eligibility. If the woman fails to apply, prenatal care ends on the last day of the month after the month of the presumptive eligibility determination. If she applies within the required time limit, her presumptive eligibility continues through the day on which a determination of her continued eligibility is made.[62,n]

Colorado law has established a particularly innovative pilot program to publicly fund prenatal care for undocumented women. Colorado's House Bill 1076, enacted June 1, 2000, enumerates the compelling reasons for providing undocumented women with prenatal care. Specifically, the state's General Assembly recognized that (1) access to prenatal care by undocumented women in Colorado is inadequate; (2) lack of prenatal care results in a high rate of low-birth-weight infants, contributing significantly to infant mortality and childhood disabilities; (3) children with low birth weights are more likely to develop health problems during their lifetimes; (4) many conditions can be prevented through prenatal care, including mental retardation, cerebral palsy, and blindness; (5) every dollar spent on prenatal care yields approximately $2 in savings by reducing neonatal complications; and (6) prenatal care benefits the public health by providing an opportunity to identify and treat communicable diseases.[62] The enacted "prenatal care for undocumented women pilot program" mandates that the state contract with managed-care organizations to provide prenatal care for undocumented women who qualify for Emergency Medicaid.[63] Colorado was the first, and may be the only, state to implement this type of program.

On the other hand, some states acted quickly pursuant to the Welfare Reform Act's passage to establish regulations consistent with the federal law in limiting benefits for undocumented immigrants. For example, California issued emergency regulations rendering undocumented immigrants ineligible for state or local public benefits. When public health organizations filed suit against the state, arguing that promulgating emergency regulations to hastily comply with federal law was an abuse of discretion, a California Court of Appeal held that the emergency regulations should be enforced. The Court reasoned that because California's program providing state funding for undocumented immigrants' prenatal care—a subject over which federal government has plenary jurisdiction—was rendered immediately illegal by the Welfare Reform Act, prompt compliance with the federal law justified the emergency regulations.[64] The Court specifically held that the state did not abuse its discretion in issuing emergency regulations because the state lacked the time to promulgate regular regulations before the Welfare Reform Act went into effect.

Practice Pointers

An important determinant of the extent of the services that may be provided to Artel and his children under the facts presented in Case Study 5 depends on the state in which Artel and his family reside. This is due primarily to provisions of the Welfare Reform Act, which generally restricts undocumented immigrants' access to state and locally funded health services. If Artel's family lives in a state that has enacted a law that affirmatively rejects the Welfare Reform Act's restrictive provisions, then obtaining the needed vaccinations and other physical and mental health services for which Artel and his children may otherwise be eligible presents no real problem.

An entirely different conclusion is reached if Artel's family lives in a state that *has not* enacted a law that affirmatively rejects the Welfare Reform Act's restrictive provisions. Under these circumstances, Artel's family may be entitled only to needed health services specifically delineated under the Welfare Reform Act or to health services not otherwise covered by the Act. For example, one type of health service that undocumented immigrants may receive includes public health assistance for vaccinations. Thus, the health department may provide Artel's child with needed vaccinations. Whether the department may provide Artel's child with other physical and mental health services will depend on the nature of those needed services. For example, although the case study does not specify what these other needed services include, if Artel's child required hospitalization or treatment for an emergency medical condition, or treatment for a communicable disease (e.g., TB infection or positive skin test), then the health department may provide such services.

Moreover, Artel and his family may be eligible for *federally* funded benefits or programs that are not subject to the Welfare Reform Act, including benefits or services enumerated in the discussion section above. Careful screening by health department staff of the needs of persons such as Artel and his family, and matching those needs to available federal programs, may help offset some of the restrictions imposed by the Welfare Reform Act.

Nonetheless, undocumented immigrants' eligibility for public health services does not necessarily ensure access to or use of these services. Other significant barriers may contribute to underutilization of public health services by undocumented immigrants, including language and cultural differences or misunderstandings, as well as the lack of knowledge about or familiarity with public health programs. Fear of apprehension by immigration authorities may also contribute to underutilization of public health services by undocumented immigrants. The fear of apprehension may be heightened because federal law prohibits state and local governments from restricting their staff from reporting to the U.S. Department of Justice's Immigration and Naturalization Service the immigration status of persons with whom they may come into contact. To address the more general problem of underutilization of health services by undocumented immigrants, public health officials may consider educational programs for the undocumented immigrant community about their eligibility for emergency, nonemergency, and preventive health services. Undocumented immigrants also should be reassured that they cannot be deported solely for seeking and receiving publicly funded health services.

Additionally, the health department director might review his state's policies and application forms to determine whether they obstruct or facilitate undocumented immigrants' access to services. To encourage undocumented immigrants to access available and needed public health services without fear of reporting or deportation, neither application and enrollment forms nor health department staff should require social security numbers, immigration status, or unnecessary documentation if this information is not otherwise required by law or essential to providing such services.

CONCLUSION

Unquestionably, public health intervention may provide untold benefits for many persons. However, providing needed health services for some of these persons may require that public health professionals carefully consider laws outside those generally considered "public health law." In fact, public health laws may fail to either improve or sustain intervention for the most needful or vulnerable among our society, those whom we include in special populations. Outside of public health practice and the laws specifically intended to support such practice exists a body of laws that are implicated when special populations are at issue. Some of these laws, although generally applicable, may appear to significantly limit the work of public health practice, such as laws that constrain the sharing of protected health information under most circumstances; in these cases, public health professionals must act quickly and prudently to conform their practice to new and changing civil liberties and other rights that are accorded to persons in the pursuit of competing values such as privacy. At the same time, public health professionals should recognize that these competing values are generally carefully balanced and, in the case of confidentiality of health information, will permit public health professionals to vigorously pursue the health and well-being of a larger society when those interests are deemed more important.

Other laws, such as those that unduly limit the eligibility of undocumented immigrants to certain public benefits, may be so onerous that little if anything can mitigate the law's impact on the health and welfare of undocumented immigrants. However, public health professionals can take solace in the many exceptions to the restrictions on public benefits for undocumented immigrants, and most of these exceptions are crafted in response to concerns that no person—not even those who are accorded fewer civil rights than others—be denied services that are considered vital to preventing disease and promoting public health. In this regard, special populations may best be served by public health practitioners making every effort to ensure that persons in need are identified, carefully evaluated, and referred to the programs that are available.

Notes

[a] Medical Practice Act, Physician–Patient Communication, states that "communications between one licensed to practice medicine, relative to or in connection with any professional services as a physician to a patient, is confidential and privileged and may not be disclosed except as provided in this section."

[b] But cf. *Africa v. Vaughn*, Civil Action No. 96–649, 1996 U.S. Dist. LEXIS 17339, at *7–8 (E.D. Pa. Nov. 22, 1996) (commenting, in denying an inmate's First Amendment claim resulting from 10-week confinement in restrictive housing for refusing tuberculosis rest, that prison authorities may not "indefinitely segregate an asymptomatic inmate who refuses on religious grounds to take a tuberculosis skin test").

[c] The element of "dangerousness" as a criterion for commitment obtained its initial dimensions in the U.S. Supreme Court's decision in *O'Connor v. Donaldson*, 422 U.S. 563 (1975). There, the Court stated that "a State cannot constitutionally confine without more a non-dangerous individual who is capable of surviving safely in freedom by himself or with the help of . . . family or friends." *Ibid* at 576. The Court left unsaid what it meant by "non-dangerous" and even stated that it would "not decide whether, when, or by what procedures" a state may justify confinement to prevent a person's injury to the public, ensure the person's own survival or safety, or to alleviate or cure his or her illness. *Ibid* at 573–4. Judging by the wide range of what states have construed as "dangerousness," state legislatures and courts have had to devise their own definitions. See, for example, Fla. Stat. Ann. § 397.052(1)(a)(2) (requiring that a petition to involuntarily treat a drug-dependent person shall allege that the drug-dependent person "[h]as lost the power of self-control with respect to the use of such controlled substance"); see generally: Hafemeister and Amirshahi, *supra* note 5, at 49–50 (providing other examples of how the term "dangerousness" resulting from drug dependency is defined by various state statutes). See, for example, Minn. Stat. Ann. § 253B.02(2)(b) (providing that substantial likelihood of physical harm can be demonstrated by recent attempts or threats to physically harm herself or others, evidence of recent serious physical problems, or failure to obtain necessary food, clothing, shelter, or medical care); see generally Garcia & Keilitz, *supra* note 4, at 426–37 (listing drug-dependency civil commitment statutes and criteria for commitment). The "clear and convincing" standard of proof for commitment purposes was established as a constitutional minimum in the U.S. Supreme Court's decision in *Addington v. Texas*, 441 U.S. 418, 431, 433 (1979).

[d] Prison officials do not necessarily violate the Eighth Amendment for every failure to test for infectious diseases. See, for example, *Doe v. Wigginton*, 21 F.3d 733, 738–39 (6th Cir. 1994), and *Feigley v. Fulcomer*, 720 F.Supp. 475, 481 (M.D. PA. 1989) (*not screening prisoners for HIV infection in the absence of indication of risk does not violate other prisoners' Eighth Amendment rights*).

[e] See also *Harris v. Thigpen*, 941 F.2d 1495, 1501 (11th Cir. 1991) (concluding that

Alabama's law mandating the testing of all prisoners for sexually transmitted diseases, including testing for HIV, does not violate prisoners' U.S. Constitutional or statutory rights).

f See also *Davidson v. Kelly*, No. 96–2066, 1997 U.S. App. LEXIS 33796 (2nd Cir. Nov. 24, 1997) (finding no Eighth Amendment, due process, or equal protection violation where an inmate was placed in keeplock for 3 days after refusing tuberculin testing. Religious objections also have been the basis for challenging mandatory tuberculin testing. Unlike prison privileges such as visitation, the right to freely exercise one's religion is carefully regarded by the courts because the right is considered a fundamental civil liberty that is retained by individuals notwithstanding their imprisonment. For example, in *Williams v. Scott*, No. 97–1223, 1998 U.S. App. LEXIS 6556 (7th Cir. Mar. 26, 1998), an inmate sued a number of prison employees, claiming that his federal constitutional right to freely exercise his religion were violated when he was placed in "restrictive medical separation" for approximately 1 month for refusing to take a purified protein derivative (PPD) test to determine his latent TB status. The inmate argued that his Muslim religious tenants did not permit the injection of "unnatural substances" into his body and that, as an alternative, he had offered to undergo a chest radiograph. The inmate also alleged that while in medical separation he was denied regular visits, telephone calls, showers, and recreation. The inmate believed that he and others of his faith who also had refused PPD testing were placed in medical separation on the basis of their religious beliefs rather than, as argued by prison officials, on their refusal to undergo testing. The court sided with prison officials and stated that prison officials need only demonstrate that their decision to segregate was rationally related to a proffered and legitimate government interest and concluded that prison officials' objective of "protecting other prisoners from an outbreak of TB" that may be posed by prisoners who refuse tuberculin testing was just such an interest.

g Generally, for a characterization of "deliberately indifferent," evidence must show that prison officials—including medical professionals—knew of and disregarded an excessive risk to inmate health and safety on the basis of their awareness of facts on which an "inference could be drawn that a substantial risk of serious harm exists" and that such an inference was made. *Farmer v. Brennan*, 511 U.S. 825, (1994) U.S. LEXIS 4274, at *25 (June 6, 1994). A "serious medical need" is a need that has been diagnosed by a physician as mandating treatment or a need that is so obvious that even a lay person would easily recognize the necessity for a doctor's attention. *Riddle v. Mondragon*, 83 F.3d 1197, 1202 (10th Cir. 1996) (citing *Laamon v. Helgemoe*, 437 F.Supp. 269 [D.C. N.H. 1977].

h An undocumented immigrant is an immigrant who is not a U.S. citizen and who has entered the United States (or has remained) without the proper documentation and who does not have legal status for immigration purposes. Approximately 20% of the immigrant population is undocumented. See Figures 7 and 8 in The Kaiser Commission on Medicaid and the Uninsured. *Immigrants' Health Care: Coverage and Access* (August, 2000).

i For example, TB rates among immigrants have remained constant, while rates among citizens have declined considerably. Undocumented immigrants are particularly vulnerable to TB partly because of the high concentration of undocumented migrant farm workers; substandard living conditions of many undocumented immigrants; and malnourishment. See Johns KA, Varkoutas C. The tuberculosis crisis: the deadly consequence of immigration policies and welfare reform. *J Contemp Health Law Policy* 1998;15:101, 115. Many public health leaders consider immigration the primary force behind the TB resurgence in the late twentieth century. See Martin JA. 89 Proposition 187, tuberculosis and the immigration epidemic. *Stanford Law Policy Rev* 1996;7:89, 90 (noting that for the first time in more than 50 years, the number of TB incidents is increasing in the United States).

ʲ The court reasoned that if under *Roe v. Wade* (410 U.S. 113 [1973]) a fetus lacks constitutional protections to ensure it an opportunity to be born, then it must also lack constitutional protections to ensure it an opportunity for good health after birth.

ᵏ An emergency medical condition is defined as the sudden onset of a medical condition—including labor and delivery—manifesting itself by acute symptoms of sufficient severity such that the absence of immediate medical attention could reasonably be expected to result in placing the person's health in serious jeopardy; serious impairment to bodily function; or serious dysfunction of any bodily organ or part. See 42 U.S.C. § 1396(v)(3) (2001).

ˡ The uncompensated care obligation of Hill-Burton facilities lasts for 20 years after the date of the federal grant. Facilities with uncompensated care obligations are required to post notices—which must be easy to read and printed in languages other than English if a significant part of the community has limited English proficiency—explaining their obligation.

ᵐ "Presumptive eligibility," in the context of state laws providing public funds for undocumented immigrants' prenatal care, generally means that income-eligible pregnant immigrants will be presumed eligible for prenatal care until they are determined to be ineligible because of their undocumented status.

ⁿ Under this regulation, an undocumented immigrant could remain presumptively eligible for prenatal care for at least 2 months. For example, if her initial visit and application for services were on March 1, she would by law have until April 30 to apply for continued eligibility. As an undocumented immigrant, she could probably use prenatal services numerous times (i.e., weekly prenatal visits to a qualified provider's office) before her continued eligibility is determined.

References

1. Wing KR. The power of the state governments in matters affecting health care. In: *The Law and the Public's Health*, 5th ed. Chicago: Health Administration Press, 1999: pp. 19–44.
2. California Business and Professions Code § 2878 (2001) (Vocational Nursing, Disciplinary Proceedings).
3. Texas Revised Civil Statutes, article 4495b, § 5.08(a) (1999) (Medical Practice Act, Physician–Patient Communication).
4. North Dakota Century Code 43 17 31(13) (1999) (Physicians and Surgeons, Grounds for Disciplinary Action).
5. 225 Illinois Compiled Statutes Annotated 65/15-50 (1999) (Advanced Practice Nurses, Grounds for Disciplinary Action).
6. Annotated Code of Maryland § 14-5A-17(a)(12) (2001) (Respiratory Care Practitioners).
7. 10 New York Codes, Rules and Regulations § 405.7(b)(13), (c)(13) (1998) (Hospitals—Minimum Standards, Patient Rights).
8. 45 C.F.R. § 160 *et seq.* (2001).
9. 42 C.F.R. § 482.25 (b)(3) (2001).

10. 42 U.S.C. Service § 290dd-2(a) (2001).
11. 42 C.F.R. § 2.20 (Confidentiality of Alcohol and Drug Abuse Patient Records, Relationship to State laws).
12. Florida Statutes Annotated § 397.0518(1) (2001).
13. California Welfare & Institutions Code § 3106.5 (2001).
14. Florida Statutes Annotated § 397.052(a)(1) (2001).
15. Oregon Revised Statutes § 426.005(2) (2001).
16. Hafemeister TL, Amirshahi AJ. Civil commitment for drug dependency: the judicial response. *Loyola Law Rev* 1992; 26:39–104.
17. *Jackson v. Indiana*, 406 U.S. 715, 731, 738 (1972).
18. *Addington v. Texas*, 441 U.S 418, 423, 425, 432 (1979).
19. *State v. Smith*, 692 P.2d 120, 122–4 (1984) (criteria of commitment for drug addicts same as criteria for commitment as with other mental disorders).
20. Florida Statutes Annotated § 397.052(1)(a)(2) (2001).
21. Minnesota Statutes Annotated § 253B.02(2)(a) (2001).
22. Florida Statutes Annotated § 397.052(1) (2001).
23. California Welfare & Institutions Code § 3050 (2001).
24. *Estelle v. Gamble*, 429 U.S 97, 103 (1976).
25. *DeGidio v. Pung*, 920 F.2d 525, 533 (8th Cir. 1990).
26. *Jolly v. Coughlin*, 76 F.3d 468 (2d Cir. 1996), No. 95-2589, 1996 U.S. App. LEXIS 1757, at *24–25 (affirming lower court's grant of preliminary injunction to plaintiff inmate who argued for release from medical keeplock imposed for refusing screening test for latent TB).
27. *Jacobson v. Massachusetts*, 197 U.S. 11 (1905).
28. *Funtanilla v. Campbell*, No. 96-15439, 1996 U.S. App. LEXIS 22581 (9th Cir., Aug. 12, 1996).
29. *Perkins v. Kansas Department of Corrections*, 165 F.3d 803, 811 (10th Cir. 1999).
30. 42 U.S.C. § 1395dd (2001).
31. Phillips PE. Adding insult to injury: the lack of medically-appropriate housing for the homeless HIV-Ill. *Univ Miami Law Rev* 1991; 45:567–615 (citing a study by Sutherland AR. Health care for the homeless. Issues Sci Technol 1988:79).
32. Kuszler PC. Balancing the barriers: exploiting and creating incentives to promote development of new tuberculosis treatments. *Washington Law Rev* 1996; 71:919–67.
33. Rothstein MA. Legal Analysis of the Institute of Medicine Recommendations to Expand Testing for and Treatment of Latent Tuberculosis 1. 2001. Unpublished report.
34. CDC. Update from the Research and Evaluation Branch. In: *TB Notes No. 2, 2000.* Atlanta: CDC, National Center for HIV, STD, and TB Prevention, Division of Tuberculosis Elimination, 2000:1-1. Available at http://www.cdc.gov/nchstp/tb/notes/TBN_2_00/reb.htm. Accessed December 18, 2001.
35. Advisory Committee for the Elimination of Tuberculosis. Tuberculosis control laws—United States, 1993. *MMWR* 1993;42(RR-15).
36. Federal Interagency Forum on Child and Family Statistics. *America's Children: Key National Indicators of Well-Being, 2001.* Washington, DC: National Institute of Child Health and Human Development, 2001.
37. Child Nutrition Act of 1966, 42 U.S.C. § 1786 (2001).
38. U.S. Department of Agriculture. *Coordination Strategies Handbook: A Guide for*

WIC and Primary Care Professionals. Washington, DC: Health Systems Research, Inc., 2000.

39. Lipsky M, Thibodeau MA. Domestic food policy in the United States. *J Health Politics Policy L* 1990;15:319–39.

40. Hutchinson J, Langlykke K. Adolescent maltreatment: youth as victims of abuse and neglect. In: *Maternal and Child Health Technical Information Bulletin.* Arlington, VA: National Center for Education in Maternal and Child Health, 1998.

41. U.S. Department of Health and Human Services. *Healthy People 2010.* Available at http://www.health.gov/healthypeople. Accessed November 5, 2001.

42. 42 U.S.C. §§ 670–679 (2001) (Adoption and Safe Families Act of 1997).

43. 42 U.S.C. § 3751 (2001) (Child Abuse Prevention and Enforcement Act).

44. U.S. Department of Health and Human Services. News from HHS agencies. Available at http://www.hhs.gov/news/press/. Accessed November 5, 2001.

45. U.S. Department of Health and Human Services, Administration for Children and Families. National Clearinghouse on Child Abuse and Neglect Information. Available at http://www.calib.com/nccanch/. Accessed November 5, 2001.

46. Oregon Health Division. Prevention of Child Abuse and Neglect. Available at http://www.ohd.hr.state.or.us/ccfh/cfhna.htm. Accessed November 5, 2001.

47. Drake SB. America's newcomers: health care issues for new Americans, In: Tomasi LF, ed. *In Defense of the Alien.* No. 17. New York: Center for Migration Studies, 1994: pp. 35–41.

48. *Takahashi v. Fish and Game Commission,* 334 U.S. 410, 419 (1948).

49. *Matthews v. Diaz,* 426 U.S. 67 (1976).

50. Welfare Reform Act, Pubic Law No. 104–193, 110 Stat. 2105 (1996) (codified in scattered sections of 42 U.S.C.).

51. Personal Responsibility and Work Opportunity Reconciliation Act of 1996 (codified at 8 United States Code § 1621 [2001]).

52. Stubbs E. Welfare and immigration reform: refusing aid to immigrants. *Berkeley Womens Law J* 1997;12:151–7.

53. *Lewis v. Thompson,* F.3d, 2001 WL 540528 (2nd Cir., decided May 22, 2001)

54. 8 U.S.C. § 1611(b)(1)(C) (2001).

55. 8 U.S.C. § 1611(b)(1)(B) (2001).

56. 42 U.S.C. § 1396a *et seq.* (2001) (detailing federal requirements for Medicaid).

57. 42 U.S.C. § 1395dd (2001) (detailing the requirements of EMTALA).

58. 42 U.S.C. § 291c (2001).

59. *Hines v. Davidowitz,* 312 U.S. 52, 66 (1941).

60. Chang C. Immigrants under the new welfare law: a call for uniformity, a call for justice. *UCLA Law Rev* 1997;45:205–81.

61. 468 NAC Ch. 4, § 001 (2000).

62. 2000 Colorado House Bill No. 1076, as enacted June 1, 2000.

63. Colorado Revised Revised Statutes Annotated § 26-4-203 (West 2001).

64. *Doe v. Wilson,* 57 Cal. App. 4th 296, 311, 67 Cal. Rptr. 2d 187, 198 (1997).

III

THE LAW IN CONTROLLING AND PREVENTING DISEASES, INJURIES, AND DISABILITIES

12

Integrating Genomics into Public Health Policy and Practice

LAURA M. BESKOW, MARTA GWINN,
AND MARK A. ROTHSTEIN

The Human Genome Project, an ongoing collaborative effort to unravel the mysteries of human DNA, has generated high expectations among scientists and the public. Rapid advances in human genetics and accompanying technologies (such as "gene chips") are expected to bring about major new developments in medicine and public health. Dr. Francis Collins, Director of the National Human Genome Research Institute, envisions a future where disease prevention and treatment advice are tailored to patients' genotypes, with such advice taking the form of more frequent or earlier medical surveillance, lifestyle or dietary modifications, or targeted drug therapy.[1] Collins and McKusick predict that genetic assessment of individual disease risks and responses to drugs will reach mainstream health care as soon as the next decade.[2]

Along with excitement about the prospect of tailored interventions, however, there is some uncertainty. What do gene discoveries—seemingly announced daily—mean for public health? Until recently, the field of genetics had been confined largely to the realm of rare disorders caused by mutations in single genes. Even so, the public health community included genetics components in some of its work, experiencing noteworthy successes in birth defects prevention, newborn screening for inborn errors of metabolism, and development of genetic services capacity. Today, the mounting accomplishments of the Human Genome Project call for reassessment of the role of genomics in every condition of public

245

health interest. Virtually all human disease results from the interaction between genetic susceptibility factors and the environment, broadly defined to include any exogenous factor—chemical, physical, infectious, nutritional, social, or behavioral. This concept of gene–environment interaction may help explain why, for example, some health-conscious individuals with "acceptable" cholesterol levels suffer myocardial infarctions at 40 years of age while others seem immune to heart disease despite years of smoking, poor diet, and lack of exercise. Unraveling the complex interplay between genes and the environment will lead to better understanding of the biologic basis of disease and to new avenues for improving health and preventing disease. (We use the term *genomics* to denote this expanded view of genes and gene products within a whole system of genes and environmental factors.)

Fulfilling this promise represents an ambitious public health leadership agenda. An immense gap exists between the scientific products of the Human Genome Project and our ability to use genetic information to benefit health, and bridging this gap requires a wide range of public health activities. For example

- Public health research is needed to translate information about genes and DNA sequences into knowledge about genetic susceptibility to disease and the interactions between these susceptibilities and modifiable risk factors.
- The public health community must help formulate policies that promote the secure and appropriate use of genetic information.
- Public health professionals must work with other health-care sectors to ensure that valid genetic tests are available and accessible—especially in underserved populations—and to ensure that people have access to proven interventions.
- Public health has an important role in facilitating communication and education about genomics among all stakeholders, including health professionals; the general public; patients; scientists; policy makers; and pharmaceutical, biotechnology, and insurance industry personnel.
- Public health also has a crucial role in evaluating the impact and cost effectiveness of integrating genomics into health promotion and disease prevention programs.

Newborn screening, or more generally mandatory mass screening, is one paradigm for the integration of genomics into public health. Another is the mandatory *offering* of genetic tests, such as laws in California (§125050–125110) requiring that all pregnant women (before a certain point in gestation) be provided information about prenatal screening for birth defects of the fetus. However, for common, complex diseases, the gene–environment interactions involved will most often increase a person's risk for disease but not definitively predict whether he or she has, or will get, the disease. Likewise, environmental interventions based on genotype may help reduce risk but not necessarily prevent or treat the disease. Thus, rather than mandatory screening, another paradigm for the integration of genomics into public health could be similar to that suggested by Dr. Collins, which is to provide individuals *who wish to know* with information about their personal genetic susceptibilities, together with tailored risk-reduction advice. Pharmacogenomics, the science of understanding the correlation between an individual's genetic makeup and his or her response to drug treatment, represents another potentially widespread application of DNA-based testing. Thus, while programs such as newborn screening will continue to be an important and valuable public health activity, other models may exist for future prevention programs involving genomics, particularly those focused on common, complex diseases.

Integrating genomics into public health research, policy, and practice raises many of the same legal issues discussed throughout this book. Although the addition of a genetic component to these activities does not necessarily change the fundamental legal considerations, society invests enormous power in the concept of genetics. Misplaced ideas of genetic determinism (a person's future is defined and fixed by his or her genetic makeup) and genetic reductionism (all traits, health problems, and behaviors are attributable to genetics) have significant negative implications for public health and prevention messages.[3] In addition, genetics and its applications in the name of "public health" bear the historical onus of eugenics, a movement that included racial hygiene laws in Nazi Germany as well as forced sterilization, antimiscegenation laws, and restrictive immigration policies in the United States and around the world.[4] Early experiences with adult screening for sickle cell disease also portend issues that must be faced in the application of genetic knowledge.[5] These programs were sometimes offered without providing proper education, consent, and follow up, and, as a result, carriers who were identified (and who had no risk of developing the disease) suffered stigmatization and discrimination.[6]

Previous commentators have addressed ethical, legal, and social issues associated with genetic testing,[7,8] and with genetic research.[9,10] This chapter focuses on selected legal issues that arise with the integration of genomics into public health policy and practice.

LEGAL AUTHORITIES

The promise of genetic information is tempered by several concerns about its misuse, and these concerns have been the subject of a variety of legislative activities. The National Conference of State Legislatures provides a regularly updated compilation of state genetic laws related to a number of issues, such as adoption, genetic engineering and cloning, criminal law and forensics, employment, insurance, research and medical testing, paternity, and privacy.[11] Here we highlight as examples two categories of such legislative activities: those aimed at genetic discrimination in employment and those involving health insurance at state and federal levels. Concerns about discrimination in insurance and employment may be of particular public health importance because fear of discrimination may prevent individuals from seeking genetic counseling or testing that could benefit their health or from participating in valuable genetic research.[12]

State Level

Employment

In 2000, the American Management Association surveyed 2133 human resources managers about workplace medical testing of employees. When presented with a specific definition of genetic testing, only seven (0.3%) respondents answered that their firms performed such testing.[13] Substantially greater proportions reported testing for susceptibility to workplace hazards and taking family medical histories (15.8% and 18.1%, respectively).

Over half the states have enacted laws prohibiting genetic discrimination in employment.[11] All of these ban discrimination based on genetic test results, and all prohibit genetic discrimination in hiring, firing, or terms of employment. Some also cover information about genetic testing, family history, or inherited characteristics. For example, North Carolina (§95-28.1A) prohibits employment discrimination "on account of the person's having requested genetic testing or counseling services, or on the basis of genetic information obtained concerning the person or a member of the person's family." The statute defines "genetic information" as "information about genes, gene products, or inherited characteristics that may derive from an individual or a family member." Many of these laws also prohibit employers from requesting or requiring genetic information, performing genetic tests, or obtaining genetic information. In New York (§296.19[a]), for example, it is unlawful for employers to (1) directly or indirectly solicit, require, or administer a genetic test to a person as a condition or employment; or (2) buy or otherwise acquire the results or interpretation of an individual's genetic test results or to make an agreement with an individual to take a genetic test or provide genetic test results.

Health insurance

Twenty-nine states prohibit health insurers from seeking, requiring, or using genetic information to determine eligibility for insurance, and 38 states forbid rating, canceling, or denying insurance on the basis of genetic information.[11] Maryland law (Ins §27-909) does both, forbidding insurers, nonprofit health service plans, and health maintenance organizations from (1) using a genetic test, the results of a genetic test, genetic information, or a request for genetic services, to reject, deny, limit, cancel, refuse to renew, increase the rates of, affect the terms or conditions of, or otherwise affect a health insurance policy or contract; and (2) requesting or requiring a genetic test, the results of a genetic test, or genetic information for determining whether to issue or renew health benefits coverage. State health insurance laws are preempted by the Employee Retirement Income Security Act (ERISA) (29 U.S.C. Chap. 18) to the extent that they attempt to regulate employer-based group health plans. Thus, the main value of the state laws is to prohibit discrimination in individual health insurance.

Hall and Rich[14] recently evaluated whether these types of laws reduce the extent of genetic discrimination by health insurers. From data collected at multiple sites, they found almost no well-documented cases of health insurers either asking for or using presymptomatic genetic test results in their underwriting decisions either before or after these laws had been enacted or in states with or without these laws. They concluded, however, that such laws have made it less likely that insurers will use genetic information in the future and that, although insurers and agents are only vaguely aware of the laws, the laws have shaped industry norms and attitudes about the legitimacy of using this information. The authors also noted that the instances of adverse health insurance consequences they did uncover concerned payment for genetic services (e.g., genetic counseling, testing, prevention services) rather than the availability and pricing of health insurance. Payment for genetics-related services is an important barrier to access that genetic discrimination laws do not address.

Federal Level

Although a number of bills have been introduced over the last decade, no federal legislation has yet been passed directly related to genetic discrimination in individual insurance coverage or in employment. The 107th Congress (2001–2002) introduced several such bills (e.g., H.R.602, S.318) that would prohibit health plans and insurers from discriminating on the basis of protected genetic information and also make discrimination because of protected genetic information unlawful. These bills define "protected genetic information" as (1) information about an individual's genetic tests, (2) information about genetic tests of family members of the individual, or (3) information about the occurrence of a disease or disorder in family members.

Aside from specific legislation, however, other federal antidiscrimination laws apply to genetics. These include

- An executive order signed by President Clinton in February 2000 banning discrimination in federal employment on the basis of genetic information.[15]
- The Americans with Disabilities Act of 1990 (ADA) (Pub. L. 101–336), which covers individuals who have a physical or mental impairment that substantially limits a major life activity, have a record of such an impairment, or are regarded as having such an impairment. The Equal Employment Opportunity

Commission (EEOC) has issued an interpretation of the ADA stating that entities that discriminate against individuals on the basis of genetic information are regarding those individuals as having impairments.[16] This interpretation is not binding on the courts, however, and subsequent case law casts doubt on whether it would be upheld. In *Sutton v. United Airlines, Inc.,*[17] the Supreme Court held that in determining the severity of an impairment under the ADA, the condition must be considered in its mitigated state, such as with eyeglasses or medications. Significantly, the Court reasoned that Congress intended the ADA's coverage to be limited to the 43 million Americans Congress estimated as having severe disabilities. According to the Court, if individuals with "mitigated" impairments were included, the coverage would greatly exceed that figure. If similar reasoning were applied to asymptomatic individuals at genetically increased risk of disease, then the conclusion would be that they also are not covered under the ADA. In 2001, the EEOC settled its first court action challenging the use of workplace genetic testing when a U.S. railway company agreed to stop requiring genetic testing of employees who file claims for carpal tunnel syndrome.[18]

• The Health Insurance Portability and Accountability Act of 1996 (HIPAA) (Pub. L. 104-191) prohibits employer-based group health plans from using any health status-related factor, including genetic information, as a basis for denying or limiting eligibility for coverage or for charging an individual more for coverage (see Chapter 8). HIPAA also limits exclusions for pre-existing conditions and states explicitly that genetic information in the absence of a current diagnosis shall not be considered a pre-existing condition.

LEGAL ISSUES AND CONTROVERSIES

A key question in crafting legislative approaches that promote the appropriate use of genomics is whether genetic information should be dealt with separately or as part of measures intended to address health information more broadly. This controversy has important implications for the integration of genomics into public health surveillance activities.

Genetic Exceptionalism

The challenge of defining the term *genetic* is one of the conceptual difficulties arising from genetic exceptionalism—the practice of treating genetic information as different from other kinds of health information and affording it special privacy and security. Theoretically, anything from the results of a DNA test to routine observations about sex, eye color, and blood type could be classified as genetic information. Narrow legislative definitions (e.g., "the results of DNA analysis") may not achieve desired policy goals, such as protecting individuals from genetic discrimination because they do not apply, for example, to family health history. On the other hand, broad definitions (e.g., "information about genes, gene products, or inherited traits") may impede important medical and public health activities. Gostin and Hodge[19] present an analysis of the extent to which genetic information is the same as, or different from, other health information and conclude that it is not so different as to legally and ethically justify special status.

Michigan created the Michigan Commission on Genetic Privacy and Progress in 1997 to advise the governor and legislature on specific issues in genetics. In its final report,[20] the Commission recommended that any legislation should consider genetics in the context of medical issues as a whole, and thus privacy protections should encompass all confidential medical information. It also recommended limiting legislation to areas in which professional standards and codes of ethics are insufficient to protect the public good and individual rights and avoiding legislation that inappropriately prohibits or hinders beneficial genetic testing and research.

In response to this report, Michigan passed a number of laws that addressed such issues as informed consent before performance of a genetic test (§333.17020), as well as genetic discrimination in employment (§37.1201) and insurance (§500.3407b). In these laws, *genetic test* is defined as "the analysis of human DNA, RNA, chromosomes, and those proteins and metabolites used to detect heritable or somatic disease-related genotypes or karyotypes for clinical purposes," and *genetic information* is defined as "information about a gene, gene product, or inherited characteristic derived from a genetic test." These definitions are similar to those suggested by other expert groups.[8,21] Michigan does not, however, have laws that afford special privacy protections to genetic information, beyond laws already covering professional–patient interactions, research confidentiality, and general medical privacy. It also does not provide for property rights in genetic samples or information, although patients have rights to access medical information.

Public Health Surveillance

One of the primary functions of public health is public health surveillance. By collecting and analyzing information about the occurrence of disease, epidemiologists can determine the likely cause of adverse health events and point the way for prevention and early intervention. As more becomes known about the relation between genetic and environmental factors in the etiology of complex disorders, obtaining genetic information from exposed and affected populations may be an important part of comprehensive public health surveillance. Regardless of whether the addition of genetic information to surveillance activities is considered qualitatively or merely quantitatively different, the issue is whether it is lawful for governmental agents to require the collection of this new information.

Legal challenges to government collection of health information usually involve constitutional claims such as illegal search and seizure, equal protection, and due process (see Chapter 7). Under all of these constitutional theories, the courts balance the public's interest in obtaining the health information against the individual's interest in preventing disclosure. An important consideration is the possible harm to the individual that could result from disclosure of private information. "Though the actual risk of social harm directly caused by surveillance is low, perceived risks (and higher actual threats arising in other settings) can create a context in which public health data collection is politically problematic or resisted by subjects."[22] Reducing public anxiety about disclosure of health information is an inexact enterprise, but the following measures undoubtedly would help:

1. Enacting strong health privacy legislation that limits the uses of the information to public health purposes, secures the records from improper access by unauthorized parties, provides that the information must be kept and used in the least identifiable form consistent with public health purposes, and provides severe penalties for violations
2. Educating the public about the existence and provision of such health privacy legislation
3. Enacting laws that prohibit unreasonable health-based discrimination by private and public sector entities.

PRACTICE CONSIDERATIONS

The public health community has an important role to play in translating genetic discoveries into opportunities to improve health and prevent disease in ways that maximize the benefits of using genetic information, minimize the risks, and conserve health-care resources. Law and policy related to public health programs and strategies, human resources, scientific and technical considerations, and consumer and financial interests will be important tools in carrying out this role. Newborn screening, professional licensure, and oversight of genetic tests are examples of areas in which the application of law and genomics already intersect.

Newborn Screening

Newborn screening for genetic disorders began in the 1960s, made possible by new technology for collecting blood samples and a simple, inexpensive laboratory test to screen for phenylketonuria (PKU). Because PKU screening was slow to become part of routine medical care, children's advocates pressed for state legislation that eventually led to newborn screening in all 50 states and the District of Columbia.[23] Statewide screening programs were launched without a full assessment either of the validity of the screening test or of the utility of the dietary intervention to prevent mental retardation in children with PKU. Nevertheless, newborn screening for PKU is now generally acknowledged as a public health success.

Nearly all of the 4 million infants born in the United States each year are screened for PKU and from 2 to 10 other disorders. State health departments are responsible for carrying out newborn screening as mandated by state laws or regulations. In the absence of federal guidelines, the numbers and types of screening tests performed have varied from state to state and over time as tests have been added and subtracted from state laboratory screening panels.[24] This lack of uniformity and the advent of new screening technology[25,26] led the federal Health Resources and Services Administration to ask the American Academy of Pediatrics to form a Newborn Screening Task Force. In August 2000, the Task Force published recommendations that called on federal and state public officials, health-care providers, and advocacy groups to work together to develop up-to-date guidelines for newborn screening programs while addressing key ethical, legal, and social issues.[27,28] These issues include informed consent, the confidentiality of screening results, the use of residual blood samples for research, and the need for heightened public and professional awareness of the capacity and limitations of newborn screening programs.

State policies on parental consent for newborn screening vary widely. Maryland has a voluntary newborn screening program, Wyoming requests informed consent, and Massachusetts has developed an informed consent process for a pilot study of newborn screening for cystic fibrosis.[27] In all other states, newborn screening is mandatory, although most states permit parental refusal. The Task Force report recommended that "additional approaches to informing and educating parents be studied further."[27]

Many state programs added newborn screening for sickle cell anemia in the 1980s, drawing renewed attention to the issue of confidentiality of screening test results.[29] More recently, the growth of electronic databases for newborn screening and other public health records has added another dimension to this issue.[30] Attempts to better coordinate and evaluate infant and child health programs have led to increased integration of information systems that were formerly largely independent. Data linkage and sharing require new methods for safeguarding confidentiality.[27]

Residual samples from newborn screening programs have become recognized as a rich resource for research studies. These samples represent a truly population-based "biobank," which can be used to develop new knowledge by identifying affected persons from medical records and retrieving their stored samples for testing.[31] Even without personally identifying information, these samples are useful for population-based genotype frequency studies. However, no general consensus exists on the use of residual newborn screening samples for research. A policy statement published in 1996 outlined some of the issues and presented guidelines,[32] but debate on this topic continues.

Professional Licensure

Ensuring a competent public and personal health-care workforce is a vital service of public health. Because most health professionals were trained before the advances in genomics brought about by the Human Genome Project, few have the education or experience necessary to participate effectively in this rapidly emerging field. For example, Giardiello and colleagues[33] studied the clinical use of commercial *APC* gene testing for familial adenomatous polyposis (FAP). They found that only 18.6% of patients received genetic counseling before the test, and only 16.9% provided written informed consent. Physicians misinterpreted the test results in 31.6% of cases, giving patients false assurance that they did not have FAP when in fact their results were inconclusive.

A number of efforts are ongoing to promote genetic education among clinical[33] and public health[34] professionals. A template of key data elements that should be made available to health professionals about a genetic test, for example, in the form of a fact sheet, has also been proposed.[35] However, as the number of DNA-based tests proliferate, one area that may receive increasing attention is licensure of genetic counseling professionals—professionals who will aid people in making decisions about genetic testing, as well as help them interpret and respond to the results. The American Board of Genetic Counselors certifies genetic counselors, but medical billing processes typically prohibit reimbursement for unlicenced professionals. Thus, payors are billed for genetic counseling visits according to physician service codes, which are often poor indicators of the service delivered as well as more expensive than if billed directly.[36]

The rationale for licensure of genetic counselors is severalfold. First, it may help protect public health and safety by defining the scope of practice, setting minimum standards for qualifications and conduct, and providing mechanisms for continuing education, performance monitoring, and disciplinary action. By restricting use of the title "genetic counselor," licensure can also protect the public by helping it identify qualified professionals. Second, licensure may increase the supply of trained genetic counselors. Although the rapid commercialization of genetic tests may drive up the *need* for genetic counselors, actual *demand* may not equal this perceived need because of reimbursement constraints. Allowing direct reimbursement for genetic counseling services could help reinforce the legitimacy of the profession and attract high-quality candidates to the field. Finally, assuming that supply does in fact increase so that availability is not a barrier, licensure may facilitate access to genetic counseling services through insurance coverage and possibly through reduced costs because physician service codes are avoided.

California became the first state to enact a licensure bill (SB 1364) in September 2000, followed by Utah (SB 59) in March 2001; New York has licensure bills pending (AB2360, SB2471). One important issue for such legislation is: Who is eligible for licensure? In many cases, genetic counseling requires the ability to elicit and interpret family history; provide information about the risks and benefits of genetic testing; interpret and explain results and options; and provide counseling, emotional support, and referral with regard to complex psychosocial issues. The California law calls for licensure of master's level genetic counselors and doctoral level clinical geneticists and restricts use of the title "genetic counselor" to those who have applied for and obtained a license. However, it allows for genetic counseling to be provided by a "physician, a certified advance practice nurse with a genetics specialty, or other appropriately trained licensed health care professional." This highlights the importance of ensuring that all health professionals have an appropriate level of genomics competence.

Licensure may be one important step in meeting the need for qualified genetic counseling professionals. At the same time, genetic counseling is traditionally founded on a "low throughput" model; it is generally a time-intensive, one-on-one process, often oriented toward the analysis of family pedigrees for highly penetrant genetic mutations. Advances in genomics will bring about high throughput genetic testing for multiple, lower penetrance gene variants associated with increased risk for common diseases. A significant need, which public health professionals can help fill, will exist for innovative products using a variety to media to help raise general genomic literacy, as well as educational tools that can be used in primary care and other settings.

Oversight of Genetic Tests

The level of oversight of genetic tests has significant medical, social, ethical, legal, economic, and public policy implications, and the system of oversight can greatly affect individuals who undergo testing, who provide tests, and who develop tests.[21] Genetic and nongenetic tests are accorded the same level of oversight, which occurs primarily through the Clinical Laboratory Improvement Amendments (CLIA) (42 C.F.R. 493), the Federal Food, Drug, and Cosmetics Act (21 U.S.C. 301), and, during investigational stages, Federal Policy for the Protection of Human Subjects (45 C.F.R. 46, 21 C.F.R. 50 and 56). Most new genetic tests are developed and provided as clinical laboratory services, which are referred to as in-house tests or "home brews." The Food and Drug Administration (FDA) has indicated that it has legal authority to regulate such tests as medical devices but has elected not to do so as a matter of enforcement discretion, in part because the number of such tests is estimated to exceed the agency's review capacity.[37,38] However, the Secretary's Advisory Committee on Genetic Testing (SACGT), chartered in 1998 to advise the U.S. Department of Health and Human Services, has recommended that all new genetic tests be reviewed by the FDA before they are used for clinical or public health purposes[21] and is developing additional recommendations to assist the FDA with this review.

SACGT also recommended that CLIA regulations be augmented to provide more specific provisions for ensuring the quality of laboratories conducting genetic tests. CLIA has requirements for certifying laboratories in such areas as cytology and microbiology, but a specialty category of genetics does not currently exist. A revision of CLIA has been proposed that would recognize a genetic testing specialty area and address issues related to accuracy and reliability of test results, informed consent, confidentiality, counseling, and clinical appropriateness.[39]

Although these regulations and standards are being developed at a national level, state and local public health programs must be prepared to undertake additional activities to recommend when and how genetic information could be applied to improve health and prevent disease in their own communities. This involves assessing the state's own medical, epidemiologic, and economic data about diseases for which genetic tests are available; the readiness and training of health professionals; the adequacy of state laws to protect the public and ensure access; laboratory proficiency; and infrastructure capacity.

EMERGING ISSUES

Given the rapidly evolving nature of genetic discovery, almost every issue could be classified as "emerging." These include the commercialization and patenting of genetic materials, reproductive rights and decision making, human cloning, and genetic modification of food and microorganisms.

One emerging issue that could significantly affect environmental health, drug safety, and risk assessment is toxicogenomics. Toxicogenomics is the study of how genomes respond to environmental stressors. Scientists in this field are using powerful new tools, such as microarray and proteomics technologies, to assess changes in gene expression on a genomewide basis, providing a global perspective about how an organism responds to a specific stress, drug, or toxicant.[40] According to the National Center for Toxicogenomics,[40] toxicogenomics could help resolve three major scientific problems:

1. *Understanding biologic responses to environmental stressors and identifying agents that are a significant risk to human health.* Toxicologists rely largely on extrapolation from animal studies when predicting human re-

sponses to potential toxins. Toxicogenomics may help scientists gain insights into pathways of toxicity and their mechanisms, leading to better models for extrapolation, fewer animal studies, and faster conclusions.

2. *Improving exposure assessment.* Use of mRNA signatures may make possible identification of the agent (class) and dose to which a person has been exposed. Protein markers could also be used to detect presymptomatic, environmentally induced disease. Thus, surveillance programs could be implemented in humans and animals in areas where exposure and/or contamination are suspected.

3. *Identifying susceptibility factors that influence an individual's response to environmental agents.* This information could be used to predict interindividual variation in response to drugs or environmental toxicants.

These potential outcomes raise several legal issues. First, discussions about genetics and employment often focus on the possibility of employers excluding individuals from employment on the basis of predictive genetic information, for example, information about future cancer risk, where the concern is excess health-care costs. Toxicogenomics presents the possibility that individual risk could be identified before toxic exposure and used to protect worker health.[41] Actions that might be taken in response to such information include increased medical monitoring to measure the early effects of exposure, more personal protection equipment or environmental controls to reduce exposure levels, and administrative controls such as limiting exposure times. Thus, the primary discrimination issue arising in these examples is whether the employer could require testing over employee objections. State laws vary on whether employers can lawfully require or even request that an individual take a job-related genetic test.

Another approach used in the beryllium industry[42] is for the employer to pay for the tests, which employees can take on a completely voluntary basis. The results are returned only to the employee, who alone decides whether to accept any genetically heightened risk.

A second application of toxicogenomics is in setting environmental health regulations. Standards could differ from one location to the next on the basis of the genotypes of the population in the area, which may be correlated with race or ethnicity. For example, suppose a smelter is located adjacent to an Indian reservation. Also suppose evidence exists that individuals with a certain genetic marker are at increased risk from environmental pollutants and that marker happens to be present at a very high rate in the members of the tribe. Such a scenario raises a number of questions: To what extent should genetic variation affect environmental standards? Should a new, more restrictive environmental standard be adopted for this particular area? Or should the same restrictive standard apply everywhere? Should individuals be urged to undergo susceptibility testing before locating in a certain area?

A significant challenge for toxicogenomics will be to reconcile the nondirective stance traditionally associated with genetics with the directiveness sometimes found in public health practice. Because of eugenics and other abuses in the first part of the twentieth century, geneticists today offer patient-centered services that attempt to respect individual autonomy. In contrast, public health programs often focus on population rather than individual health, and some use governmental power to compel actions to protect health. Therefore, political and public support for integrating genomics into public health policies and programs will depend on accommodating the nondirectiveness that an ethical approach to genomics requires.

CONCLUSION

Advances in human genetics are expected to revolutionize medicine and public health, leading to new understandings of underlying disease processes—including gene–environment interactions associated with common chronic diseases—and to new avenues for prevention and treatment. Realizing this potential requires the integration of genomics into a wide range of public health research, policy, and practice activities. This integration does not give rise to fundamentally new or different legal challenges than those public health professionals generally encounter; rather, genetic information adds a variable to the already complex interplay between medicine, public health, and health law.

Here we reviewed evolving legal authorities aimed at reducing the misuse of genetic information, including examples of state and federal legislative activities related to insurance and employment discrimination. These activities highlight the need to enact strong measures to protect better the privacy of all health information, while not impeding the core public health function of collecting and deploying information critical to the health of communities. Genetic information is already an integral part of public health practice in the area of newborn screening and, as we move beyond the realm of rare, single-gene disorders, the system of oversight for genetic tests and the need for widespread professional and public education about genomics present challenges for public health practitioners. Issues continue to emerge along with rapid advances in genetics and genetic technology, and these must be addressed as we work to understand the appropriate use of genetic information in medicine, public health, and society.

ACKNOWLEDGMENTS

This project was supported under a cooperative agreement from the Centers for Disease Control and Prevention through the Association of Teachers of Preventive Medicine.

References

1. Collins FS. Shattuck lecture—medical and societal consequences of the Human Genome Project. *N Engl J Med* 1999;341:28–37.
2. Collins FS, McKusick VA. Implications of the Human Genome Project for medical science. *JAMA* 2001;285:540–4.
3. Rothenberg KH. Breast cancer, the genetic "quick fix," and the Jewish community. *Health Matrix J Law-Med* 1997;7:97–124.
4. National Reference Center for Bioethics Literature. *Eugenics—Scope Note 28.* Available at http://www.georgetown.edu/research/nrcbl/scopenotes/sn28.htm. Accessed June 29, 2001.
5. Phoenix DD, Lybrook SM, Trottier RW, Hodgin FC, Crandall LA. Sickle cell screening policies as portent: how will the Human Genome Project affect public sector genetic services? *J Natl Med Assoc* 1995;87:807–12.
6. Billings PR. Human genetic complexity. *GeneLetter.* May 2001. Available at http://www.geneletter.com/05-01-01/prn_editorial.html. Accessed July 27, 2001.
7. Andrews LB, Fullarton JE, Holtzman NA, Motulsky AG, eds. *Assessing Genetic Risks: Implications for Health and Social Policy.* Washington, DC: National Academy Press, 1994.
8. Holtzman NA, Watson MS, eds. *Promoting Safe and Effective Genetic Testing in the United States: Final Report of the Task Force on Genetic Testing.* Baltimore: Johns Hopkins University Press, 1998.
9. American Society of Human Genetics. Statement on informed consent for genetic research. *Am J Hum Genet* 1996;59:471–4.
10. National Bioethics Advisory Commission. *Research Involving Human Biological Materials: Ethical Issues and Policy Guidance,* vol. I and II. Rockville, MD: National Bioethics Advisory Commission, 1999.
11. National Conference of State Legislatures. Genetic Technologies Project. *NCSL Genetics Tables.* Available at http://www.ncsl.org/programs/health/genetics/charts.htm *(click on "Public User").* Accessed June 29, 2001.
12. Lapham EV, Kozma C, Weiss JO. Genetic discrimination: perspectives of consumers. *Science* 1996;274:621–4.
13. American Management Association. *Workplace Testing: Medical Testing. A 2000 AMA Survey.* Available at http://www.amanet.org/research/summ.htm. Accessed May 5, 2001.
14. Hall MA, Rich SS. Laws restricting health insurers' use of genetic information: impact on genetic discrimination. *Am J Hum Genet* 2000;66:293–307.
15. National Archives and Records Administration. Executive Orders Disposition Tables: William J. Clinton—2000. Executive Order No. 13145 To Prohibit Discrimination in Federal Employment Based on Genetic Information. Available at http://www.nara.gov/fedreg/eo2000.html. Accessed May 4, 2001.
16. Equal Opportunity Employment Commission. 2 EEOC Compliance Manual, §§ 902-45 (March 14, 1995), reprinted in *Daily Lab Rep* 1995 (Mar. 16), at E-1, E-23.
17. *Sutton v. United Airlines, Inc.,* 527 U.S. 471 (1999).
18. Gottlieb S. US employer agrees to stop genetic testing. *BMJ* 2001;322:449.
19. Gostin LO, Hodge JG. Genetic privacy and the law: an end to genetics exceptionalism. *Jurimetrics* 1999;40:21–58.
20. Michigan Commission on Genetic Privacy and Progress. *Final Report and Recom-*

mendations, February 1999. Available at http://www.mdmh.state.mi.us/mcgpp/ mcgpp.htm. Accessed May 22, 2001.

21. Secretary's Advisory Committee on Genetic Testing. *Enhancing the Oversight of Genetic Tests: Recommendations of the SACGT.* Available at http:// www4.od.nih.gov/oba/sacgt/gtdocuments.html. Accessed May 17, 2001.

22. Burris S, Gostin LO, Tress D. Public health surveillance of genetic information: ethical and legal responses to social risk. In: Khoury MJ, Burke W, Thomson EJ, eds. *Genetics and Public Health in the 21st Century.* New York: Oxford University Press, 2000: pp. 527–46, 535.

23. Paul DB. The history of newborn phenylketonuria screening in the U.S. (Appendix 5). In: Holtzman NA, Watson MS, eds. *Promoting Safe and Effective Genetic Testing in the United States: Final Report of the Task Force on Genetic Testing.* Available at http://www.nhgri.nih.gov/ELS/TFGT_final/#QUALITY. Accessed April 1, 2002.

24. National Conference of State Legislatures. *Newborn Genetic, Metabolic, and Other Disease Screening.* Available at http://www.ncsl.org/programs/health/screen.htm (click on "Public User"). Accessed July 24, 2001.

25. CDC. Using tandem mass spectrometry for metabolic disease screening among newborns: a report of a work group. *MMWR* 2001; 50(RR-3):1–34.

26. McCabe ERB, McCabe LL. State-of-the-art for DNA technology in newborn screening. *Acta Paediatr* 1999; (Suppl 432):58–60.

27. American Academy of Pediatrics. Serving the family from birth to the medical home. Newborn screening: a blueprint for the future—a call for a national agenda on state newborn screening programs. *Pediatrics* 2000;106(2 Pt 2):389–422.

28. Mitka M. Medical news and perspectives: neonatal screening varies by state of birth. *JAMA* 2000;284:2044–6.

29. Andrews LB. Overview of legal issues. *Pediatrics* 1989;83(5 Pt 2):886–90.

30. Goodman KW. Bioethics and health informatics: an introduction. In: Goodman KW, ed. *Ethics, Computing and Medicine.* Cambridge: Cambridge University Press, 1998: pp. 1–31.

31. Norgaard-Pedersen B, Simonsen H. Biological specimen banks in neonatal screening. *Acta Paediatr* 1999; (Suppl 432):106–9.

32. Therrell BL, Hannon WH, Pass KA, et al. Guidelines for the retention, storage, and use of residual dried blood spot samples after newborn screening analysis: statement of the Council of Regional Networks for Genetic Services. *Biochem Mol Med* 1996; 57:116–24.

33. Giardiello FM, Brensinger JD, Petersen GM, et al. The use and interpretation of commercial APC gene testing for familial adenomatous polyposis. *N Engl J Med* 1997;336:823–7.

34. National Coalition for Health Professional Education in Genetics. *Core Competencies in Genetics Essential for All Health-Care Professionals.* Available at http:// www.nchpeg.org/news-box/corecompetencies000.html. Accessed May 5, 2001.

35. CDC. *(b). Genomics competencies for the public health workforce.* Available at http: //www.cdc.gov/genetics/training/competencies/default.html. Accessed June 29, 2001.

36. 65 *Federal Register* 77631.

37. Vance A. Licensing genetic counselors holds promise for higher quality, more cost-effective service for patients. *GeneLett* Nov. 2000. Available at http:// www.geneletter.com/11-01-00/features/prn_licensing.html. Accessed May 17, 2001.

38. Statement by Mary K. Pendergast, Deputy Commissioner and Senior Advisor to the Commissioner, Food and Drug Administration, Department of Health and Human

Services, before the Subcommittee on Technology, Committee on Science, U.S. House of Representatives. September 17, 1996. Available at http://www.house.gov/science/mary_pendergast.htm. Accessed July 28, 2001.

39. Gutman S. The role of Food and Drug Administration regulation of in vitro diagnostic devices—applications to genetics testing. *Clin Chem* 1999;45:746–9.
40. National Center for Toxicogenomics. *NCT Overview—Impact.* Available at http://www.niehs.nih.gov/nct/concept.htm. Accessed June 29, 2001.
41. Mohr S, Gochfeld M, Pransky G. Genetically and medically susceptible workers. *Occup Med* 1999;14:595–611.
42. Bartell SM, Ponce RA, Takaro TK, Zerbe RO, Omenn GS, Faustman EM. Risk estimation and value-of-information analysis for three proposed genetic screening programs for chronic beryllium disease prevention. *Risk Anal* 2000;20:87–99.

13

Vaccination Mandates: The Public Health Imperative and Individual Rights

KEVIN M. MALONE AND ALAN R. HINMAN

In 1796, Edward Jenner demonstrated that inoculation with material from a cowpox (vaccinia) lesion would protect against subsequent exposure to smallpox. This began the vaccine era, although it was nearly 100 years until the next vaccine (against rabies) was introduced. In the twentieth century, many new vaccines were developed and used, with spectacular impact on the occurrence of disease. The Centers for Disease Control and Prevention (CDC) declared vaccinations to be one of the 10 great public health achievements of the twentieth century.[1,2]

This chapter describes the impact of vaccines in dramatically reducing infectious diseases in the United States, the role of mandatory vaccination in achieving that impact, and the constitutional basis for these mandates. The chapter also briefly reviews the federal government's role in immunization practices.

BACKGROUND

Concept for Community Disease Prevention

Garrett Hardin's classic essay *The Tragedy of the Commons*[3] describes the challenges presented when societal interest conflicts with the individual's interest. Hardin notes the incentives present when the cattle of a community are commingled in a common pasture. At capacity, each owner still has an incentive to add additional cattle to the common because even though the yield from each animal decreases with the addition of more cattle, this decrease is offset for the individual owner by the additional animal. With this incentive, individual owners continue to add cattle to the commons to reap their individual benefit, leading to the inevitable failure of the common from overgrazing. The community interest in maximizing food production, therefore, can be achieved only by placing controls on the interests of the individual owners in favor of those of the community.

Analogously, a community free of an infectious disease because of a high vaccination rate can be viewed as a common. As in Hardin's common, the very existence of this common leads to tension between the best interests of the individual and those of the community. Increased immunization rates result in significantly decreased risk for disease. Although no remaining unimmunized individual can be said to be free of risk from the infectious disease, the herd effect generated from high immunization rates significantly reduces the risk for disease for those individuals. Additional benefit is conferred on the unimmunized person because avoidance of the vaccine avoids the risk for any adverse reactions associated with the vaccine. As disease rates drop, the risks associated with the vaccine come even more to the fore, providing further incentive to avoid immunization. Thus, when an individual in this common chooses to go unimmunized, it only minimally increases the risk of illness for that individual, while conferring on that person the benefit of avoiding the risk of vaccine-induced side effects. At the same time, however, this action weakens the herd effect protection for the entire community. As more and more individuals choose to do what is in their "best" individual interest, the common eventually fails as herd immunity disappears and disease outbreaks occur. To avoid this "tragedy of the commons," legal requirements have been imposed by communities (in recent times, by states) to mandate particular vaccinations.

Vaccine Safety and Effectiveness

Vaccines are safe and effective. However, they are neither perfectly safe nor perfectly effective. Consequently, some persons who receive vaccines will be injured as a result, and some persons who receive vaccines will not be protected. Most adverse events associated with vaccines are minor and involve local soreness or redness at the injection site or perhaps fever for a day or so. Rarely, however, vaccine can cause more serious adverse events. Whether an adverse event that occurs after vaccination was caused by the vaccine or was merely temporally related and caused by some totally independent (and often unknown or unidentified) factor is often difficult to ascertain. This is particularly problematic during infancy, when a number of conditions may occur spontaneously. In a given instance, determining whether vaccine was responsible may be impossible.[4] Particularly when dealing with rare events, large-scale case–control studies or reviews of comprehensive records of large numbers of infants may be necessary to ascertain whether those who received a vaccine had a higher incidence of the event than those who did not. The CDC operates an extensive linked database involving several large health-maintenance organizations. This Vaccine Safety Datalink project includes more than 6 million persons (approximately 2% of the U.S. population) and has proved invaluable for attempting to determine causality.[5]

Decisions about use of vaccines are based on the relative balance of risks and benefits. This balance may change over time. For example, recipients of oral polio vaccine (OPV) and their close contacts have a risk of developing paralysis associated with the vaccine of 1 in approximately every 2.4 million doses of vaccine distributed. This risk is small and was certainly outweighed by the much larger risk for paralysis from wild polioviruses at the time they were circulating in the United States. However, because wild polioviruses no longer circulate in the United States and the risk of importation of wild viruses has been greatly reduced by the global effort to eradicate polio, the balance has shifted. There has not been a case of paralysis in the United States from indigenously acquired wild poliovirus since 1979, and the entire Western Hemisphere has been free from wild poliovirus circulation since 1991.[6] The Advisory Committee on Immunization Practices (ACIP), an advisory group to the CDC, recommended, in 1997, that children should receive a sequential schedule with two doses of inactivated polio vaccine (IPV) (which carries no risk for paralysis but has slightly less effect in preventing community spread of wild poliovirus), followed by two doses of OPV. In 2000, the recommendation was made to switch to an all-IPV regimen.[7]

An important characteristic of most vaccines is that they provide both individual and community protection. Most of the diseases against which we vaccinate are transmitted from person to person. When a sufficiently large proportion of individuals in a community is immunized, those persons serve as a protective barrier against the likelihood of transmission of the disease in the community, thus indirectly protecting those who are not immunized and those who received vaccine but are not protected (vaccine failures). One commentator has suggested that a social contract exists among parents to immunize their children not only to provide them individual protection, but also to contribute to the protection of other children who cannot be immunized or for whom the vaccine is not effective.[8] The proportion of the population that has to be immune to provide this "herd immunity" varies according to the infectiousness of the agent. For poliomyelitis, that proportion is considered to be on the order of 80%, whereas for measles it exceeds 90%.

When a community has a high level of vaccination, an individual might decide to not be vaccinated to avoid the small risk for adverse events while benefitting from the vaccination of others. Of course, if a sufficient number of individuals make this decision, the protection levels in the community decline, the herd immunity effect is lost, and the risk of transmission rises.

Impact of Vaccines

The introduction and widespread use of vaccines have profoundly affected the occurrence of several infectious diseases. Smallpox was eradicated from the world—onset of the last naturally occurring case was in 1977—and vaccination against smallpox stopped. Poliomyelitis is on the verge of eradication (the last indigenous case in the United States associated with wild virus occurred in 1979, and only 20 to 30 countries were still reporting transmission as of mid-2001).

Because approximately 11,000 infants are born every day in the United States, the need to ensure that children continue to be protected is ongoing. In addition, a continuing threat exists of importation of disease from other countries. In the United States, infants and young children are currently vaccinated against 11 diseases: diphtheria, *Haemophilus influenzae* type b, hepatitis B, measles, mumps, pertussis, poliomyelitis, rubella, *Streptococcus pneumoniae*, tetanus, and varicella.[9] In states with high risk for hepatitis A, children are also vaccinated against this disease. With the exception of tetanus, each of these diseases is spread from person to person by direct contact or by aerosol droplet transmission. Most of the diseases historically have had very high incidence in school-aged children because of the high potential for transmission in the congregate setting. With more children in preschool programs, outbreaks have occurred at earlier ages. In contrast, hepatitis B has its highest incidence in young adulthood as a result of transmission through sexual contact or needle sharing. Tetanus is acquired by contamination of wounds and is not transmitted from person to person. Table 13–1 shows the representative annual morbidity (typically, average morbidity reported in the 3 years before introduction of the vaccine) in the twentieth century and the number of cases reported in 2000 for diseases against which children have been routinely vaccinated.[10] Most diseases have declined by 99% or more (pneumococcal disease and varicella are not reportable conditions) and are at all-time lows. Vaccination coverage in 19–35-month-old children is at an all-time high (Table 13–2).[11]

Modern Government Role in Immunization

Vaccines are subject to licensure in the United States by the Food and Drug Administration (FDA) following studies that address safety and efficacy.[12,13] With declining vaccine production capacity in the United States, in 1986 Congress approved the National Childhood Vaccine Injury Act (NCVIA).[14] This comprehensive law established the National Vaccine Program within the U.S.

TABLE 13–1. Comparison of Twentieth Century Annual Morbidity* and Current Morbidity of Vaccine-Preventable Diseases of Children in the United States

DISEASE	TWENTIETH CENTURY ANNUAL MORBIDITY	2000†	PERCENTAGE DECREASE
Smallpox	48,164	0	100
Diphtheria	175,885	4	99.99
Measles	503,282	81	99.98
Mumps	152,209	323	99.80
Pertussis	147,271	6755	95.40
Polio (paralytic)	16,316	0	100
Rubella	47,745	152	99.70
Congenital rubella syndrome	823	7	99.10
Tetanus	1314	26	98.00
Haemophilus influenzae type b and unknown (<5 years)	20,000	167	99.10

*Typical average during the 3 years before vaccine licensure.
†Provisional data.

TABLE 13–2. Vaccination Coverage Levels Among Children Aged 19–35 Months in the United States, 2000

VACCINE, DOSES	COVERAGE (%)
DTP, 3	94.1
DTP, 4	81.7
Polio, 3	89.5
Hib, 3	93.4
MMR, 1,	90.5
Hepatitis B, 3	90.3
Varicella	67.8
Combined series	
4 DTP/3 polio/1 MMR	77.6
4 DTP/3 polio/1 MMR/3 Hib	76.2
4 DTP/3 polio/1 MMR/3 Hib/3 Hep B	72.8

DTP, diphtheria and tetanus toxoids and pertussis vaccine; Hib, *Haemophilus influenzae* type b vaccine; MMR, measles-mumps-rubella vaccine; Hep B, hepatitis B vaccine.

Department of Health and Human Services to coordinate and oversee all activities within the U.S. government related to vaccine research and development, vaccine-safety monitoring, and vaccination activities. In addition, the Act established the National Vaccine Injury Compensation Program (VICP) to compensate for injuries associated with routinely administered childhood vaccines (42 U.S.C. §§ 300aa-10–300aa-23). At least some of the decline in the number of vaccine producers in the United States had been attributed to liability costs. The VICP effectively removes this as a significant consideration.

Acknowledging that vaccines, as with any medication, are not without risk to the patient, that vaccines, unlike other medications, are a medical intervention generally given to healthy individuals, and that vaccination has benefits beyond the individual by significantly benefitting the public health through creation of herd immunity, the VICP was established to shift the monetary costs of vaccine injuries away from vaccine recipients and manufacturers. Using a vaccine injury table and a simplified administrative process through the U.S. Court of Federal Claims, this no-fault system is designed to fairly compensate children and their families (along with adult recipients of these vaccines) for the costs associated with the rare injuries related to vaccination. An excise tax on each dose of covered vaccine funds the compensation program.

Individuals alleging vaccine injury must go through the VICP before filing any tort actions against the administering health-care provider or the vaccine manufacturer. If the judgment of the court is accepted, further actions against the provider and manufacturer are barred. Even if the judgment is declined, the NCVIA significantly narrows the scope of any tort action against the manufacturer. Since the inception of the VICP, few individuals have chosen to reject the judgment of the court and file suit against the provider or manufacturer. Thus, liability costs of the vaccine manufacturers have dropped dramatically since the establishment of the VICP.

With the product liability incentive for vaccine improvement substantially reduced by the existence of the VICP, the role of the government in monitoring vaccine safety becomes more prominent. Beyond post-licensure surveillance requirements of the FDA, the NCVIA also established the Vaccine Adverse Event Reporting System (VAERS), which requires reporting of adverse events by vaccination providers (42 U.S.C. § 300aa-25). Providers must also record lot numbers of vaccines administered. Furthermore, various federal agencies, including the CDC's National Immunization Program, have expanded vaccine-safety activities. In addition, with diminished liability costs, more pharmaceuticals have entered the vaccine production arena with the resultant competition leading to further vaccine improvements and development of new vaccines against other diseases.

The NCVIA also seeks to improve the knowledge level of parents through its requirement that the CDC produce vaccine information materials for mandatory distribution by providers to patients or parents before administration of VICP-covered vaccines (42 U.S.C. § 300aa-26). Through these materials, called Vaccine Information Statements, parents are informed about the schedules for administration of the vaccines, are alerted to contraindications that dictate against administration to particular individuals, and are informed about potential adverse reactions to look for to encourage timely medical intervention, as needed.

Most children in the United States receive their vaccinations in the private sector, from pediatricians or family physicians. A significant minority receive vaccinations in the public sector, typically from local health departments. There is considerable variation around the country.[15] At current prices, the cost for vaccines alone (irrespective of physician fees) is approximately $600 in the private sector (CDC, unpublished data). Most employer-based insurance plans now cover childhood vaccinations.

Since 1962, the federal government has supported childhood vaccination programs through a grant program administered by the CDC.[16] These "317" grants, named for the authorizing statute, support purchase of vaccine for free administration at local health departments and support immunization delivery, surveillance, and communication and education. As of 2000, the CDC purchased over half the childhood vaccine administered in the United States through two federally overseen, state-administered programs. In addition to the 317 program, in 1994 the Vaccines for Children (VFC) [17] program began, under which all Medicaid-eligible children, all children who are uninsured, all American Indian and Alaska Native children, and insured children whose coverage does not include vaccinations (with limitations on the locations where this last group can receive VFC vaccine) qualify to receive routine childhood vaccines at no cost for the vaccine. The VFC program operates in both public health clinics and private provider offices. The 317 grant program provides additional vaccines to the states for administration to adults and to children who do not qualify for VFC vaccine. Additional federal assistance for vaccination is provided by the Children's Health Insurance Program through expanded Medicaid eligibility for low-income children.[18] Many states use state funds to purchase additional quantities of vaccine.

The ACIP determines the vaccines to be administered in the VFC program and the schedules for their use. In addition, the ACIP issues recommendations for use of adult and pediatric vaccines in the United States and, generally in coordination with the American Academy of Pediatrics and the American Academy of Family Physicians, establishes a recommended schedule for administration of routine childhood vaccines. The ACIP recommendations are often considered by states as they determine which vaccinations to mandate for school attendance.

To assist parents in complying with the often complex vaccine schedules, many states and localities, with the assistance of the CDC and professional organizations, have established vaccination registries to send parents reminders when vaccines are due. In a mobile era when families move often and frequently change health-care providers, these registries also help avoid over-vaccination and ensure catch-up vaccination when needed.[19]

School and Daycare Vaccination Laws

School vaccination laws have played a key role in the control of vaccine-preventable diseases in the United States. The first school vaccination requirement was enacted in the 1850s in Massachusetts to prevent smallpox transmission in schools.[20] By the beginning of the twentieth century, nearly half of the states had requirements for children to be vaccinated before they entered school. By 1963, 20 states, the District of Columbia, and Puerto Rico had such laws, with a variety of vaccines being mandated.[21] However, enforcement was uneven.

In the late 1960s, efforts were undertaken to eradicate measles from the United States. Transmission in schools was recognized as a significant problem.[22] In the early 1970s, states that had school vaccination laws for measles vaccine had measles incidence rates 40% to 51% lower than states without such laws.[23] In 1976 and 1977, measles outbreaks in Alaska and Los Angeles, respectively, led health officials to strictly enforce the existing requirements.[24] Advance notice was given that the laws were to be enforced, and major efforts were undertaken to ensure that vaccination could be easily obtained. In Alaska, on the announced day of enforcement, 7418 of 89,109 students (8.3%) failed to provide proof of vaccination and were excluded from school. One month later, fewer than 51 students were still excluded. No further cases of measles occurred.[25] In Los Angeles, approximately 50,000 of 1,400,000 students (<4%) were excluded; most were back in school within a few days, and the number of measles cases dropped precipitously. These experiences demonstrated that mandatory vaccination could be enforced and was effective.

Because of declining vaccination levels in children, a nationwide Childhood Immunization Initiative was undertaken in 1977 to raise vaccination levels in children to 90% by 1979. An important component of this initiative was to support enactment and enforcement of school vaccination requirements. During a 2 year period, more than 28 million records were reviewed, and children in need were vaccinated.[26]

An analysis of six states that strictly enforced comprehensive laws (affecting all grades) beginning with the 1977–1978 school year compared with the rest of the country showed that in the 1975–1976 school year, they had comparable incidence rates of measles. However, in the 1977–1978 school year, the six

states that strictly enforced the laws had incidence rates less than half those of
the rest of the country; and in the 1978–1979 school year, the incidence rates
were less than one tenth those of the rest of the country.[27] An analysis of states
with the highest and lowest incidences of measles in 1979–1980 found that states
with the lowest incidence rates were significantly more likely to have laws covering the entire school population (rather than just first entrants) and more likely
to be strictly enforcing the laws.[28]

By the 1980–1981 school year, all 50 states had laws covering students
first entering school. In most states, these laws affected children at all grade
levels, as well as those involved in licensed preschool settings. Some of the
laws specified the particular vaccines required (and the numbers of doses of
each); others authorized the State Health Officer (or public health board) to
designate which vaccines (and doses) were required, often after a public rule-
making process.

As of the 1998–1999 school year, all states but four (Louisiana, Michigan,
South Carolina, and West Virginia) had requirements covering all grades from
kindergarten through 12th grade. In all states, the District of Columbia, and
Puerto Rico, the requirements covered daycare centers; in 48 states (all but Iowa
and West Virginia), the requirements covered Head Start programs. Thirty states,
the District of Columbia, and Puerto Rico had some requirements for college
entrance. The requirements covered diphtheria toxoid and polio, measles, and
rubella vaccines in all 50 states; 49 states required tetanus toxoid, 46 required
mumps vaccine, 44 required pertussis vaccine, and 28 required hepatitis B
vaccine.[29]

Since 1981, vaccination levels in school entrants have been 95% or higher
for diphtheria and tetanus toxoids and pertussis vaccine (DTP), polio vaccine,
and measles vaccine. All states require vaccination for children attending licensed daycare centers and as a result such children have vaccination levels
90% or higher. Nonetheless, overall levels in preschool children have not been
as high, as manifested by the resurgence of measles that occurred during 1989–
1991, primarily affecting unvaccinated preschool-aged children.[30] Levels in
preschool-aged children have recently been raised to their currently high levels
as a result of major efforts (and major infusions of resources) directed at this
population.[15]

The Task Force on Community Preventive Services is an independent
body carrying out evidence-based reviews of the literature to assess the claims
that preventive interventions directed to populations are effective. One of
the 17 interventions reviewed for vaccine-preventable diseases was mandatory vaccination requirements. The Task Force found that sufficient evidence
existed to demonstrate the effectiveness of these requirements in increasing
vaccine coverage, thereby reducing disease incidence, and so recommended
their use.[31]

Historical Context

Duffy's description of smallpox vaccination in early American history highlights both the significant positive public health impact of vaccines and the ongoing challenges that this success presents[20]:

Smallpox . . . was the great scourge of the American colonies until the introduction of inoculation or variolation, and the subsequent discovery of vaccination in 1796 relegated it to minor importance among the great epidemic diseases. As memories of the horrifying outbreaks of smallpox gradually faded, and a generation appeared which had had little contact with its victims, vaccination was neglected, and the incidence of smallpox began to rise. Beginning in the 1830s its attacks gradually intensified, and by the time of the Civil War the disorder was once again a serious problem.

By chance, the rise of smallpox coincided with the enactment of compulsory school attendance laws and the subsequent rapid growth in the number of public schools. Since the bringing together of large numbers of children clearly facilitated the spread of small-pox, and since vaccination provided a relatively safe preventive, it was natural that com-pulsory school attendance laws should lead to a movement for compulsory vaccination. . . ."

Many other childhood diseases for which vaccines were developed also fre-quently occurred in school-based outbreaks; consequently, when polio and mea-sles vaccines were introduced in 1955 and 1963, respectively, adding them to the list of requirements for school entry was a logical consideration. The 1963 survey of state laws found that, of 20 states with requirements, 18 included smallpox, 11 included diphtheria, 10 included polio, 7 included tetanus, and 5 included pertussis. Measles requirements were soon added. By 1970, 20 states required measles vaccination, and by 1983 all 50 states did.[32]

LEGAL AUTHORITIES—CONSTITUTIONAL BASIS OF MANDATORY VACCINATION

Police Power

The first state law mandating vaccination was enacted in Massachusetts in 1809; in 1855, Massachusetts became the first state to enact a school vaccination re-quirement. The constitutional basis of vaccination requirements rests in the po-lice power of the state. Nearly 100 years ago, the U.S. Supreme Court issued its landmark ruling in *Jacobson v. Massachusetts,*[33] upholding the right of states to compel vaccination. The Court held that a health regulation requiring small-pox vaccination was a reasonable exercise of the state's police power that did not violate the liberty rights of individuals under the Fourteenth Amendment to the U.S. Constitution. The police power is the authority reserved to the states by the Constitution and embraces "such reasonable regulations established di-rectly by legislative enactment as will protect the public health and the public safety"[a] (197 U.S. at 25, 25 S.Ct. at 361).

In *Jacobson*, the Commonwealth of Massachusetts had enacted a statute that authorized local boards of health to require vaccination. Jacobson challenged his conviction for refusal to be vaccinated against smallpox as required by regulations of the Cambridge Board of Health. While acknowledging the potential for vaccines to cause adverse events and the inability to determine with absolute certainty whether a particular person can be safely vaccinated, the Court specifically rejected the idea of an exemption based on personal choice.[b] To do otherwise "would practically strip the legislative department of its function to [in its considered judgment] care for the public health and the public safety when endangered by epidemics of disease" (197 U.S. at 37, 25 S.Ct. at 366). The Court elaborated on the tension between personal freedom and public health inherent in liberty: "The liberty secured by the Constitution of the United States to every person within its jurisdiction does not import an absolute right in each person to be, at all times and in all circumstances, wholly freed from restraint. There are manifold restraints to which every person is necessarily subject for the common good. On any other basis organized society could not exist with safety to its members" (197 U.S. at 26, 25 S.Ct. at 361).

School Vaccination Laws

The Supreme Court in 1922 addressed the constitutionality of childhood vaccination requirements in *Zucht v. King*.[34] The Court denied a due process Fourteenth Amendment challenge to the constitutionality of city ordinances that excluded children from school attendance for failure to present a certificate of vaccination holding that "these ordinances confer not arbitrary power, but only that broad discretion required for the protection of the public health"[c] (260 U.S. at 177, 43 S.Ct. at 25).

More recently, in the face of a measles epidemic in Maricopa County, Arizona, the Arizona Court of Appeals rejected the argument that an individual's right to education would trump the state's need to protect against the spread of infectious diseases short of confirmed cases of measles in the particular school. Given the nature of the spread of measles and the lag time in getting laboratory confirmation of cases, the court in *Maricopa County Health Department v. Harmon*[35] was satisfied that it is prudent to take action to combat disease by excluding unvaccinated children from school when there is a reasonably perceived, but unconfirmed, risk for the spread of measles (156 Ariz. at 166, 750 P.2d at 1369). Although the court considered the right to education under Arizona's constitution, the decision is instructive in showing the reach of the police power to ensure the public health. The court in *Maricopa* specifically noted that *Jacobson* did not require that epidemic conditions exist to compel vaccination (156 Ariz. at 166, 750 P.2d at 1369).

Parens Patriae

Further authority to compel vaccination of children comes under the doctrine of *parens patriae* in which the state asserts authority over child welfare. In the 1944 case of *Prince v. Massachusetts*,[36] which involved child labor under an asserted right of religious freedom, the U.S. Supreme Court summarized the doctrine, noting that

Neither rights of religion nor rights of parenthood are beyond limitation. Acting to guard the general interest in youth's well being, the state as *parens patriae* may restrict the parent's control by requiring school attendance, regulating or prohibiting the child's labor, and in many other ways. Its authority is not nullified merely because the parent grounds his claim to control the child's course of conduct on religion or conscience. Thus, he cannot claim freedom from compulsory vaccination for the child more than for himself on religious grounds. The right to practice religion freely does not include liberty to expose the community or the child to communicable disease or the latter to ill health or death.[d] (321 U.S. at 166–7, 64 S.Ct. at 442)

LEGAL ISSUES AND CONTROVERSIES—EXEMPTIONS TO MANDATORY VACCINATION

Although vaccines are safe and effective, they are neither perfectly safe nor perfectly effective. Some persons who receive vaccines will have an adverse reaction, and some will not be protected. In developing vaccines, the challenge is to minimize the likelihood of adverse effect while maximizing effectiveness. Some people have medical conditions that increase the risk for adverse effect, and therefore they should not receive vaccines. Recognizing this fact, all state vaccination laws provide for exemptions for persons with contraindicating conditions.

The religious beliefs of some people are in opposition to vaccination, and other people oppose vaccination on other grounds, including philosophic. In addition, some persons are not opposed to all vaccines but oppose the concept of mandatory vaccination or mandates for specific vaccines. In the latter case, they may believe they (or their children) are not at risk for a particular disease or that, if contracted, the disease is not severe. If the disease in question is uncommon (as is the case in the United States today for most vaccine-preventable diseases), they might not be willing to undertake any level of risk of adverse effect.

Forty-eight states allow religious exemptions (all but Mississippi and West Virginia), and 15 (California, Colorado, Idaho, Louisiana, Maine, Michigan, Minnesota, New Mexico, North Dakota, Ohio, Oklahoma, Utah, Vermont, Washington, and Wisconsin) permit philosophic exemptions[29] (RH Snyder, National Immunization Program [NIP], CDC, personal communication). The criteria for allowing these exemptions vary greatly. Some states require membership in a recognized religion,[e] whereas others merely require an affirmation of religious (or philosophic) opposition. Nationwide, fewer than 1% of school entrants have medical, religious, or philosophic exemptions to mandatory vaccination. Seven states had more than 1% with exemptions in the 1997–1998 school year (*Colorado, Michigan*, Oregon, South Dakota, *Utah, Washington*, and West Virginia [those with philosophic exemptions are italicized]). Michigan had the highest level of exemption at 2.3% (RH Snyder, NIP, CDC, personal communication.). However, in some communities, the levels of exemptors may be as high as 5%. In 1995, 84% of California schools had fewer than 1% of students with exemptions, but 4% of schools had 5% or more with exemptions (NA Smith, Immunization Program, California Department of Public Health, personal communication).

Thirteen outbreaks of measles were identified during 1985–1994 in religious groups opposing vaccination. These outbreaks resulted in more than 1200 cases and 9 deaths. Outbreaks of polio (in the 1970s), pertussis, and rubella have been documented among Amish groups.[37] Salmon et al.[38] found that persons with religious or philosophic exemptions were 35 times more likely to contract measles than were vaccinated persons during 1985–1992. They also found that persons living in communities with high concentrations of exemptors were themselves at increased risk for measles because of increased risk for exposure.

Rota et al.[39] studied the processes required to obtain religious and philosophic exemptions to school vaccination laws and found an inverse correlation between the complexity of the exemption process and the proportion of exemptions filed. None of 19 states with the highest level of complexity in gaining exemptions had more than 1% of students exempted compared with 5 of 15 states with the simplest procedure. In these latter states, less effort was required to claim a nonmedical exemption than to fulfill the vaccination requirement.

Is There a Constitutional Right to a Religious Exemption from Mandatory Vaccination?

Challenges to mandatory vaccination laws based on religion or philosophic belief have led various courts to hold that no constitutional right exists to either religious or philosophic exemptions.

First Amendment[f] free exercise clause

Freedom to believe in a religion is absolute under the First Amendment. However, freedom to act in accordance with one's religious beliefs "remains subject to regulation for the protection of society."[40] The U.S. Supreme Court in the 1963 case of *Sherbert v. Verner*[41] established a balancing test for determining whether a regulation violated a person's First Amendment right to free exercise of religion. The test, which prevailed until 1990, required the government to justify any substantial burden on religiously motivated conduct by a compelling government interest and by means narrowly tailored to achieve that interest (374 U.S. at 406–8, 83 S.Ct. at 1795–6).

Notwithstanding the state's power as *parens patriae*, instances occur in which a parent's claim of religious freedom under the Free Exercise Clause will prevail, as in *Wisconsin v. Yoder*.[42] *Yoder* involved a challenge by Amish parents of a Wisconsin law that required formal education of children to age 16 years. The parents asserted that formal schooling beyond the eighth grade would gravely endanger the free exercise of their religion because of their belief that the values taught in higher education, including the exposure to worldly influences, are in marked variance with Amish values and the Amish way of life. While acknowledging the state's interest in universal education, the U.S. Supreme Court, in applying the *Sherbert* compelling interest test, rejected Wisconsin's argument of a compelling state interest in requiring formal education of the Amish beyond eighth grade given the strong religious interference of such a requirement and the fact that the Amish provided adequate alternative informal vocational education. The Court in *Yoder* articulated its application of the compelling interest test as follows. "[W]here fundamental claims of religious freedom are at stake," the Court will not accept a state's "sweeping claim" that its interest in compulsory education is compelling; "despite its admitted validity in the generality of cases, we must searchingly examine the interests that the State seeks to promote . . . and the impediment to those objectives that would flow from recognizing the claimed Amish exemption" (406 U.S. at 221, 92 S.Ct. at 1536).

Little recent case law directly addresses the existence of a First Amendment free exercise right to a religious exemption from mandatory vaccination because 48 states have provided by statute for religious exemptions to school vaccination laws.[29] However, dicta in both *Sherbert*[43] and *Yoder*[44] referring to the *Jacobson* and *Prince* decisions clearly indicate that on both *parens patriae* and police power grounds the U.S. Supreme Court sees a compelling state interest in mandating vaccination of children because of the health threat to the community and to the children themselves. With little practical alternative to vaccination to avoid or be a disease risk (e.g., inability to avoid contact with other persons, except for those totally isolated from society), mandatory vaccination of all school children should also meet the "narrowly tailored" criterion of *Sherbert*.

In addition, in a case that predates the *Yoder* decision and enactment of a statutory religious exemption by Arkansas, the Arkansas Supreme Court in *Wright v. DeWitt School District*[45] held that no First Amendment right existed to a religious exemption given the state's compelling interest in mandating vaccination under its police power to protect the public health.[g] (238 Ark. at 913, 385 S.W.2d at 648). Significantly, the U.S. Supreme Court in *Yoder* referenced the *Wright* decision in dicta regarding cases in which the health of the child or public health are at issue, with the implication that a vaccination mandate providing no religious exemption would meet the compelling state interest test (406 U.S. at 230, 92 S.Ct. at 1540–1).

Whether a vaccination law that does not provide for religious exemptions would meet the compelling state interest test is essentially moot now because of a U.S. Supreme Court ruling that significantly lowers the bar for states to prevail. In its 1990 decision in *Employment Div., Dept. of Human Resources of Oregon v. Smith,*[46] the Supreme Court rejected the compelling interest test and established a new standard that holds that "the right of free exercise does not relieve an individual of the obligation to comply with a 'valid and neutral law of general applicability on the ground that the law proscribes (or prescribes) conduct that his religion prescribes (or proscribes)' " (494 U.S. at 879, 110 S.Ct. at 1600 [quoting *United States v. Lee*, 455 U.S. 252, 263, n. 3, 102 S.Ct. 1051, 1058, n. 3 (1982)]).

Congress attempted to legislatively override the ruling in *Smith* by enacting the Religious Freedom Restoration Act of 1993 (RFRA), which reestablished the compelling interest test as the standard for considering the constitutionality of free exercise claims.[47] However, the U.S. Supreme Court in *City of Boerne v. Flores*[48] struck down RFRA, holding that Congress had exceeded its constitutional authority in implementing the statute (521 U.S. at 510–37, 117 S.Ct. at 2160–72). Thus, the *Smith* standard is the current law. Whether judged under the neutral law of general applicability test of *Smith* or the compelling interest test of *Sherbert*, it is reasonable to conclude that there is no First Amendment free exercise right to an exemption from mandatory vaccination requirements.

Is a Statutory Religious Exemption Constitutional?

With no First Amendment free exercise right to a religious exemption, the next question is whether the states have the discretion to allow such exemptions by statute. The court decisions are mixed. The Establishment Clause[h] of the First Amendment establishes the constitutional limits within which a state may accommodate a religious exemption to a law of general application, including whether such an exemption is allowed and how inclusively the exemption must be defined. As noted above, 48 states have provided by statute for religious exemptions to school vaccination laws.[29]

In *Brown v. Stone,*[49] the Mississippi Supreme Court struck down the religious exemption that appeared in the Mississippi school vaccination statute, holding that the statutory religious exemption violated the Equal Protection Clause of the Fourteenth Amendment because it would "require the great body of school children to be vaccinated and at the same time expose them to the hazard of associating in school with children exempted under the religious exemption who had not been immunized" (378 So.2d at 223). Thus, the *Jacobson* argument comes full circle. The fact that no vaccine confers immunity on all vaccinees illustrates the point that even persons who comply with vaccination statutes can be placed at increased risk by exposure to individuals never vaccinated because of exemptions.

First amendment—establishment clause

Most challenges to religious-based vaccination exemptions have been decided by the courts on establishment grounds and concern the inclusiveness of such exemptions rather than their existence. The U.S. Supreme Court in *Lemon v. Kurtzman*,[50] a case involving state supplementation of parochial school salaries, defined a three-pronged test for determining whether a state religious accommodation complies with the Establishment Clause: "First, the statute must have a secular legislative purpose; second, its principal or primary effect must be one that neither advances nor inhibits religion; finally, the statute must not foster 'an excessive government entanglement with religion' " (403 U.S. at 612–3, 91 S.Ct. at 2111 [citation omitted] [quoting *Walz v. Tax Commission*, 397 U.S. 664, 674, 90 S.Ct. 1409, 1414 (1970)]).

Scope of statutory exemptions—sincerely held religious belief

In *Sherr v. Northport-East Northport Union Free School District*,[51] the plaintiffs had been denied an exemption under the state's religious exemption statute by the school district because, although they claimed religious opposition to vaccination, they were not "bona fide members of a recognized religious organization" whose teachings oppose vaccination, as required by New York law (672 F.Supp. at 84 [quoting subsection 9 of N.Y. Pub. Health L. § 2164]). The U.S. District Court for the Eastern District of New York found that New York's limitation of the religious exemption violated both the Establishment and Free Exercise clauses of the First Amendment.

The court found that this limitation violated the Establishment Clause by running afoul of at least the last two prongs of the *Lemon* test: (*1*) by inhibiting the religious practices of individuals who oppose vaccination of their children on religious grounds but are not members of a religious organization recognized by the state and (2) by restricting the exemption to "recognized religious organizations" requires that the government involve itself in religious matters to an inordinate degree through such government approval (672 F.Supp. at 89–90). In addition, the court held that the limiting language violated the Free Exercise Clause because no compelling societal interest existed to justify the burden placed on the free religious exercise of "certain individuals while other persons remain free to avoid subjecting their children to a religiously objectionable medical technique because they may belong to a particular religious organization to which the state has given a stamp of approval" (672 F.Supp. at 90–1). There "surely exist less restrictive alternative means of achieving the state's aims than the blatantly discriminatory restriction . . . the state has devised" (672 F.Supp. at 91). Striking down New York's limitation, the court found that "sincerely held religious beliefs" in opposition to vaccination, whether or not as part of a recognized religion, should suffice (672 F.Supp. at 98).

Do Statutory Religious Exemptions Encompass Philosophic Opposition?

Strength of convictions aside, defining "religious" belief can be difficult, and understanding its implications for philosophic exemptions that a state may or may not wish to voluntarily confer is a challenge. As the Supreme Court noted in *Yoder*: "to have the protection of the Religion Clauses, the claims must be rooted in religious belief" (406 U.S. at 215, 92 S.Ct. at 1533). Decisions by the U.S. Supreme Court in two conscientious objector cases indicate that a bright line may not always exist between the religious and the philosophic and that at least some amount of philosophic opposition to vaccination may rise to the level of being religious and therefore incorporated into a voluntarily conferred religious exemption, regardless of whether the state explicitly provides for a philosophic exemption.[k] In *United States v. Seeger*[52] and *Welsh v. United States,*[53] the Court interpreted "religious," as it appeared in a federal statutory religious-based conscientious objector exemption from military conscription, very expansively to extend beyond traditional religious beliefs. *Seeger* defined the test as "[a] sincere and meaningful belief which occupies in the life of its possessor a place parallel to that filled by the God of those admittedly qualifying for the exemption" (380 U.S. at 176, 85 S.Ct. at 859). The Court elaborated in *Welsh*: "to be 'religious' . . . this opposition . . . [must] stem from . . . moral, ethical, or religious beliefs about what is right and wrong and that these beliefs be held with the strength of traditional religious convictions" (398 U.S. at 340, 90 S.Ct. at 1796).

However, the *Welsh Court* clarified that "moral, ethical, or religious principles" do not incorporate "considerations of policy, pragmatism, or expediency" (398 U.S. at 342–3, 90 S.Ct. at 1798). *Yoder* provides further illumination: "A way of life, however virtuous and admirable, may not be interposed as a barrier to reasonable state regulation of education if it is based on purely secular considerations. . . . [T]he very concept of ordered liberty precludes allowing every person to make his own standards on matters of conduct in which the society as a whole has important interests. Thus, if the Amish asserted their claims because of their subjective evaluation and rejection of the contemporary secular values accepted by the majority, much as Thoreau rejected the social values of his time and isolated himself at Walden Pond, their claims would not rest on a religious basis. Thoreau's choice was philosophical and personal rather than religious, and such belief does not rise to the demands of the Religion Clauses" (406 U.S. at 215–6, 92 S.Ct. at 1533). Thus, the court in *Mason v. General Brown Central School District*[54] rejected fear of the possible side effects from vaccination, although based on strong convictions, as rising to the level of religious beliefs because of evidence that the plaintiff's beliefs were "simply an embodiment of secular chiropractic ethics" (851 F.2d at 51–2). *Mason*, and similar decisions, indicate that the expansive religious interpretation of *Seeger* and *Welsh* should not be read too broadly.

Impact of Evolving Privacy Rights

Finally, the general concept of a liberty interest in bodily integrity was first articulated by then-Judge, later Justice, Cardozo in *Schloendorff v. Society of New York Hospital*: "Every human being of adult years and sound mind has a right to determine what shall be done with his own body" regarding medical needs.[55] Recognition by the courts in recent years of a liberty right, or right to privacy, in medical decision making emanating from the due process clause of the Fourteenth Amendment and noted most prominently by the U.S. Supreme Court in its 1973 decision *Roe v. Wade*[56] might be used as the basis of a claimed privacy right by a college student subject to mandatory vaccination. However, the Court in *Roe,* referencing *Jacobson,* noted that the medical privacy right is not unlimited and must be balanced against important state interests in regulation (410 U.S. at 154, 193 S.Ct. at 727). More recently, in dicta in the 1990 "right to die" case of *Cruzan v. Director, Missouri Dept. of Health,*[57] the U.S. Supreme Court again acknowledged the viability of the *Jacobson* holding, leading to the conclusion that, as long as the public health need for widespread vaccination exists, the courts will not recognize a privacy right to refuse state-mandated vaccination and will uphold the police power of states to mandate vaccination.

PRACTICE CONSIDERATIONS AND EMERGING ISSUES

As new vaccines have been introduced and recommended for universal use in infants and children, states have responded by expanding the scope of their vaccination laws. Vaccination laws were first enacted to control epidemic diseases. Now they are also used to increase coverage with vaccines that are deemed important to protect the public's health even in the absence of epidemics. This practice is increasingly becoming subject to challenge, particularly with vaccines such as the varicella vaccine. Varicella is typically a mild disease in children, although nationwide it accounts for more than 50 deaths each year. Some parents have argued that no compelling state interest exists in preventing this disease. With hepatitis B vaccine, the argument has been that most hepatitis B occurs in adults whose sexual or drug-using behavior puts them at risk and that school children should not be forced to be vaccinated against a disease that often results from voluntary behavior of adults.

Publicity about adverse events alleged to be caused by vaccine fuels controversy about the wisdom or necessity of requiring vaccination, particularly in the absence of visible threat from disease. In the 1970s, concern about the possibility of pertussis vaccine causing sudden infant death syndrome or infantile spasms led to debate about pertussis vaccination requirements, even though studies showed that the vaccine caused neither event.[58] More recently, concern about the possibility that measles-mumps-rubella vaccine (MMR) might cause autism has led to congressional hearings and challenges to requirements for this vaccine.[59] Persons opposed to vaccination have extensively used the Internet to communicate their beliefs.

Of course, the appearance of new adverse events caused by vaccines further feeds the controversy. The occurrence of intestinal intussusception after administration of the recently licensed rotavirus vaccine led to withdrawal of the vaccine and lent some support to the arguments of those opposed to vaccination.[60]

CONCLUSION

School vaccination requirements have been a key factor in the prevention and control of vaccine-preventable diseases in the United States. Their constitutional basis rests in the police power of the state as well as in the *parens patriae* doctrine. No constitutional right exists to either a religious or philosophic exemption to these requirements, although most states allow religious exemptions and several allow philosophic exemptions. The courts have generally upheld these exemptions. Most litigation regarding exemptions has focused on the scope of the exemption, with courts holding that religious exemptions may not be limited to members of organized religions but rather must allow all who have sincerely held religious beliefs in opposition to vaccination to qualify. "Religious" may be defined broadly enough to incorporate some amount of philosophic opposition but should not be interpreted to bring purely secular-based "philosophic" opposition to vaccination within the meaning of religion.

With the increasing numbers of vaccines being introduced and the generally low level of visible threat from disease, continued challenges to school vaccination requirements are expected. School vaccination laws continue to play a central role in avoiding "the tragedy of the commons" by preventing disease through high vaccination coverage. These laws can be expected to be upheld by the courts as long as the balance of protecting the public health is achieved by mandating such requirements.

Notes

[a] Compulsory vaccination is not beyond the police power without arbitrariness or extreme injustice under particular facts. (See note b regarding medical-based exemption). In *Jacobson*, the Court—in addition to holding that providing for compulsory vaccination is within the police power of a state—also held that such authority may be delegated to a local body (197 U.S. at 25, 25 S.Ct. at 361).

[b] In dicta, the Court in *Jacobson* indicated, however, that there would be a liberty right to an exemption based on known medical contraindication "to protect the health and life of the individual concerned" (197 U.S. at 39, 25 S.Ct. at 366). (Dicta is discussion in a court decision that addresses an issue outside the direct facts presented by the case and therefore outside the court's holding and thus is of no precedential value in directing future court decisions.)

ᶜ See also *Brown v. Stone* (378 So. 2d 218, 222–3) (Miss. 1979), *cert. denied* 449 U.S. 887 (1980) for discussion regarding the logical nexus between mandatory vaccination and school attendance: "overriding and compelling public interest . . . [in] exclusion of a child until such immunization has been effected, not only as a protection of that child but as a protection of the large number of other children comprising the school community and with whom he will be daily in close contact in the school room."

ᵈ See also *In re: Christine M.*, 157 Misc.2d 4, 595 N.Y.S.2d 606 (N.Y. Fam. Ct. 1992) in which the court, citing *Prince*, held that a father's knowing failure to have his child vaccinated against measles in the midst of a measles outbreak, and not qualifying for a statutory religious exemption, caused the child to be a "neglected child" under state law. However, the court declined to order vaccination because the measles outbreak had ended by then and the child was not yet old enough to be subject to the school attendance law.

ᵉ But see discussion regarding holding in *Sherr* striking down state religious exemption requirement that an individual be a "bona fide member of a recognized religious organization."

ᶠ The First Amendment to the U.S. Constitution states in pertinent part, "Congress shall make no law respecting an establishment of religion, or prohibiting the free exercise thereof. . . ." The Free Exercise and Establishment Clauses have been held applicable to the States through the Due Process Clause of the Fourteenth Amendment.[40]

ᵍ See also *Cude v. State*, 237 Ark. 927, 377 S.W.2d 816 (Ark. 1964) (upholding ruling of neglect and appointment of temporary guardian to consent to vaccination of children despite parents' good faith religious beliefs in opposition).

ʰ See note f, above.

ⁱ See also *Davis v. State*, 294 Md. 379, 451 A.2d 107 (Md. 1982), which held that limiting religious exemption to children whose parents were "members" (as statute provided) or "adherents" (as health department regulation further attempted to narrow the qualification) of a "recognized church or religious denomination" opposing vaccination violated the Establishment Clause. On the basis of rules of statutory construction in Maryland, the court severed the offending religious exemption from the statute and upheld the conviction of Davis under the remaining statute that compelled vaccination (294 Md. at 382–5, 451 A.2d at 114–5). Rules of statutory construction vary so that in the *Sherr* case the court struck down the limiting "bona fide members of a recognized religious organization" language but otherwise upheld the religious exemption. In addition, the court enjoined enforcement of the "bona fide" language as to one of the two sets of plaintiffs, who otherwise qualified, and further enjoined the state from enforcing the offending language in the future (672 F.Supp. at 97–9).

ʲ The court in *Sherr*, having noted the constitutional infirmity of the "bona fide" limitation under the other two prongs of *Lemon*, did not resolve whether the "bona fide" portion of the religious exemption possessed a secular purpose as required under the first prong. However, in dicta, the court noted that the legislature may have had a number of secular purposes for adopting such language, including "as a guard against claims of exemption on the basis of personal moral scruples or unsupported fear of vaccinations, as a means of allowing certain exemptions without risking lessened effectiveness of the state's inoculation program due to the granting of a large number of exemptions, or perhaps because of the difficulties inherent in devising a legally workable definition of religion" (672 F.Supp. at 89).

ᵏ Fifteen states provide a separate philosophic exemption to school attendance vaccination laws, in addition to religious exemptions[29] (RH Snyder, NIP, CDC, personal communication).

References

1. CDC. Ten great public health achievements—United States, 1900–1999. *MMWR* 1999;48:241–3.
2. CDC. Impact of vaccines universally recommended for children—United States, 1900–1998. *MMWR* 1999;48:243–8.
3. Hardin G. The tragedy of the commons. *Science* 1968;162:1243–8.
4. ACIP. Update: vaccine side effects, adverse reactions, contraindications, and precautions. Recommendations of the Advisory Committee on Immunization Practices (ACIP). *MMWR* 1996;45(RR12):1–35.
5. Chen RT, DeStefano F, Davis RL, et al. The Vaccine Safety Datalink: immunization research in health maintenance organizations in the USA. *Bull WHO* 2000;78:186–94.
6. Robbins FC, de Quadros CA. Certification of the eradication of indigenous transmission of wild poliovirus in the Americas. *J Infect Dis* 1997;175(Suppl 1):S281–5.
7. ACIP. Poliomyelitis prevention in the United States. Updated recommendations of the Advisory Committee on Immunization Practices (ACIP). *MMWR* 2000; 49(RR05):1–22.
8. Freed GL, Katz SL, Clark SJ. Safety of vaccinations: Miss America, the media, and public health. *JAMA* 1996;276:1869–72.
9. CDC. Recommended childhood immunization schedule—United States, 2001. *MMWR* 2001;50:7–10, 19.
10. CDC. Provisional cases of selected notifiable diseases, week ending December 23, 2000. *MMWR* 2001;49:1164, 1167, 1173.
11. CDC. National, state, and urban area vaccination coverage levels among children aged 19–35 months—United States, 2000. *MMWR* 2001;50:637–41.
12. Section 351 of the Public Health Service Act, 42 U.S.C. § 262.
13. 21 U.S.C. §§ 321 *et seq.* (Federal Food, Drug and Cosmetic Act).
14. 42 U.S.C. §§ 300aa-1 *et seq.* (National Childhood Vaccine Injury Act).
15. Orenstein WA, Hinman AR, Rodewald LE. Public health considerations—United States. In: Plotkin SA, Orenstein WA, eds. *Vaccines*, 3rd ed. Philadelphia: WB Saunders, 1999: 1006–32.
16. Section 317 of the Public Health Service Act, 42 U.S.C. § 247b.
17. Section 1928 of the Social Security Act, 42 U.S.C. § 1396s.
18. 42 U.S.C. §§ 1397aa–1397jj.
19. National Vaccine Advisory Committee. *Development of Community- and State-Based Immunization Registries.* Approved January 12, 1999. Available at http://www.cdc.gov/nip/registry/nvac.htm. Accessed December 26, 2001.
20. Duffy J. School vaccination: the precursor to school medical inspection. *J Hist Med Allied Sci* 1978;33:344–55.
21. Hein FV, Bauer WW. Legal requirements for immunizations: a survey of state laws and regulations. *Arch Environ Health* 1964;9:82–5.
22. Sencer DJ, Dull HB, Langmuir AD. Epidemiologic basis for eradication of measles in 1967. *Public Health Rep* 1967;82:253–6.

23. CDC. Measles—United States. *MMWR* 1977;26:101–9.
24. Orenstein WA, Hinman AR. The immunization system in the United States—the role of school immunization laws. *Vaccine* 1999;17:S19–24.
25. Middaugh JP, Zyla LD. Enforcement of school immunization law in Alaska. *JAMA* 1978;239:2128–30.
26. Hinman AR. A new U.S. initiative in childhood immunization. *Bull Pan Am Health Org* 1979;13:169–76.
27. CDC. Measles and school immunization requirements—United States. *MMWR* 1978; 27:303–4.
28. Robbins KB, Brandling-Bennett AD, Hinman AR. Low measles incidence: association with enforcement of school immunization laws. *Am J Public Health* 1981;71: 270–4.
29. CDC. State immunization requirements, 1998–1999. Atlanta: U.S. Department of Health and Human Services, CDC, 1999.
30. National Vaccine Advisory Committee. The measles epidemic: the problems, barriers, and recommendations. *JAMA* 1991;266:1547–52.
31. Task Force on Community Preventive Services. Recommendations regarding interventions to improve vaccination coverage in children, adolescents, and adults. *Am J Prev Med* 2000;18(1S):92–6.
32. CDC. *State Immunization Requirements.* Atlanta: CDC, 1970, 1983.
33. *Jacobson v. Massachusetts,* 197 U.S. 11, 25 S.Ct. 358 (1905).
34. *Zucht v. King,* 260 U.S. 174, 43 S.Ct. 24 (1922).
35. *Maricopa County Health Department v. Harmon,* 156 Ariz. 161, 750 P.2d 1364 (Ariz. Ct. App. 1987).
36. *Prince v. Massachusetts,* 321 U.S. 158, 64 S.Ct. 438 (1944).
37. Hinman AR. How should physicians and nurses deal with people who do not want immunizations? *Can J Public Health* 2000;91:248–51.
38. Salmon DA, Haber M, Gangarosa EJ, et al. Health consequences of religious and philosophical exemptions from immunization laws: individual and societal risk of measles. *JAMA* 1999;282:47–53.
39. Rota JS, Salmon DA, Rodewald LE, et al. Processes for obtaining nonmedical exemptions to state immunization laws. *Am J Public Health* 2001;91:645–8.
40. *Cantwell v. Connecticut,* 310 U.S. 296, 303–4, 60 S.Ct. 900, 903 (1940).
41. *Sherbert v. Verner,* 374 U.S. 398, 83 S.Ct. 1790 (1963).
42. *Wisconsin v. Yoder,* 406 U.S. 205, 92 S.Ct. 1526 (1972).
43. 374 U.S. at 402–3, 83 S.Ct. at 1793.
44. 406 U.S. at 229–30, 233–4, 92 S.Ct. at 1540–42.
45. *Wright v. DeWitt School District,* 238 Ark. 906, 385 S.W.2d 644 (Ark. 1965).
46. Employment *Div., Dept. of Human Resources of Oregon v. Smith,* 494 U.S. 872, 110 S.Ct. 1595 (1990).
47. 42 U.S.C. §§ 2000bb-2000bb-4 (Religious Freedom Restoration Act of 1993).
48. *City of Boerne v. Flores,* 521 U.S. 507, 117 S.Ct. 2157 (1997).
49. *Brown v. Stone,* 378 So. 2d 218 (Miss. 1979), *cert. denied* 449 U.S. 887 (1980).
50. *Lemon v. Kurtzman,* 403 U.S. 602, 91 S.Ct. 2105 (1971).
51. *Sherr v. Northport-East Northport Union Free School District,* 672 F.Supp. 81 (E.D.N.Y. 1987).
52. *United States v. Seeger,* 380 U.S. 163, 85 S.Ct. 850 (1965).
53. *Walsh v. United States,* 398 U.S. 333, 90 S.Ct. 1792 (1970).
54. *Mason v. General Brown Central School District,* 851 F.2d 47 (2d Cir. 1988).

55. *Schloendorff v. Society of New York Hospital*, 211 N.Y. 125, 129, 105 N.E. 92, 93 (N.Y. 1914).
56. *Roe v. Wade*, 410 U.S. 113, 193 S.Ct. 705 (1973).
57. *Cruzan v. Director, Missouri Dept. of Health*, 497 U.S. 261, 278, 110 S.Ct. 2841, 2851 (1990).
58. Hinman AR. The pertussis vaccine controversy. *Public Health Rep* 1984;99:255–9.
59. Institute of Medicine. *Measles-Mumps-Rubella Vaccine and Autism. Report by the Immunization Safety Review Committee, Institute of Medicine*. Washington, DC: National Academy Press, 2001.
60. CDC. Withdrawal of rotavirus vaccine recommendation. *MMWR* 1999;48:1007.

14

Control of Foodborne Diseases

KEVIN FAIN AND JEREMY SOBEL

Successes in controlling foodborne diseases, due in large part to public health laws, rank among the great achievements of public health during the past 100 years. At the beginning of the twentieth century, infectious foodborne diseases, including typhoid fever, tuberculosis, botulism, and scarlet fever, were leading causes of mortality in the United States. The passage of the Pure Food and Drug Act and the Meat Inspection Act in 1906 signified the government's new role in ensuring the safety of the nation's food supply. During the next half-century the implementation of various food-safety laws, as well as the related advances in science and technology, resulted in new food-protection measures, such as milk pasteurization and the inspection and improved sanitization of slaughter plants, canneries, and other processing factories. These measures, along with better farm animal care and improved living standards and personal hygiene, dramatically decreased the societal costs of foodborne diseases. In 1900, the incidence of typhoid fever in the U.S. population was about 100 per 100,000 persons; by 1950, this rate had dropped to 1.7 per 100,000 persons.[1]

From 1950 to 2000, food safety laws, along with scientific understanding and technologic capabilities, continued to evolve. Despite these improvements, however, foodborne diseases continue to cause significant burden in the United States at the beginning of the twenty-first century. Approximately 76 million cases of foodborne illness now occur each year in the United States, including

323,000 hospitalizations and 5200 deaths. The economic cost may be as high as $24 billion per year.[2]

Government agencies at the federal, state, and local levels are charged with the responsibility of applying food-safety laws. These agencies generally fall within two distinct categories: "public health nonregulatory agencies" (or "public health agencies"), which are usually responsible for disease control through surveillance and investigation of individual cases of illness and outbreaks of disease, as well as the scientific research into the host- and pathogen-specific risk factors for foodborne diseases; and "food-safety regulatory agencies" (or "regulatory agencies"), which are usually responsible for drafting and enforcing food-safety requirements with respect to the processors and handlers of food. Food-safety regulatory agencies, by ensuring the safety of the nation's food supply, are also responsible for protecting the public health. However, the specific duties and responsibilities of these types of agencies differ. These differences between public health and regulatory agencies stem from their respective enabling statutes and legal authorities. The duties of public health agencies generally focus on the human illness that results from foodborne pathogens, while the duties of regulatory agencies generally focus on the behavior of the regulated entities and the food products themselves.

Despite these differences in duties and responsibilities, the goals of public health and regulatory agencies complement each other. Public health officials use surveillance reports of foodborne illness from physicians and laboratories to identify and investigate specific cases and outbreaks of illness. These investigations aim to identify a contaminated food so that it can be removed from circulation. Additionally, public health officials may identify unsafe practices at various stages of the human food chain, from the farm to the dinner table, that allowed the contamination and suggest ways in which these practices can be corrected. Regulatory agencies promulgate and enforce regulations that aim to ensure the safety of food along the extremely complex human food chain, which includes the farm, animals and their feed, slaughterhouses, packing and processing plants, transport vehicles, storage and retail facilities, and commercial food establishments. Ensuring compliance entails, among other things, inspection of facilities and testing of product. In turn, the surveillance by public health agencies for human illness and outbreaks then indicates whether these regulations accomplish their intended purpose of disease reduction. Rapid changes in the food supply constantly produce new modes of contamination, which require vigilant disease surveillance and investigation and frequent adjustment of the regulatory framework.[3]

Like all laws, public health law governing the prevention of foodborne disease is shaped by the political process. Participants in this process include the agricultural sector, the food industry, consumer and public interest groups, and academic and professional health associations. Not surprisingly, the promulgation, application, and interpretation of food-safety laws reflect both the interplay of expert scientific opinion and the goals of various political interests. Additionally, coordination of food-safety activities between government agencies at the federal, state, and local levels shapes the application of these laws in a specific setting, such as an outbreak investigation. The jurisdictions of different food-safety agencies, both public health and regulatory, intersect at times, and the division of authority at these intersection points may be subject to interpretation.

These federal, state, and local agencies, both regulatory and nonregulatory, face significant challenges in ensuring food safety because of the complexity of the scientific and political issues that shape food safety laws, as well as the logistical difficulties in quickly and effectively conducting outbreak investigations. To the extent that these agencies can interpret and apply their relevant authorities collaboratively, their efforts to protect the public health will be optimized, particularly in the context of specific outbreak investigations.

LEGAL AUTHORITIES

Various federal, state, and local authorities implement the statutes, regulations, and codes that govern food safety.

Federal Authorities

At the national level, some of the agencies charged with ensuring the safety of the nation's food supply include the Food and Drug Administration (FDA) and the Centers for Disease Control and Prevention (CDC) (both within the U.S. Department of Health and Human Services [DHHS]), the U.S. Department of Agriculture (USDA), and the U.S. Environmental Protection Agency (EPA). These agencies together administer the following food-safety laws: the Federal Food, Drug, and Cosmetic Act (FFDCA),[4] the Public Health Service Act,[5] the Federal Meat Inspection Act,[6] the Poultry Products Inspection Act,[7] the Egg Products Inspection Act,[8] and the Federal Insecticide, Fungicide, and Rodenticide Act.[9] The FDA, USDA, and EPA exercise their authority primarily as food-safety regulatory agencies, while the CDC exercises its authority primarily as a public health nonregulatory agency.

These national regulatory agencies exercise their authority over food safety at three general stages along the farm-to-table continuum: on the farm itself, during subsequent processing of the food, and at distribution. On the farm, the FDA has authority over the safety of food, feed, and animals, including over live food animals (e.g., cattle) before they go to slaughter. Additionally, the

Animal Plant Health Inspection Service (APHIS) of the USDA has the authority to protect plant and animal health on the farm and to ensure the safety of animal vaccines. The EPA has authority over pesticide use on the farm.

The FDA has authority over all food processing, except the slaughter and processing of domesticated meat and poultry and certain egg products, over which the Food Safety Inspection Service (FSIS) of the USDA exercises jurisdiction. Thus, the FDA and the USDA can have authority over different parts of a processing plant that make both meat/poultry and non-meat/non-poultry products. For example, the FDA will inspect the cheese pizza line at a facility, while the USDA will inspect the pepperoni pizza line at that facility. Furthermore, the EPA sets limits for pesticide residues in food (so-called "tolerances"), which the FDA and USDA then enforce. Additionally, under the Agriculture Marketing Act, both the USDA and the U.S. Department of Commerce run inspection programs for food quality (such as for "Grade A" rankings) at processing facilities.[10] At the post-processing stage, the FDA has authority over the labeling, transportation, storage, and retail sale of all food. In practice, however, states handle the regulation of retail establishments, such as restaurants and groceries. The USDA shares authority with the FDA over the labeling, transportation, storage, and retail sale of meat, poultry, and certain egg products. In practice, however, the FDA generally defers to the USDA on these matters.[11]

These agencies exercise their food-safety authority primarily by inspecting facilities (and on some occasions, farms) involved in the production and distribution of food products, as well as approving chemical substances and establishing tolerances in food for those substances (such as pesticides by the EPA and food additives by the FDA). These inspections allow the agency to determine whether the facility or farm, as well as the food product at issue, complies with applicable legal requirements. These inspections can focus on the product itself by sampling and testing for foodborne pathogens.

In the arena of foodborne diseases, the CDC functions as an expert scientific agency providing consultative support to state health departments. The CDC exercises its authority as a public health agency by monitoring the number and causes of various types of foodborne diseases in the United States using data submitted voluntarily by state health departments; by assisting, on request, state health departments investigating outbreaks of disease in humans; and by making recommendations for disease prevention. Other than the rarely exercised power to quarantine emigrants with communicable diseases and the inspection of international cruise ships, the CDC does not exercise regulatory authority, particularly with respect to farms, facilities, and food product. CDC investigations of disease outbreaks, which include the acquiring of records of human illness, are performed at the request of the states. To exercise effectively its surveillance and investigation authority, the CDC relies on the cooperation of state and local health agencies in providing data on human illness and inviting the CDC to conduct specific investigations of such illness. In practice, in an outbreak affecting residents of several states, the CDC plays an indispensable role in coordinating the investigation and analyzing and interpreting the data needed to guide public health action, including regulatory action.

State and Local Authorities

State and local agencies also play an important role in protecting the nation's food supply. These agencies, both regulatory and public health, share numerous responsibilities with the above-described federal agencies in exercising food safety authority. For example, numerous states have laws governing the processing and distribution of food product that are similar to laws administered by the FDA and the USDA.[12] Thus, investigators in these states will conduct investigations of facilities, including the sampling and testing of food products, that are also inspected by the FDA and the USDA. Furthermore, as noted above, although the FDA has jurisdiction over restaurants, groceries, and other retail food establishments, the agency generally defers to state and local agencies to enforce its own food codes against these establishments through inspections.

The FDA has issued a model food code that it encourages state and local agencies to adopt and enforce with respect to the retail establishments within their respective jurisdictions.[13] Additionally, the FDA has entered into cooperative agreements with states that allow state and local heath agencies to inspect shellfish and milk processors. Finally, unlike the CDC, state and local public health agencies exercise the authority to collect information about ill persons for disease surveillance and to directly investigate outbreaks of human illness along the farm-to-table continuum, from interviewing patients to inspecting implicated food processing facilities.[14] Under the health codes of some states, the state health department can seize foods that threaten human health.[15]

The FDA as an Example of a Food-Safety Regulatory Agency

An analysis of the FDA's regulatory authority provides a useful framework in considering relevant legal issues facing federal, state, and local food-safety agencies. The FDA is charged with implementing the FFDCA, as well as various parts of other statutes, such as the Public Health Service Act and the Egg Products Inspection Act. The FFDCA is the primary authority by which the FDA exercises authority over foods, and the statute sets forth applicable standards for food safety. (The USDA operates under a separate act and therefore has a somewhat different framework, history, and operating culture.) The statute, 21 U.S.C. § 402, defines certain categories of food as "adulterated." Furthermore, the statute, 21 U.S.C. § 301, sets forth those acts that are prohibited. 21 U.S.C. § 301(a) prohibits the introduction of adulterated food into interstate commerce, and 21 U.S.C. § 301(k) prohibits any act that results in the adulteration of food while it is held for sale after shipment in interstate commerce. These two provisions, working together, cover the stages of the farm-to-table continuum from the food producer to the retailer. However, the statute requires interstate commerce for the FDA to exercise jurisdiction. This requirement supplements the interstate commerce requirement of the U.S. Constitution, which limits all federal regulatory agencies' jurisdiction.[16] Food produced, distributed, and consumed wholly within one state does not, therefore, fall under the jurisdiction of the FDA pursuant to the FFDCA.

Food is deemed to be "adulterated" under the act, 21 U.S.C. § 402(a)(1), if it "bears or contains any poisonous or deleterious substance which may render it injurious to health." This provision applies to the presence in food of pathogens, such as *Salmonella* and *Listeria*, that cause illness in humans. Additionally, a food is deemed adulterated under 21 U.S.C. § 402(a)(2) if it bears or contains a food additive or pesticide chemical residue above those tolerances established by the FDA and the EPA, respectively, as safe for use in food. Furthermore, food is deemed adulterated under 21 U.S.C. § 402(a)(3) if it "consists in whole or in part of any filthy, putrid, or decomposed substance, or if it is otherwise unfit for food." This provision applies to the presence in food of excreta from rodents or insect fragments, for example.

The above provisions focus on the condition of the food product itself. The definition of adulterated food also includes the conditions of manufacturing and handling of the food product. Food is deemed adulterated under 21 U.S.C. § 402(a)(4) if "it has been prepared, packed, or held under insanitary conditions whereby it may have become contaminated with filth, or whereby it may have been rendered injurious to health." This provision applies where a food processor, retailer, or other establishment has failed, for example, to maintain a clean facility or to handle product at the proper temperatures.

If an individual or a farm or facility commits a prohibited act under 21 U.S.C. § 301 with respect to a food that is adulterated under 21 U.S.C. § 402, then such an act is subject to legal penalties and enforcement action under the FFDCA. These remedies allow the FDA to enforce the legal requirements of those programs that it is charged by statute to administer. The agency, for example, can pursue criminal action under 21 U.S.C. § 303(a) against an individual or company for any violations of its statute, such as the introduction by a farm or facility of food that is adulterated because of the presence of filth, contamination by a substance that may render it injurious to health, or the inadequate processing and handling of food by the facility. These criminal remedies, as punitive measures, are intended to punish individuals and companies for their past violative behavior.

The FDA can also pursue civil remedies, such as an injunction under 21 U.S.C. § 302, against individuals and companies that commit a prohibited act under 21 U.S.C. § 301, for example, for the distribution of adulterated food. An injunction action is based on the FDA's evidence of past food contamination or inadequate food handling practices at the defendant's facility. However, the goal of an injunction is forward-looking in that the FDA seeks an order from a federal district court that would require a violative facility's operations to cease until the FDA determines that the facility, by addressing its inadequacies, is ready to resume operations. The FDA pursues injunction actions when, for example, a current and definite health hazard (such as food with *Listeria*) exists; or chronic violative practices exist that, although not having produced a clear health hazard, have not yet been corrected.[17] If the FDA concludes from an inspection that an immediate shutdown of the facility is warranted, then the agency may seek more expedient relief in the form of a preliminary injunction or temporary restraining order from a court. Thus, an injunction action is a tool that the FDA can wield to ensure that a facility or farm does not continue to distribute adulterated food.

Additionally, the FDA may pursue civil remedies with respect to the violative product itself. For example, in an injunction proceeding, the FDA may also legally seek an immediate recall of product when the agency has concluded that such product may injure the health of consumers. Furthermore, the statute provides in 21 U.S.C. § 304 for the civil remedy of seizure of an adulterated food "when introduced into or while in interstate commerce or while held for sale (whether or not the first sale) after shipment in interstate commerce." A seizure action allows the FDA to remove from the farm-to-table continuum a specific lot of food that consists of filth or is contaminated by a substance that is injurious to health or has been processed or handled under insanitary conditions. A seizure action is an "in rem" proceeding against the adulterated food itself in which the U.S. Marshal's Office typically holds the product in its protective custody until the federal district court decides the outcome of the case and the product's disposition. The applicable rules of procedure provide for individuals with any property interest in the food, known as "claimants," to enter the case against the government and argue for the release of the goods.[18] Typically, if the court rules that the food is "adulterated," then the court will order destruction of the food.[19]

State agencies are not limited by the jurisdiction requirement of the FFDCA for interstate commerce. Furthermore, in some instances the enforcement tools available to the states can be swifter. For example, the state law of Florida authorizes its food-safety agency to issue a temporary "stop-sale" order, without the necessity of a court order, to immediately detain product.[19]

In applying the statutory adulteration standard, the FDA has implemented regulations that set forth in more detail the legal requirements for facilities that process foods. Specifically, the regulations at 21 C.F.R. Part 110 specify the requirements of "current good manufacturing practice" in manufacturing, packing, and holding human food. The provisions of this regulation require, among other things, that food facilities maintain clean equipment and grounds, as well as ensure that their employees maintain good sanitation practices.[20] Additionally, the FDA has enacted specific regulations for the seafood industry at 21 C.F.R. Part 123. The core of these regulations requires each seafood firm to maintain and follow a Hazard Analysis and Critical Control Point Plan (HACCP plan) to ensure that seafood is held, processed, and shipped at proper temperatures and times to prevent contamination by food pathogens.[21]

The firm must identify in its HACCP plan the relevant food safety hazards that are reasonably likely to occur during the storage, processing, and shipping of its product and identify the "critical control points" designed to control these hazards that could be introduced in the processing plant environment.[22] Furthermore, the firm must identify the "critical limits" that must be met at these points to prevent contamination by food pathogens and monitor production for these limits.[22] For example, the processors of ready-to-eat crabmeat will typically set specific minimum and/or maximum times and temperatures for the cooking and handling of product. Finally, the FDA has enacted similar regulations with respect to specific food products, such as juice,[23] low-acid canned foods,[24] and acidified food.[25]

The FDA also has enacted procedures and standards for the recall of adulterated product at 21 C.F.R. Part 7. A recall is advantageous to the FDA because it allows the agency to ensure the immediate withdrawal of a dangerous food from the marketplace without taking the various legal steps and procedures to ensure a court-ordered seizure. Although these regulations allow the FDA to request the immediate recall of a food product with a pathogen, this action is, ultimately, voluntary on the part of the firm. However, the regulations also authorize the FDA to issue public notice of its recall requests, which can persuade firms to comply by focusing public scrutiny on the firm's response.[26]

The FDA periodically inspects regulated facilities to ensure that they follow the relevant statutory and regulatory requirements.[27] Typically, these inspections are initiated by the FDA as part of its routine inspection program rather than by the discovery of human illness that has resulted from pathogens in food handled or processed by the facility. During these inspections FDA investigators observe and record the processing and handling of food products, as well as take product and environmental samples to be tested by FDA laboratories for filth and pathogens, among other things. If a facility fails to maintain adequate sanitary conditions at the plant or if samples of product test positive for filth or pathogens, then the FDA can consider its options for bringing enforcement actions for civil or criminal relief. The FDA may also request that a firm immediately recall violative product.

LEGAL ISSUES AND CONTROVERSIES

Most of the legal issues and controversies in the realm of food safety have arisen in the context of enforcement actions brought by regulatory agencies against members of industry or their product. The FDA, in particular, brings numerous seizure actions each year against adulterated food, including product that has tested positive for a pathogen, as well as injunction actions against food processors that distribute adulterated food under 21 U.S.C. § 402(a)(1) and fail to follow good sanitary practices under 21 U.S.C. § 402(a)(4). The FDA has faced two general types of challenges in these actions: factual and legal.

First, claimants in seizure actions and defendants in injunction actions have previously challenged the adequacy of the FDA's sampling and testing methods in detecting the pathogen or the accuracy of its inspectional findings at the facility in question. Thus, the FDA has developed internal guidance for its investigators to follow in collecting samples of food, documenting the chain of custody from the time of collection to the time of testing, and recording the testing of product and the results.[28] Additionally, the FDA ensures that the tests used at its regional laboratories are accepted throughout the scientific community as valid methods.[29] These procedures help to ensure the accuracy and validity of the test results in each individual case, as well as the sufficiency of evidence under the Federal Rules of Civil Procedure. Furthermore, these procedures ensure that the FDA handles the sampling and testing uniformly across the food industry.

While conducting an inspection, FDA investigators accompany a responsible individual at the facility in observing all of the relevant manufacturing and processing functions.[30] The investigators take detailed notes and photographs of the sanitary conditions. At the conclusion of the inspection, the investigator notes all observed violations of good manufacturing practices at the facility, such as failure to maintain clean equipment or lack of controls to ensure adequate cooking time and temperature. At the conclusion of the investigation the investigator will list these violations in a written report and review them with the facility's responsible individual, who then verifies and signs the report.[31] These steps help ensure that the FDA is prepared to support the factual bases of its cases with sufficient evidence.

Second, claimants in seizure actions and defendants in injunction actions often challenge whether the FDA's inspectional findings and test results, even if accurate and valid, actually show that the food in question is adulterated under the applicable legal standard. The courts have considered many such issues related to the presence of pathogens in food and insanitary conditions at food facilities. For example, courts have considered the scope of 21 U.S.C. § 402(a)(1) in defining an adulterated food as a "poisonous or deleterious substance which may render it injurious to health." Courts have held specifically that the presence of a pathogen in a food product, such as *Salmonella*, satisfies this definition, even though the pathogen's harmful effects can be avoided by proper cooking and handling.[32,33] Furthermore, to satisfy this legal standard, courts have found that the agency does not have to identify any individuals who have become sick as a result of eating the contaminated product at issue.[34]

Furthermore, courts have considered what proof is required when the FDA has brought an adulteration claim under 21 U.S.C. § 402(a)(4) on the basis of its findings of insanitary conditions at a facility. Courts have held that the FDA is not required to show that any individual food product would be injurious to health (i.e., by the presence of a contaminant, such as *Salmonella*). Instead, the FDA must show only that the insanitary conditions at a facility are such that they are reasonably likely to result in the production of contaminated food product.[35–37]

This standard, by placing the burden on the food processor to maintain sanitary conditions at all stages and locations of production, provides greater protection for the consumer in preventing the reasonable possibility of contamination. By shifting the focus of inquiry from specific product test results to the general conditions at a plant, this statutory standard allows the FDA to bring enforcement actions in circumstances where a real probability exists of future harm to the consumer but no specific evidence of contamination or incidences of human illness have been documented. This legal requirement is also helpful to the FDA in protecting the public health because, as a practical matter, the agency has neither the resources nor the time to test a representative sample of every product lot that is distributed each day from a food facility for a pathogen.

This legal analysis concerning the FDA's adulteration standard demonstrates that the agency's primary focus and authority is preventing contamination of food product before distribution. Thus, a significant part of the FDA's food-safety programs are based on its inspection of facilities and testing of product to determine industry compliance with the relevant legal standards applicable to that facility and product. Of course, the effectiveness of the statute in protecting the public depends on the compliance by industry and the efficiency and resources of the FDA's enforcement programs. The effectiveness of the public health system in investigating and determining the causes of foodborne disease outbreaks is a key to identify circumstances in which the statutes themselves or their enforcement still permit food contamination and require updating.[38–40] With the nation's recent heightened focus on bioterrorism issues following the events of September 2001, the FDA's food-safety budget has increased significantly.[41]

The agency has adopted this forward-looking approach in its HACCP regulations, such as for seafood. These regulations, 21 C.F.R. Part 123, as described briefly above, are intended to provide additional protection to the consumer by requiring seafood facilities to establish written critical control points in an HACCP plan for the various steps in processing (such as cooking, preparing, and packing) and to record the relevant critical control point measurements (such as actual times and temperatures) for each batch of product at the various stages. The failure to follow these HACCP requirements, in itself, constitutes an insanitary condition that causes the food to be adulterated under 21 U.S.C. § 402(a)(4).[42] The USDA has also implemented similar regulations requiring HACCP plans for meat packers, with dramatic results.[43]

During FDA inspections under the HACCP program, the investigator focuses much time reviewing the records to ensure compliance with the firm's HACCP plan. These HACCP regulations ease the burden on the regulatory agency to conduct inspections because the burden lies on each individual firm to ensure that the food product will not become contaminated by following its individual HACCP plan. The FDA has recently begun to initiate injunction proceedings against various seafood firms that have repeatedly failed to follow such plans.[44]

PRACTICE CONSIDERATIONS

Using Epidemiologic Data as the Basis of Regulatory Actions

In the outbreak setting, an epidemiologic investigation can provide strong scientific evidence linking illness to a particular food.[45] The strength of the association, in terms of its probability of being true and not a statistical fluke, are quantifiable. Epidemiologic analysis involves the assessment of the various possible exposures to a pathogen in individual patients in an outbreak. Laboratory results can sometimes confirm such an epidemiologic association between an exposure and a disease. For example, in an outbreak investigation, the isolation of indistinguishable pathogens from a patient sample and from an implicated food confirms the statistical association.[38,46–51] However, the agent responsible for an outbreak may not be isolated from or identified in the implicated food for several reasons: Some organisms and toxins are difficult or impossible to detect in food using available methods; agents may have been reduced or eliminated from food samples by freezing, temperature abuse, or overgrowth by other microorganisms; and in many outbreaks samples of implicated foods no longer exist.

If epidemiologic data obtained from the study of an illness in humans implicate a specific type of food or food producer, then food-safety regulatory agencies can initiate or participate in a "traceback" investigation. Successful tracebacks typically depend on an epidemiologic assessment of traceback data to optimally link the human illness findings with food distributor records and plant or farm evaluation. Public health agency epidemiologists and regulatory agency investigators at this stage often negotiate informally the details of their interaction.

In some outbreak investigations, cases of human illness may still be occurring when a suspected food is identified by epidemiologic methods, so quick public health action is necessary to end the outbreak. Such action may entail issuing a press release that warns the public to avoid consuming a specific food, requesting a product recall, or initiating legal action to shut down a production facility. Strong epidemiologic data that implicate a contaminated food vehicle can be the basis for rapid, targeted, and carefully applied control measures to prevent further illness and death, even without laboratory confirmation.

For example, in 1997, an outbreak of *Escherichia coli* O157:H7 infections caused 70 illnesses, including 14 cases of hemolytic uremic syndrome and one death. Epidemiologic data strongly linked these illnesses with consumption of a particular brand of unpasteurized apple juice. State, local, and CDC investigators concluded that the most effective response would be to warn the public and recall the implicated juice. Because of the FDA's authority in regulating food products, such as the juice at issue, the investigators presented their findings and conclusion to FDA staff in an emergency session. The FDA then issued public notice of the suspect apple juice and requested that the manufacturer recall immediately all lots of the juice. The manufacturer complied with the FDA's request. Later, laboratory tests confirmed the epidemiologic findings by isolating indistinguishable strains of *E. coli* O157:H7 in patient samples and in the implicated juice. This sequence of events demonstrates successful regulatory action that was based on the use of epidemiologic data.[38] The CDC's and the FDA's prompt actions in responding to the outbreak probably prevented additional cases of illness and possibly deaths.

However, despite the success of such multiple agency efforts, the potential remains for inefficiency when public health and regulatory agencies act on epidemiologic data in exigent circumstances. Such inefficiency is caused, in large part, by the legal and administrative divisions of authority between public health and regulatory agencies for the pursuit of outbreak investigations, particularly for the use of epidemiologic data. As a result of these limitations and the exigency of circumstances, government officials at various agencies often must implement ad hoc procedures in coordinating each individual outbreak investigation and the use of epidemiologic data. Both public health and regulatory agencies might be able to act more quickly and coordinate more effectively their responses if these agencies would collaborate prospectively in developing specific guidelines for the shared use of epidemiologic data in certain types of investigations.[52,53]

Coordinating Outbreak and Traceback Investigations

In an outbreak of foodborne disease, a traceback investigation attempts to determine the source of the disease by tracking the food vehicle to its origins to determine the source of contamination. Investigators often review the records of vendors, shippers, producers, and processors involved in handling the implicated food and may inspect their facilities. These activities are within the jurisdiction of local, state, and federal government regulatory agencies that exercise authority over the particular industries. Because the traceback is often an integral part of the outbreak investigation, epidemiologists can and should participate in the traceback investigation.

Analysis of the epidemiologic data, combined with the results of the traceback and environmental investigation, can allow the investigators to determine where contamination is likely to have occurred—at the distributor, processing facility, or farm. Relevant information gathered in the course of a traceback investigation includes the volume of food produced at a facility or farm and the area in which it was distributed; other foods that might contain the contaminated ingredient of a multi-ingredient food; the growth, production, or transportation stages at which contamination may have occurred; and the specific practice or circumstance that allowed for contamination. For example, in an investigation of a multistate outbreak of *Salmonella* serotype Agona from toasted oats cereal, traceback was facilitated by epidemiologists determining the dates of production of contaminated cereal from cereal boxes collected at patients' homes.[47] These findings are relevant both to control the acute outbreak and to identify and ultimately change farming, production, or transport processes that allowed for food contamination.[54]

Because of the need to provide continuity between the epidemiologic data and the product information, the respective responsibilities of public health and regulatory agencies overlap. Agencies often handle this overlap by making ad hoc arrangements in each circumstance. Public health epidemiologists may be invited to accompany regulatory investigators in the field or go under the authority of state agencies. Otherwise, they must await a written report from the regulatory agency, which typically is issued months after the investigation and may not address all of their concerns. Optimally, epidemiologists from either the public health or regulatory agency participate personally and directly in the traceback investigation. One approach to maximize the effectiveness of such outbreak investigations in controlling foodborne diseases would be to establish a standing group of investigators from regulatory agencies whose principal responsibility is outbreak investigation to work with public health epidemiologists on traceback investigations.

Sharing Information about Products and Producers Among Investigators

Public health officials at the CDC and state and local health departments must know the identity and brand names of suspected foods to confirm or dismiss the role of those foods in an outbreak investigation. For example, in investigating an outbreak in which ground meat is suspected, health officials will often identify stores at which patients purchased meat and may then request the help of regulatory agencies to assist in tracing the suspect meat to the distributor(s) and the processor. Brand name identities are necessary to determine whether the implicated meat indeed came from the same source and, if so, to focus the investigation on implicating or excluding that particular source as the cause of the outbreak. Public health officials have a strong incentive not to publicly identify prematurely any foods generically or by brand name because this identification might bias members of the public being questioned in the course of the investigation about foods they consumed, resulting in the failure to reach scientifically valid results. Regulatory agencies frequently obtain production records, distribution information, and other documents related to food products from members of industry. These agencies are not generally legally prohibited from disclosing the identity of products in communicating with other federal agencies during an outbreak investigation, although such disclosure is usually conditioned on the satisfaction of certain requirements.[55]

On the other hand, these regulatory agencies are limited by specific confidentiality rules that prohibit them from sharing certain other types of information with officials from other agencies, such as a public health agency, who are not bound by these rules.[55,56] For example, the FFDCA and other laws generally prohibit the FDA from disclosing trade secret information to the public, including other government agencies outside of the DHHS.[57,58] Furthermore, these laws prohibit the FDA from disclosing confidential commercial information to state and local government agencies that fail to satisfy certain conditions.[56,58] The FDA may happen to observe and record such information during its inspection of facilities, such as the method of processing a specific food, and thus may share such information with state and local public health agencies only if such conditions are satisfied. This information can be critical for public health agencies in identifying a specific source of pathogen and cause of contamination.

Similarly, the ability of public health and regulatory agencies to share information with each other may be asymmetric. Public health agencies are generally allowed pursuant to their laws to share any information with other agencies after removing the names and other personal identifiers of individuals. Regulatory agencies, on the other hand, may be reluctant to share any information that potentially constitutes part of a legal enforcement action, particularly a criminal case against an industry member. For example, in a 1999 investigation of an outbreak of *E. coli* O157:H7 in patrons of a national fast-food chain, the CDC suspected that ground beef had been contaminated and requested that the USDA determine the distribution of meat from the processor. The USDA dispatched a large team of investigators to the meat-processing facility, where initial findings reportedly suggested a violation of law. After becoming involved in the case, the USDA would not share data on its findings because of its concern with compromising evidence in a potential criminal case (CDC, unpublished data, 1999). Similar incidents have occurred for investigations pursued by CDC and FDA and by other regulatory agencies. These scenarios are a prime example of different interests driving government agencies with broadly complementary, but at times divergent, missions. Public health agencies can sometimes negotiate with regulatory agencies to obtain a limited sharing of their information, but the resulting delays in reaching such agreements can compromise implementation of appropriate public health responses. More explicit authority for agencies to share such information in these circumstances could assist in the conduct of outbreak investigations.

Laboratory Testing Issues

Another practical issue facing food-safety agencies with legal implications involves laboratory testing of food or environmental specimens and use of the results in public health investigations or enforcement actions. In the case of regulatory agencies, laboratory testing is generally conducted in U.S. government or other authorized laboratories. The FDA has issued information about international requirements for the testing of product by foreign laboratories.[59] In the context of enforcement litigation, regulatory agencies, such as the FDA, would not usually rely on a foreign laboratory's results because of the procedural requirements applicable to the sampling and testing of evidence, particularly when the product has not been in that agency's custody and control. In a multinational outbreak of *Salmonella* Agona in the early 1990s, a public health laboratory in the United Kingdom identified the pathogen at issue in the suspected food. FDA could not rely on the laboratory results because these findings were not from a U.S. government or other authorized laboratory.

A related issue involves the effect of a regulatory agency's choice of laboratory tests, based on its goals for such testing, on the investigations and related actions of public health agencies. For example, the finding of *Salmonella* serotype Enteritidis in eggs, poultry, or the environment at a poultry farm is typically sufficient to trigger regulatory action, regardless of whether human illness resulted. Therefore, agency laboratories in many instances do not further subtype *Salmonella* Enteritidis isolates in these samples, although such subtyping may help confirm the epidemiologic link between eggs from the farm and illness in the humans who consumed them. This subtyping is important to epidemiologic investigators because the findings confirm the validity of the epidemiologic methods and may contribute further to the understanding of the mechanisms of contamination and transmission.

Federal Agency Regulation of Farms: Effect of Interstate Commerce Requirement

Finally, the regulatory status of farms that are identified as the possible source of contaminated food, where no interstate commerce is involved, represents a potential difficulty for federal agencies in outbreak investigations. If an epidemiologic investigation identifies a farm as the possible source of an outbreak, investigation of the farm would be important so that any problem on the farm can be identified and corrected, and such information subsequently could be used to prevent similar contamination events on other farms. Where no interstate commerce has occurred—that is, eggs from the farm have not been shipped across a stateline—jurisdiction over the farm may rest solely with the state agriculture department. The resources of some state agricultural departments, which can be politically influenced as a result of their contradictory dual role of both promoting and regulating agriculture, may limit their effectiveness in carrying out investigations.

In one example, epidemiologic investigation of a statewide outbreak of *Salmonella* Enteritidis infections strongly implicated eggs from a cooperative supplied by five chicken farms.[60] The state agriculture department was asked to perform microbiologic testing on the farms to confirm the source of the outbreak. A standardized, validated FDA protocol for such sampling existed; however, the state agriculture department obtained less than 5% of the number of samples required in the FDA protocol. Tests on these samples did not detect *Salmonella*, and the state agriculture department announced that the epidemiologic findings were thereby invalidated. The subsequent discovery of interstate commerce in the suspected eggs triggered federal jurisdiction and allowed the FDA to investigate and sample the farms more thoroughly, which showed heavy contamination at one of these egg farms. In another example, a commercial dairy was implicated in a multistate outbreak of *Salmonella* serotype Typhimurium infections from contaminated milk. The dairy had passed regular inspections by the state agriculture department. However, FDA inspectors then found gross violations of the sanitary code sufficient to close the dairy.[61]

EMERGING ISSUES

Implications of the Changing Locus of Outbreaks and Public Health Legal Authority

The locus of legal authority for public health agencies is at the local and state levels. This focus was specified when most foodborne disease prevention measures were local because food was produced mostly within individual states, and disease outbreaks typically occurred in small groups of people who knew each other, so the outbreaks were readily detectable. However, in the opening years of the twenty-first century, food safety issues are increasingly national—and even international—because of extensive international food trade, the consolidation of food manufacturing and processing, and the widespread distribution of food products. These conditions have resulted in large, diffuse outbreaks affecting persons in many states and even countries. These outbreaks may be difficult to detect at the state level because the diffuse distribution of ill persons may result in initially imperceptible increases in infections.

Additionally, differences in state public health laws may impede response to foodborne disease. For example, individual states determine which diseases must be reported by laboratories and physicians and in turn voluntarily report these cases to the CDC. Even though an estimated 27% of deaths from foodborne disease in the United States result from *Listeria monocytogenes*, this infection is not reportable in 13 states. Two large outbreaks of *L. monocytogenes* resulting from contaminated commercially produced hot dogs were detected only through collation of surveillance data from several states because cases were spread over many states with no geographic clustering and occurred over several months.[62,63]

Another difficulty facing public health authorities is that reporting of food-borne disease outbreaks is voluntary. Although such voluntary reporting is widely practiced, no standard exists for the immediate reporting by states to the CDC of outbreaks that may extend beyond one state or even beyond the national borders (suggestive features would include a large number of infected persons within a state, wide geographic distribution of cases, involvement of travelers, implication of a food imported into or exported from the involved state, or relation to a dining facility near a state border). Rapid, efficient investigation of the growing number of multistate outbreaks would be facilitated by uniform rapid reporting standards. As foodborne disease outbreaks become less of a local and more of a national or international phenomenon, consideration should be given to appropriately revising the public health legal structure. Such restructuring might be considered a public health corollary of the authority of federal regulatory agencies under the interstate commerce clause of their respective enabling statutes—when events affecting human health extend beyond a single state or extend to the international arena, they would fall under the jurisdiction of federal public health agencies, rather than the individual states alone.

Food Disparagement Laws

Another emerging issue for the regulation of food safety involves the passage of a unique class of state laws that restrict discussion of food safety issues. These so-called food disparagement laws enacted in the 1990s in 13 states make persons legally liable for asserting that certain foods are unsafe for human consumption.[64] These laws burden critics of foods with the requirement that they demonstrate that their claims are backed by scientific data of high reliability. Thus, for several reasons, these laws are restrictive in a manner unparalleled in the United States. First, the food disparagement laws cover generic classes of products, such as "perishable foods," rather than the product of an individual enterprise. Second, the laws require the critic to demonstrate not simply good faith in his or her information but rather satisfy a uniquely high standard of proof. One of the most far-reaching of these laws is in Colorado.[65] Under its provisions, critics are subject to criminal prosecution for food disparagement. Although these laws exist in a minority of states, they exert a nationwide effect because national publishers and electronic media purveyors fear they might be sued in any such state where their publications or broadcasts are available to the public.

The best-known case involving food disparagement laws was the $10 million lawsuit by the Texan Cattlemen's Association against the television talk-show host Oprah Winfrey for her allegedly disparaging comments about hamburgers and the risk for *E. coli* O157:H7 infection.[66] Although the court dismissed the suit because the state failed to make its case under the standards of the Texas food disparagement law, the court did not question the constitutionality of the statute.

Despite its seemingly favorable outcome, this litigation illustrates the dangerous potential of food disparagement laws. These laws, in effect, can allow for the organized intimidation of any perceived critics of the food industry by the filing of multimillion-dollar lawsuits for exercising what in many other forms would be considered constitutionally protected speech. This effect is likely to inhibit most critics who lack Ms. Winfrey's resources from engaging in debate. The limitation of free public discussion on general issues of food safety can inhibit the development of sound public health policy in this area. The great public debate on food safety that resulted in the passage of the Pure Food and Drug Act in 1906 was launched by Upton Sinclair's description of unsanitary and poor working conditions in Chicago's meat-packing plants in *The Jungle*.[67] Oddly enough, under today's food disparagement laws, he may well have had difficulty finding a publisher.

Regulation of Food Production

Another crucial issue recently emerging for food safety involves the differences between agencies in regulating the production of food at the farm compared with the remaining phases of the farm-to-table continuum. Many agencies at the federal, state, and local levels generally regulate processed foods like any other consumer product subject to government regulation, such that these agencies essentially view foods contaminated by pathogens as defective products under their respective laws (such as under the FDA's adulteration provisions). FDA inspections of facilities and food products, as well as any resulting enforcement action, place the burden on the facility and individuals to comply with the law and absorb the loss of any noncompliance. When contaminated food is defined as a defective product, that is, "adulterated" under the FFDCA, then monetary losses from any destruction of condemned product, shutdown of a plant, and loss of sales are borne by the manufacturer. Thus, this burden creates a strong incentive on regulated industry to comply with regulations and produce safe foods. Similarly, restaurants are subject to licensing, regulation, inspection, and sanctions for violations by state and local agencies.

On the other hand, farms and farm produce, as broadly defined, are under a different regulatory scheme, particularly at the state level. Contamination of animal-derived foods at the level of the farm with organisms pathogenic to humans is often considered a "no-fault" event in which the state assumes the cost by indemnifying the farmer for financial losses and upgrading safety standards. Regular inspection, mandatory safety plans, and sanctions for farms are generally not widely employed by states in improving the safety of animal-derived foods. Agriculture in the United States, however, is increasingly characterized by industrial scale animal and produce production.[68,69] Thus, from a public health perspective, farm produce, as part of the farm-to-table continuum, should be treated under the law as a consumer product, just like processed food or a restaurant meal, and should be regulated with similar rigor.

CONCLUSION

Public health and food-safety regulatory agencies face many challenges today in ensuring the safety of the U.S. food supply. The emergence of new pathogens and sources of transmission, the rapidly changing practices for food production and distribution, and the practical difficulties in responding to foodborne disease outbreaks are issues that federal, state, and local government agencies must address in protecting the public health. These agencies rely on their scientific and administrative capabilities, within the boundary of their legal authorities, in crafting general programs and specific actions to handle these food-safety issues. As food-safety challenges evolve, so must agencies' legal authorities, along with their scientific and administrative capabilities. This dynamic has been illustrated during the last century by the evolution of laws, and scientific and administrative advancements, in response to emerging food-safety threats. This dynamic is likely to continue throughout the next century, as public health and food-safety regulatory agencies require new legal authorities to employ more advanced and effective scientific and administrative tools against ever-changing food-safety dangers.

References

1. CDC. Achievements in public health, 1900–1999. Safer and healthier foods. *MMWR* 1999;48:905–13.
2. Mead P, Slutsker L, Dietz V, et al. Food-related illness and death in the United States. *Emerg Infect Dis* 1999;5:607–25.
3. Swerdlow DL, Altekruse S. Foodborne diseases in the global village: what's on the plate for the 21st century. In: Schled WM, Craig WA, Hughes JM, eds. *Emerging Infections 2*. Washington, DC: ASM Press, 1998: pp. 273–94.
4. Act of June 25, 1938, Ch. 675, 52 Stat. 1040 (codified at 21 U.S.C. §§ 301–97 [2001]).
5. Act of July 1, 1944, Ch. 373, 58 Stat. 682 (codified at 42 U.S.C. §§ 201–300qq-91 [2001]).
6. Pub. L. No. 90-201, 81 Stat. 584 (1967) (codified at 21 U.S.C. §§ 601–91 [2001]).

7. Pub. L. No. 85-172, 71 Stat. 441 (1957) (codified at 21 U.S.C. §§ 451–71 [2001]).

8. Pub. L. No. 91-597, 84 Stat. 1620 (1970) (codified at 21 U.S.C. §§ 1031–56 [2001]).

9. Federal Insecticide, Fungicide and Rodenticide Act of Oct. 30, 1947, Ch. 125, 61 Stat. 163 (codified at 7 U.S.C. §§ 136–136y [2001]).

10. Act of August 14, 1946, Ch. 966, Title II, 60 Stat. 1087 (codified at U.S.C. §§ 1621–37b [2001]).

11. FDA. *Compliance Policy Guide,* Sec. 565.100 (Aug. 2000), available at http://www.fda.gov/ora/compliance_ref/cpg/default.htm. Accessed December 20, 2001.

12. California Health and Safety Code, Division 104 (Environmental Health), Part 5 (Sherman Food, Drug, and Cosmetic Laws), West's Ann. Cal. Health & Safety Code § 111150 *et seq.* (2001).

13. FDA. *Food Code* (1999). Available at http://www.cfsan.fda.gov/~dms/fc01-toc.html. Accessed December 20, 2001.

14. California Health and Safety Code, Division 101 (Administration of Public Health), Part 3 (Local Health Departments); Division 102 (Vital Records and Health Statistics); Division 104 (Environmental Health), Part 7 (Retail Food); West's Ann. Cal. Health & Safety Code (2001).

15. Florida Statutes Annotated, Title XXIX (Public Health), Chapter 381(6) (Imminent Dangers, Stop-Sale Orders), West's FSA § 381.0072 (2001).

16. U.S. Constitution, Article I, Section 8, Subsection 3.

17. FDA. *Regulatory Procedures Manual,* Chapter 6, Subchapter Injunctions (Aug. 1997). Available at http://www.fda.gov/ora/compliance_ref/rpm_new2/.

18. Federal Supplemental Rules for Certain Admiralty and Maritime Claims, Rule C.

19. 21 U.S.C. § 304(d)(1) (2001).

20. 21 C.F.R. §§ 110.10, 110.35, 110.37, and 110.40 (2001).

21. 21 C.F.R. § 123.6 (2001).

22. 21 C.F.R. § 123.6(c) (2001).

23. 21 C.F.R. Part 120 (2001).

24. 21 C.F.R. Part 113 (2001).

25. 21 C.F.R. Part 114 (2001).

26. 21 C.F.R. § 7.50 (2001).

27. FDA. *Investigations Operations Manual,* Chapter 5 (2001), available at http://www.fda.gov/ora/inspect_ref/iom/Contents/ch5_TOC.html. Accessed December 20, 2001.

28. FDA. *Investigations Operations Manual.* (2001) Chapter 4. Sampling. Available at http://www.fda.gov/ora/inspect_ref/iom/Contents/ch4_TOC.html. Accessed December 20, 2001.

29. FDA. *Laboratory Procedures Manual* (2001). Available at http://www.fda.gov/ora/science_rcf/lpm/lpmtc_dec02.html. Accessed December 20, 2001.

30. FDA. *Investigations Operations Manual* (2001). Subchapter 511, Notice of inspection. Available at http://www.fda.gov/ora/inspect_ref/iom/chaptertext/510part1.html#511. Accessed March 21, 2002.

31. FDA. *Investigations Operations Manual* (2001). Subchapter 512, Reports of observations. Available at http://www.fda.gov/ora/inspect_ref/iom/chaptertext/510part2.html#512. Accessed March 21, 2002.

32. *Continental Seafoods, Inc. v. Schweiker*, 674 F.2d 38 (D.C. Cir. 1982).

33. *United States v. 1200 Cans . . . Pasteurized Whole Eggs*, 339 F.Supp. 131 (N.D. Ga. 1972).

34. *Schweiker*, 674 F.2d at 43–4.
35. *United States v. 1200 Cans . . . Pasteurized Whole Eggs*, 339 F.Supp. at 141.
36. *United States v. International Exterminator Corporation*, 294 F.2d 270, 271 (5th Cir. 1961).
37. *Berger v. United States*, 200 F.2d 818, 821 (8th Cir. 1952).
38. Cody S, Glynn K, Farrar JA, et al. An outbreak of *Escherichia coli* O157:H7 infection from unpasteurized commercial apple juice. *Ann Intern Med* 1999;130:202–9.
39. St. Louis ME, Morse DL, Potter ME, et al., The emergence of grade A eggs as a major source of *Salmonella* Enteritidis infections: implications for the control of salmonellosis. *JAMA* 1988;259:2103–7.
40. Sivapalasingam SKA, Ying M, Frisch A, et al. A multistate outbreak of *Salmonella* Newport infections linked to mango consumption, November–December 1999 [latebreaker abstract]. In: 49th Annual Epidemic Intelligence Service (EIS) Conference. Atlanta: Centers for Disease Control and Prevention, 2000.
41. FDA. FY 2003 budget summary. p. 12. Available at http://www.fda.gov/oc/oms/ofm/budget/2003/BIB2003.pdf. Accessed May 10, 2002.
42. 21 C.F.R. § 123.6(g) (2001).
43. 9 C.F.R. Part 417 (Hazard Analysis and Critical Control Point Systems) (2001).
44. *United States v. Blue Ribbon Smoked Fish, Inc., et alia*, CV-01–3887 (CPS) (EDNY 2001).
45. Goodman RA, Buehler JW. Field epidemiology defined. In: Gregg MB, ed. *Field Epidemiology*. New York: Oxford University Press, 2002. 3 7.
46. Riley LW, Remis RS, Helgerson SD, et al. Hemorrhagic colitis associated with a rare *Escherichia coli* serotype. *N Engl J Med* 1983;308:681–5.
47. CDC. Multistate outbreak of *Salmonella* serotype Agona infections linked to toasted oats cereal. *MMWR* 1998;47:462–72.
48. Hennessy TW, Hedberg CW, Slutsker L, et al. A national outbreak of *Salmonella* Enteritidis infections from ice cream. *N Engl J Med* 1996;334:1281–6.
49. CDC. Outbreak of *Salmonella* serotype Muenchen infections associated with unpasteurized orange juice—United States and Canada, June 1999. *MMWR* 1999;48:582–5.
50. CDC. Outbreak of *Escherichia coli* O157:H7 infections associated with drinking unpasteurized commercial apple juice—British Columbia, California, Colorado, Washington. *MMWR* 1996;45:975.
51. Villar R, Macek MD, Simons S, et al. Investigation of multidrug-resistant *Salmonella* serotype Typhimurium DT104 infections linked to raw-milk cheese in Washington State. *JAMA* 1999;281:1811–6.
52. FDA. Regulatory Procedures Manual, Chapter 7, Subchapter 10. Emergency Procedures (Aug. 1997). Available at http://www.fda.gov/ora/compliance_ref/rpm_new2/ch7.html#pu. Accesses March 21, 2002.
53. FDA. *Investigations Operation Manual*, Chapter 9, Subchapter 910 Investigation of Foodborne Outbreaks (2001). Investigation of foodborne outbreaks. Available at http://www.fda.gov/ora/inspect_ref/icom/chaptertext/910.html. Accessed March 21, 2002.
54. Tauxe RV. The role of epidemiology in the detection and prevention of foodborne disease. In: *Issues in Food Safety. Proceedings of Joint Meeting of the Toxicology Forum and the Chinese Academy of Preventive Medicine*, Beijing, October 16–20, 1988. Washington, DC: Toxicology Forum, 1989:40–6.
55. FDA. Regulatory Procedures Manual, Chapter 8, Subchapter Sharing Non-Public Information with Federal Government Officials (Aug. 1997). Available at http://www.fda.gov/ora/compliance_ref/rpm_new2/8html#pur. Accessed March 21, 2002.

56. FDA. Regulatory Procedures Manual, Chapter 8, Subchapter Sharing Non-Public Information with State and Local Government Officials (Aug. 1997). Available at http:www.fda.gov/ora/compliance_ref/rpm_new2/ch8.html#purp. Accessed March 21, 2002.
57. 21 U.S.C. § 301(j); 18 U.S.C. § 1906.
58. 5 U.S.C. § 552(b)(4).
59. FDA. *Laboratory Procedures Manual*, Chapter 21.8. Review of Foreign Laboratories (2001). Available at http://www.fda.gov/ora/science_ref/lpm/lpchtr21.htm1#21.8%20 Review%20of%Foreign%20Laboratorie. Accessed March 21, 2002.
60. Sobel J, Hirshfeld AB, McTigue K, et al. The pandemic of *Salmonella* Enteritidis phage type 4 reaches Utah: a complex investigation confirms the need for continuing rigorous control measures. *Epidemiol Infect* 2000;125:1–8.
61. Olsen SJ, Ying M, Davis M, et al. Multistate outbreak of multidrug-resistant *Salmonella* serotype Typhimurium infections due to post-pasteurization contaminated milk. Abstracts of the Infectious Disease Society of America Annual Meeting, October 2001.
62. CDC. Update: multistate outbreak of listeriosis—United States, 1998–1999. *MMWR* 1998;47:1117–32.
63. CDC. Update: multistate outbreak of listeriosis—United States. *MMWR* 1999;47: 1085–6.
64. Jones EG. Forbidden fruit: talking about pesticides and food safety in the era of agricultural product disparagement laws. *Brooklyn Law Rev* 2001;66:823.
65. Colo. Rev. Stat. Ann. §§ 35-31-01 and 35-331-01 (West 1999).
66. *Texas Beef Group v. Winfrey*, 11 F.Supp. 2d 858, 864–5 (N.D. Tex. 1998), aff'd, 201 F.3d 680 (5th Cir. 2000).
67. Sinclair U. *The Jungle*. New York: Bantam Books, 1981.
68. U.S. Department of Agriculture, A.P.H.I.S. *Current trends and uncertainties for the future of agriculture*, 2000.
69. Hogue A, White P, Petter-Guard J, et al. Epidemiology and control of egg-associated *Salmonella* Enteritidis in the United States of America. Rev Sci Off Int Epiz 1997; 16:542–53.

15

Bloodborne and Sexually Transmitted Infections

EDWARD P. RICHARDS AND
GUTHRIE S. BIRKHEAD

This chapter focuses on legal tools for controlling sexually transmitted infections (STIs) and certain related bloodborne infections for which sexual transmission is important. The STIs pose difficult legal and public policy issues in public health law practice. Sex and procreation are the most intimate of human activities; thus prevention and control activities aimed at STIs present difficult privacy and personal freedom issues. Sex is also a primal biologic drive that is particularly difficult to influence or modify through rational argument and education. The second major route of transmission for some STIs is blood-to-blood contact such as that which occurs among drug users during injection of narcotics and other drugs. Drug use behaviors are complex, are wrapped in the psychology and physiology of addiction, and present similar challenges to sexual behaviors for public health prevention and control. Divisions are deep among knowledgeable professionals about the correct approach to STI control, with the greatest diversity of opinion over the control of human immunodeficiency virus (HIV) infection.

Many human diseases can be spread by sexual contact, including those caused by bacteria (e.g., bacterial vaginosis, chancroid, gonorrhea, granuloma inguinale, and syphilis), *Chlamydia* (e.g., genital chlamydia, lymphogranuloma venereum), *mycoplasma, protozoa* (e.g., trichomoniasis), and viruses (e.g., hepatitis B virus [HBV], hepatitis C virus [HCV], herpes simplex virus [HSV], HIV, and human papilloma virus [HPV]). Other diseases can be transmitted during sexual activity (e.g., phthiriasis [crab lice]) or oral-anal-genital contact (e.g., hepatitis A virus [HAV] and a myriad of enteric infections). These diseases range from simply irritating (crab lice) to fatal (HIV infection). Asymptomatic infection may occur for some or be the rule for others. Curative treatment is available for some (syphilis, gonorrhea, and some cases of chronic HBV infection) but not others (e.g., HIV infection). Early preventive therapy sometimes can prevent infection altogether (e.g., syphilis). Some STIs are associated with significant bloodborne transmission (HIV, HBV, and HCV infections). Finally, several STIs can also be transmitted from mother to child (syphilis, gonorrhea, HIV, HBV). Perinatal transmission can occur in utero, during delivery, or postpartum, for example, through breastfeeding.

This chapter focuses on the public health and legal response to four selected STIs that also are associated with significant bloodborne or perinatal transmission: HIV, gonorrhea, syphilis, and HBV. Together, these pose the key legal questions common to all STIs.

The core public health activities in STI and bloodborne infection control are (*1*) identification of index cases through public health surveillance (mandated reporting to the health department of persons with infection); (*2*) treatment and counseling of index patients; (*3*) identification, notification, prophylaxis or treatment, and counseling of sex or needle-sharing (blood-to-blood) contacts of the index patient; (*4*) mandated prevention measures (e.g., postpartum eye drops to prevent gonorrheal eye infections, mandated hepatitis B vaccination for school entry, and mandated condom availability in schools in Los Angeles, New York City, and elsewhere); (*5*) mandated education (required school curricula in some states); (*6*) mandated screening for infection (e.g., mandated prenatal screening for syphilis [not a common practice currently], HBV infection, and premarital screening for syphilis [not a common practice currently]); (*7*) closing of institutions and businesses that promote the spread of infection, such as bathhouses and crack houses; (*8*) in rare cases, detention of persons who pose a threat to the community through their unwillingness or inability to desist from unsafe practices; and (*9*) the regulation of blood and blood products to prevent the spread of STIs. Carrying out these activities demands a careful balancing between state police power and individual privacy.

LEGAL AUTHORITIES

Public health law is primarily mandated by state and local government laws. The U.S. Constitution reserved the police powers, which include the power to protect the public from communicable diseases, to the states. Congress has been pressured to pass laws allowing federal personnel to assert authority over disease outbreaks related to bioterrorism and other situations that could involve the interstate spread of disease, but Congress has not done so at this time. Constitutional law scholars and the courts are divided over whether such legislation would be constitutional.

Congress can address public health problems that involve interstate commerce or otherwise fall under other enumerated powers. For example, the Public Health Service has authority over the control of diseases that are related to interstate commerce and international shipping,[1] and the federal Food and Drug Administration (FDA) and Department of Agriculture (USDA) share some authority over foodborne illness control. The FDA's regulation of blood products and management of transfusion-related transmission of infectious agents are the only areas of significant direct federal regulation of STIs. Congress has passed anti-discrimination laws such as the Americans with Disabilities Act and privacy laws that affect some public health STI services, but Congress has not passed any national STI control legislation that preempts state authority in this area.

Outside direct regulatory authority, the federal government exercises significant control over all aspects of public health through its spending power. When Congress establishes programs such as the Ryan White CARE Act to address the health needs of HIV-infected persons, it attaches conditions to the receipt of the money and uses those conditions to control state public health services For example, the 1996 reauthorized CARE Act required states to demonstrate a "good faith effort" to conduct partner notification of spouses of persons with HIV infection as a condition for receipt of funds under Title II of the Act. Because most states depend on the federal government for a substantial part of their public health efforts, federal funding priorities often shape state public health efforts. For example, for many years the federal government provided funds for syphilis case finding and partner notification, and thus states conducted case finding and partner notification for syphilis. When HBV was recognized as a major U.S. public health problem in the 1970s, the federal government did not provide funds for case finding and partner notification, and few states funded these programs on their own—probably at least partially because "serum hepatitis," as HBV was previously known, was not widely recognized before the mid-1970s to be sexually transmitted,[2] and therefore partner notification was not used as a control strategy.

The Police Power

Control of STIs tests the limits of public health authority under the police power more than most areas of public health practice. It is critical to understand the breadth of the police power because STI control requires the state to intrude on the most intimate relationships and to collect the most private information. This chapter discusses the U.S. Constitutional limitations on state authority and how, within the constitutional limits, states have approached STI-control laws. State laws on STI control, especially HIV control, differ substantially, representing different political and epidemiologic conditions in the states. Persons implementing STI-control programs must work with lawyers in their individual state to ensure they work within that state's statutory framework.

Police powers are derived from the doctrine of societal self-defense.[3] Society has almost unlimited powers to protect itself because, in the classic Hobbesian view, life is, without society, nasty, brutish, and short. The U.S. Constitution and the state constitutions limit the power of the state and give individuals some rights against state action. When drafted, the U.S. Constitution protected individuals only from the actions of the federal government, but most of its protections were subsequently extended to the states. These protections are strongest when the state is prosecuting an individual for a crime with possible imprisonment as the punishment, and they are weakest when the state is restricting the liberty of individuals to protect others in society. The U.S. Constitution provides persons accused of a crime a right to counsel, protection from searches and seizures, right to trial by jury, and other procedural rights. These constitutional rights are the subject of popular discourse ranging from TV police shows to newspaper editorial pages and have entered the popular consciousness as applying to all persons at all times.

Most people, including many lawyers and public health professionals, are surprised to learn that individual rights are attenuated when the state acts to protect itself or its citizens from future harm, as opposed to punishing criminals or taking property for state use. When public health is threatened, a person can be detained without a trial, premises can be searched without a probable-cause warrant, and property can be destroyed without compensation. Because of the breadth of these powers, it is important that they not be abused. Public health officials may not use their police powers to accomplish nonpublic health objectives, such as clearing prostitutes from the streets before a convention, nor may they use these powers to circumvent criminal law protections. Because states criminalize many activities involved with the spread of STIs, such as prostitution, illicit drug use, and sexual activity with children under the age of consent, public health officials receiving disease reports, investigating cases, and delivering services often learn of criminal behavior. Although police officials are sometimes tempted to use public health authority to bolster criminal law enforcement, this is an unconstitutional deprivation of criminal due process rights and should be opposed by public health officials.

Protection of STI Information

Both state and federal courts have ruled that using the police power to circumvent the constitutional protections against unreasonable search and seizure is unconstitutional. For example, public health inspectors can enter private property to look for rats without procuring a criminal search warrant. If the search for vermin results in evidence of a crime, this evidence is not admissible in a criminal proceeding because there was no proper search warrant. A recent U.S. Supreme Court case applied this principle to the unconsented screening of pregnant women for drug use. The information from the screening was used to threaten the women with criminal prosecution for endangering their unborn children. The court ruled that such screening was an improper use of the public health authority, and the information could not be used by law enforcement.[4] The court was careful to distinguish this from acceptable public health testing. It found that testing would have been constitutional if the information had been used to improve the medical care of the women or their babies or for some other legitimate public health purpose.

Much of the information that public health professionals collect about STIs is not constitutionally protected. For example, if an index patient names a contact and identifies that contact as a crack dealer, that information would not be protected and could be provided to law enforcement. Doing so, however, would make carrying out many public health investigations impossible. Recognizing this, many states have laws that limit the use of information gained through public health reporting and investigations to public health purposes. Even states that do not enact this protection into a specific law recognize its importance and do not force public health officials to provide information to law enforcement agencies, except under very limited circumstances. This is important because many STI control measures rely on the voluntary cooperation of individuals with diseases or risk factors of public health interest. For example, obtaining the names of sex or needle-sharing partners of persons with HIV or HBV infection is inherently voluntary. Coercion or the threat of legal action to obtain partner names may result only in producing false names or names of nonpartners, wasting public health resources at best and confounding public health efforts at worst. Voluntary cooperation is important because public health efforts are not only reactive, for example, following up after the report of a case of disease, but also aimed at preventing future disease. Counseling a person with syphilis or HIV infection to prevent future sexual exposure to disease requires a supportive, voluntary approach to succeed.

The privacy of nonconstitutionally protected public health information depends on the specific provisions of the applicable state laws. Most of these laws, which generally provide strong protection for public health information, allow disclosure in two circumstances. First, the person who is the subject of the report may release the information in the report that concerns his or her own conduct and medical condition, although the courts limit this disclosure in many situations.[5] In contrast, at least one state—Colorado—bans the release of public health department case investigation information to the individual and thus prevents coerced release.[6] Because public health department case investigation records are not the patient's primary medical records, they do not contain information that is relevant to medical treatment that is not otherwise available to the patient. Banning the release of public health investigation data to the individual provides useful protection of records containing information about sexual activity and drug use without depriving the individual of necessary information for personal medical needs.

Second, most state public health confidentiality laws allow disclosure when necessary to serve the ends of justice. An example is the New York State HIV confidentiality statute, which permits a court-ordered release of HIV information if there exists "a clear and imminent danger to an individual whose life or health may unknowingly be at significant risk as a result of contact with the individual."[7] This exception comes into play when no other way exists to get the information, and the court determines that disclosure of the information is in the public's interest.[8,9]

State Administrative Process

Public health law is administrative law, meaning that it is enforced by state and local administrative agencies rather than by a police or sheriff's department. Although the U.S. Constitution does not explicitly provide for administrative agencies, the courts have allowed Congress to delegate its power to agencies administered by the President. All states have a similar administrative agency structure, although the extent to which that power can be delegated to an agency and type of executive and judicial oversight of agencies varies substantially among the states. Traditionally, legislatures did not specify the details of public health programs and enforcement, leaving that to the discretion of the health officer. In many states, public health statutes said little more than that the health department is directed to protect the citizens of the state from threats to the public health. Such vague delegation passes Constitutional muster because agencies need flexibility to respond to changing threats and to change their regulations as better science becomes available. The courts recognize that the expert agency staff are in a better position than the judges and the legislature to determine the details of public health practice. Thus when controversy arises over whether the public health agency has made the correct decision, the courts will defer to the agency.[10]

This deference has become more controversial with the advent of HIV infection and the growing political pressure of civil liberties organizations. In a case involving the closing of a gay bathhouse, the court reiterated that this deference to the health agency decision maker includes decisions about STI control that potentially interfere with personal freedom:

[D]efendants and the intervening patrons challenge the soundness of the scientific judgments upon which the Health Council regulation is based. . . . They go further and argue that facilities such as St. Mark's, which attempts to educate its patrons with written materials, signed pledges, and posted notices as to the advisability of safe sexual practices, provide a positive force in combatting AIDS, and a valuable communication link between public health authorities and the homosexual community. While these arguments and proposals may have varying degrees of merit, they overlook a fundamental principle of applicable law: "It is not for the courts to determine which scientific view is correct in ruling upon whether the police power has been properly exercised. The judicial function is exhausted with the discovery that the relation between means and end is not wholly vain and fanciful, an illusory pretense."[11]

Administrative Regulations and Orders

Because the statutes that delegate the authority for conducting STI control are generally broad, the details of enforcement are developed by the agency. These enforcement polices are embodied in formal regulations, promulgated under the state's Administrative Procedure Act, or in informal guidance documents and administrative orders. For example, listing HIV infection as a reportable disease subject to contact tracing may require a formal regulation subject to notice and comment (see Chapter 2). The process for reporting and contact tracing will be specified in internal health department policies that are not subject to notice and comment, although they are subject to Freedom of Information Act requests in most states.

Formal regulations and informal guidance documents apply to the population in general; they are not directed at the activities of specific individuals or institutions. Public health agencies also issue orders to specific businesses or individuals, such as an order to a restaurant to eliminate a rat infestation or face closure. When these policies and procedures apply to third parties, they are administrative orders, sometimes called "health-hold orders." Administrative orders vary in formality and specificity, with some applying to many persons rather than to one individual or institution. The bathhouse closing case discussed above is an example of an administrative order to close a facility. Administrative orders also have been used to require that arrested prostitutes be screened for gonorrhea before being released.[12] Unless restricted by a specific state statute, the federal and most state constitutions give health departments broad authority to use administrative orders without getting a court order, even when the order involves individual restrictions.

To survive a constitutional challenge in the courts, administrative orders to control STIs must[13] (*1*) Address a real problem that poses a direct threat to the public health; (*2*) Be based on a rational scientific control strategy, although there need not be scientific consensus on the strategy chosen; (*3*) Implement that strategy with the fewest restrictions consistent with the resources available and other public health policy concerns; (*4*) Include periodic program evaluation to show that that the strategy is working; and (*5*) Provide for phasing out the program when it is no longer epidemiologically sound.[13]

When the courts review administrative orders, they recognize that public health decision making is based on risk analysis, and solutions that are accepted by all members in the community are seldom clear and unambiguous. The courts do not demand perfection, and they do not require that the strategy be the least restrictive alternative, only that it be reasonably related to legitimate public health objectives.

LEGAL ISSUES AND CONTROVERSIES

Core STI public health control functions, which include primary reporting and partner notification, pose four types of legal issues: (1) invasion of privacy; (2) invasion of the person; (3) nuisance abatement (closures); and (4) regulation of interstate commerce (blood). Because legal prostitution is limited in the United States, this section does not discuss STIs as an occupational problem. Some of these issues, as they relate to requirements for proof of vaccination to attend school or as a condition of employment, and the right to perform newborn screening, do not pose special issues for STIs. This section focuses on issues that pose either special problems in STI control, such as infection reporting and partner notification, or issues not covered elsewhere, such as blood products.

The central controversy in STI law is whether STI law in particular, and public health law in general, is individual based or society based. Before the 1970s, public health law and STI control law were seen as protecting society through the control of infection in individuals. Even though some concern always existed regarding the rights of infected persons, these rights were viewed as secondary to the right of society to control the spread of disease. The patient empowerment movement starting in the 1970s, the individual autonomy model of medical care promoted by bioethicists in the 1980s, and the flooding of health departments with medical-care professionals who delivered personal medical services, such as prenatal care and indigent health care, blurred the line between personal medical care and public health. Many health directors and their staffs no longer recognize the difference between the physician–patient relationship and that of a public health enforcement officer to a disease carrier. This shift from public health to personal health law was evidenced by the failure to close bathhouses in the 1970s[14] despite the spread of HBV infection and other communicable diseases and was then reflected in the different approaches that states took to HIV-control strategies such as reporting, contact tracing, and partner notification, as well as to whether HIV-related medical information is treated differently from other medical information.

Invasion of Privacy

Almost all STI control since the 1930s has been through epidemiologic investigation, partner notification and education, and voluntary treatment and testing.

Although these methods invade personal privacy, they do not involve restrictions of the person; thus most of the legal controversies surrounding STI control have been driven by privacy concerns. Case identification through physician reports and contact investigation is the keystone of epidemiology and communicable disease control. Reporting allows the identification of infected individuals so that they can be treated (if treatment is available) and counseled in the prevention of the spread of the disease, but this is only part of the role of reporting. Reporting is critical to surveillance and enables the identification of emerging and reemerging infections; the spread of infections into new communities; changes in the incidence and prevalence of diseases in defined communities; new avenues of infection, such as the link between crack cocaine and STI; and, of increasing importance, changes in patterns of antimicrobial resistance.

The U.S. Supreme Court addressed the legality of public health reporting in *Whalen v. Roe*,[15] a case involving another controversial issue, the reporting of controlled substance prescriptions to identify physicians writing illegal prescriptions and patients seeking improper medication. This case directly confronted the claim that reporting might deter individuals from seeking diagnosis and treatment:

Unquestionably, some individuals' concern for their own privacy may lead them to avoid or to postpone needed medical attention. Nevertheless, disclosures of private medical information to doctors, to hospital personnel, to insurance companies, and to public health agencies are often an essential part of modern medical practice even when the disclosure may reflect unfavorably on the character of the patient. Requiring such disclosures to representatives of the State having responsibility for the health of the community, does not automatically amount to an impermissible invasion of privacy.

This was based on an earlier ruling upholding reporting and record keeping requirements for abortion, which is the most legally protected area in medical and public health jurisprudence.[16] In each of these cases it is assumed that the state will use reasonable measures to protect the privacy of the information it requires from negligent disclosure.

Invasion of the Person

Personal restrictions are used infrequently in STI control. Such restrictions are constitutional and were litigated in the STI landmark case *Reynolds v. Mc-Nichols*,[17] which involved an administrative order to check arrested prostitutes for gonorrhea as part of the longest running epidemiologic study and control program for gonorrhea.[12,18] These orders required prostitutes arrested as part of routine police activity to be detained until examined and/or treated for gonorrhea. The court found that this temporary detention for the diagnosis and treatment of gonorrhea was a proper response and did not violate the plaintiff's constitutional rights. This is consistent with current case law, recognizing the constitutional limits that such restrictions cannot be used as a subterfuge for criminal enforcement and that the restricted individual always has access to *habeas corpus* proceedings to review the restriction. If persons infected with an STI violate the criminal law, such as prohibitions against reckless endangerment or specific laws criminalizing the spread of STIs, they can be prosecuted by the police, who must provide them with full criminal due process protections. Such measures are not a public health action and should not involve public health personnel.

Nuisance Abatement

Public health officials have broad powers to close establishments that threaten the public health. This power has been routinely used in the past to close down houses of prostitution. Although such authority has not been employed routinely for STI control in recent times, it is within the powers of the health department as was reiterated in the St. Mark's baths case discussed earlier. However, this power has been used to close adult book stores[19] and video arcades that permit unsafe sex practices and could be used to close crack houses and other facilities that foster the unsafe use of illegal drugs. Such closing should be done by the police, however, because health departments are not staffed to deal with criminal enterprises, and involvement in police raids may undermine the credibility of the health department.

Regulation of Interstate Commerce

Bloodborne STIs raise special legal issues because they are subject to significant federal regulation under congressional power to regulate interstate commerce. Blood and blood products are classic commercial goods that are part of interstate commerce. Illegal intervenous drug use, which also spreads bloodborne STIs, is regulated because the illegal drugs pass over state lines and international boundaries. There are two classes of legal issues surrounding bloodborne infections; those that involve illegal drug use and those that result from exposure to blood and body fluids as part of medical, emergency, and custodial care. Most public health professionals agree that the U.S. policies prohibiting the use, possession, and sale of illegal drugs give very little consideration to the prevention of blood-borne infections. The often severe penalties for drug possession and the related laws on drug paraphernalia make it difficult for public health personnel to identify and work with drug users and to help them prevent transmission of communicable diseases.

Exposure to blood and body fluids in medical care, custodial care, sports, and other nonmedical settings was recognized as a potentially important risk associated with the spread of HBV in the 1970s. Concerns about HIV transmission escalated this to a high profile issue in the 1980s. Except for regulations on blood products, public health officials have acted in advisory and educating roles on managing these risks but have only a limited regulatory role. Litigation in this area has been considerable under the federal disability laws and under state tort laws, with some large judgments against health-care providers for negligence in diagnosing and treating HIV.[20] Most of the litigation has been against blood banks for failing to screen for HIV in a timely manner.[21] The provision of whole blood and blood products is an interstate business, now heavily regulated by the FDA. Although blood banks and blood products manufacturers were slow to recognize the risks posed by HBV and HIV, the combination of government regulation and private tort litigation substantially increased their sensitivity to the prevention of bloodborne infections.

PRACTICE CONSIDERATIONS

Physician and Laboratory Reporting

Reporting of communicable diseases identified through the provision of personal medical services in the private community has been a key component of public health surveillance and practice for more than 100 years. These reports first came from physicians, and as the formal system of laboratories evolved and more diseases of public health interest were diagnosed directly by laboratory tests, laboratory directors also were required to report communicable diseases. Before 1983, such reporting was not controversial, and all states had a list of more than 50 diseases and conditions, including syphilis, gonorrhea, viral hepatitis, and, later, hepatitis A and B, that required personally identified reporting.

When acquired immunodeficiency syndrome (AIDS) was recognized in 1981, states quickly instituted reporting of AIDS cases. Much information about the epidemiology of AIDS was worked out through this reporting system. AIDS reporting continued even after HIV, the virus that causes AIDS, was identified in the mid-1980s because, in the absence of treatment, such reporting can give an accurate epidemiologic picture of trends in the epidemic, albeit delayed by a number of years. AIDS case data also were used to determine federal funding formulas for AIDS care, and the AIDS case definition was borrowed and used to determine eligibility for disability compensation. Reporting of the causal agent would normally have been substituted for reporting of the diagnostic syndrome once the causal agent was identified and a test became available for it. Four of the five highest incidence states—New York, Florida, Texas, and New Jersey (but not California)—now report cases of HIV infection by patient name. A number of states use some form of reporting by unique identifier rather than by name.

Although physician reporting was not controversial until the HIV/AIDS epidemic, it was never reliable. For example, one study in the late 1970s showed that only 10% to 20% of gonorrhea cases were reported by physicians and that many physicians never reported any cases.[22] Many reasons existed for the failure to report, including administrative time and costs, which have only worsened during the last 20 years. One legal reason for the failure to report is that, except for child abuse reporting, physicians are seldom disciplined or prosecuted for failing to report communicable diseases. Public health has come to depend on laboratory reporting because it is much more effective for surveillance. Laboratories can automate the reporting process, and they are subject to certification and accreditation procedures that help ensure that they comply with the law. Physician reporting is still critical for conditions that do not have a specific laboratory diagnosis and for emerging conditions that are not yet reportable, as with the original reports of AIDS in 1981.

Involuntary Screening, Treatment, and Vaccination

At one time, involuntary screening of adults at risk for STIs was common in the United States. The principle that screening is constitutionally permissible was upheld in the *Ferguson* case discussed above, even though the case rejected the screening program at issue because it was not for public health purposes. Screening for STIs has fallen out of favor for both privacy and epidemiologic reasons, although several states still have premarital screening requirements and most states require pregnant women to be screened for syphilis. Involuntary screening is effective because it does not require the patient's consent, so the problem of patient refusal does not arise. Even if a patient refuses screening, he or she can still be screened if blood has been drawn for other purposes. In theory, patients could be forced to submit samples for screening, but this is almost never advisable for adults outside of involuntary confinement. Screening of children is less controversial and is done at birth for several conditions, including HIV infection. Although some states require neonatal screening for HIV without mandatory screening of pregnant women earlier in pregnancy, screening early in pregnancy, when HIV treatment can have the greatest benefit to the baby, is preferable.[23] This would be constitutionally acceptable, as are the existing mandatory syphilis screening programs, but no state has yet mandated such screening.

Involuntary treatment is not a major issue in STI control because of the limited amount of resistance to treatment, especially for symptomatic disease. HIV infection is more problematic, however, because it requires ongoing treatment, sometimes with substantial side effects. The only situation in which involuntary treatment for HIV infection has been raised is for pregnant women, where treatment can reduce the risk of transmission to the child. Such treatment is probably constitutional in that the courts have found that a woman's right to privacy does not include harming her fetus; however, this is controversial and is not recommended by public health experts at this time. The HBV vaccine is the only vaccine available for an STI; its use worldwide has dramatically reduced the incidence of HBV and may nearly eliminate it in future generations in the United States. Mandatory school entrance requirements for HBV vaccination are an important tool in the eventual control and potential eradication of HBV in the United States.

Contact Tracing and Partner Notification

Disease reporting provides valuable epidemiologic information, but it is only the first step in disease investigation. When epidemiologically justified, the next step is to interview the reported (index) patient to identify other potentially infected contacts. Contact tracing is legally justifiable because it is critical to elucidating the epidemiology of a disease and to mapping its spread in existing and new communities. It is usually combined with partner notification, which includes counseling the contact about testing and treatment alternatives and how to avoid the spread of the disease. Contact tracing is used extensively for tuberculosis and even for the investigation of diseases that are spread through other routes (e.g., foodborne illness), but it is most controversial for STIs because individuals must disclose intimate and sometimes illegal behavior. Individuals and businesses have no constitutional right to withhold information from public health investigators and could be ordered by a court to provide information necessary for a public health investigation. However, public health personnel always treat contact tracing and partner notification as voluntary. Even though contact tracing is sometimes criticized because people lie to investigators, it is effective in identifying core group members who are disproportionally responsible for spreading STIs.[24] When a criminal prosecution is contemplated, such as in child abuse cases, public health personnel should not be involved, and the investigation should be conducted by law enforcement personnel.

Contact information must be treated as confidential by public health personnel and cannot be released unless there is a court order or statutory authorization to do so. The more common problem is how to interview subsequent contacts without divulging the source of the information. The typical text of a public health worker's speech to a contact is, "you have been named as a contact of someone with an STI. You need to be screened and treated, if necessary." The identity of the index case is never revealed in this process. Unfortunately, if the contact has few or only one sex or needle partner, preventing the contact from guessing who must have exposed him or her is impossible. The investigator must resist all entreaties to confirm the interviewee's suspicions, but this will have little practical effect. Contact tracing raises difficult ethical questions, especially whether the interview will trigger a violent reprisal on the suspected partner.

Partner notification, separate from contact tracing for epidemiologic purposes, is used for syphilis to try to treat contacts during the 3 week incubation period and for gonorrhea to identify asymptomatic female contacts. This approach has been controversial for HIV infection because there is no cure and effective treatments were not developed until several years after the identification of the disease. However, health departments that employed partner notification found that it was justified as a very personal form of education because many contacts are not yet infected when first identified and because it helped prompt individuals to get tested and to obtain counseling about how to prevent the spread of the disease.[25,26]

Prostitution and Illegal Drug Use

Prostitution and illegal drug use are generally linked in that they involve overlapping populations on the fringe of the law and because prostitutes are often drug users. Thus, bloodborne STIs are spread through both sexual activity to get drugs and, for intravenous drugs, the use of the drugs themselves. Public health activities are complicated because both activities are illegal and because intravenous drug possession and sale carry draconian penalties under state and federal laws. Prostitutes and drug users are suspicious of government officials and will not participate in programs that might increase their chances of arrest. Laws criminalizing possession of drug paraphernalia make using effective STI control strategies such as needle exchange difficult or impossible. In many jurisdictions that do not criminalize possession and sale of needles and syringes, it may be politically difficult for health departments to provide assistance to intravenous drug users.

Legal Issues in Personal Medical Services

Health department personnel have significant immunity when performing core public health functions such as case finding, partner notification, basic STI treatment intended to protect the public, and general epidemiologic investigations. Health departments often provide personal medical services beyond these core public health functions, the most common being prenatal care. In many states, however, because there is no sovereign immunity for personal medical-care services, personnel may be exposed to medical malpractice litigation. This is further complicated when health departments use contract personnel to deliver medical services. Such personnel have few of the legal protections of a state employee. More problematically, most state laws regarding privacy of public health records do not apply to personal medical records. Health department personnel who both deliver personal medical services, such as prenatal care, and interview persons about their exposure to STIs must be careful to keep public health information, such as the identity of sexual contacts or other disease investigation information, separate from the patient's personal medical records. Thus the patient's medical record might contain the information that the patient had six sexual contacts in the last month, but it should not contain the names of the contacts. These would be maintained in a separate disease-control investigation file. This is especially important in small departments where each staff member has multiple job responsibilities.

In addition to liability concerns, personal medical services are covered by many state and federal laws such as the Americans with Disabilities Act and health-care information privacy laws that do not apply to core public health functions and disease-control investigations. The major issue unique to STI control is preventing the risk of HIV transmission, including transmission between adults or between a mother and an unborn child. Maternal transmission poses special problems because the fetus cannot protect itself. Health department personnel must take especial care to ensure that pregnant women are properly counseled about the need for HIV testing and that they are properly followed up with counseling about treatment if their test results are positive.

EMERGING ISSUES

Surveillance and Treatment for HIV Infection

As HIV treatments become more effective, and as evidence accumulates that they may also reduce the treated individual's infectivity, there is growing support for contact tracing and partner notification to ensure that individuals who are HIV infected receive treatment to protect the public as well as themselves. This will raise the issue of drug-resistant strains of HIV and whether persons with such strains should be subject to public health restrictions. It also will raise the question of whether HIV treatment should be supervised to help reduce the development of resistant strains of the virus. These issues have been addressed with multidrug-resistant tuberculosis, but for only relatively small numbers of persons compared with how many persons are infected with HIV.

HIV Vaccine

The potential for HIV vaccines in the near future opens up the possibility of vaccines becoming an important public health tool to combat the spread of HIV. Efforts to gain acceptance of an HIV vaccine, especially in minority communities that have traditionally distrusted public health efforts, will require careful attention to public perceptions and distrust of the government. If an effective vaccine becomes available, community acceptance issues will probably delay mandatory vaccination requirements for many years. HIV vaccines that are less than 100% effective, or that have dangerous side effects, will pose substantial product liability issues and may require the state to provide immunity for manufacturers.

References

1. 42 U.S.C. 264 (Regulations to Control Communicable Diseases).
2. Benenson AS, ed. *Control of Communicable Diseases in Man*, 11th ed. Washington, DC: American Public Health Association, 1970: pp. 105–10.
3. Richards EP. The jurisprudence of prevention: society's right of self-defense against dangerous individuals. *Hastings Constitutional Law Q* 1989;16:329.
4. *Ferguson v. City of Charleston*, 532 U.S. 67 (2001).
5. *Grattan v. People*, 65 N.Y.2d 243, 480 N.E.2d 714, 491 N.Y.S.2d 125 (N.Y. 1985).
6. Richards EP. Colorado public health laws: a rational approach to AIDS. *Dev ULR* 1988;65:127.
7. NYS Public Health Law Sec 2785.2. *McKinney's Consolidated Laws of New York, Annotated.* St. Paul, MN: West Publishing Co., 1993.
8. *Westchester County v. People*, 504 N.Y.S.2d 497, 498, 122 A.D.2d 1, 2 (N.Y.A.D. 2 Dept. 1986).
9. *McBarnette v. Sobol*, 610 N.Y.S.2d 460, 462, 632 N.E.2d 866, 868, 83 N.Y.2d 333, 339, 62 USLW 2623, 2623 (N.Y. 1994).
10. *Jacobson v. Massachusetts*, 197 U.S. 11 (1905).
11. *City of New York v. New St. Mark's Baths*, 130 Misc.2d 911, 497 N.Y.S.2d 979 (1986), citations omitted.
12. Potterat JJ, Rothenberg RB, et al. Invoking, monitoring, and relinquishing a public health power: the health hold order. *Sex Transm Dis* 1999;26:345–9.
13. Richards EP 3rd, Rathbun KC. The role of the police power in 21st century public health. *Sex Transm Dis* 1999;26:350–7.
14. Thompson JR. Is the United States country zero for the First-World AIDS epidemic? *J Theor Biol* 2000;204:621–8.
15. *Whalen v. Roe*, 429 U.S. 589 (1977).
16. *Planned Parenthood of Central Missouri v. Danforth*, 428 U.S. 52 (1976), at 81.
17. *Reynolds v. McNichols*, 488 F.2d 1378 (10th Cir. 1973).
18. Potterat JJ, Rothenberg R, Bross DC. Gonorrhea in street prostitutes: epidemiologic and legal implications. *Sex Transm Dis* 1979;6:58–63.
19. *Arcara v. Cloud Books, Inc.*, 478 U.S. 697 (1986).
20. *Doe v. McNulty*, 630 So.2d 825 (La. Ct. App. 4th Cir. 1993).
21. *Snyder v. American Association of Blood Banks*, 676 A.2d 1036 (1996).
22. Rothenberg R, Bross DC, et al. Reporting of gonorrhea by private physicians: a behavioral study. *Am J Public Health* 1980;70:983–6.
23. Grimes RM, Richards EP, et al. Hepatitis B, syphilis, and human immunodeficiency virus: are different approaches to prenatal screening justified? *Pediatr AIDS HIV Infect* 1997;8:98–101.
24. Hethcote HW, Yorke JA. *Gonorrhea Transmission Dynamics and Control*. Lecture Notes in Mathematics, vol 56. New York: Springer Verlag, 1984.
25. Holtgrave DR, Valdiserri RO, Gerber AR, Hinman AR. Human immunodeficiency virus counseling, testing, referral, and partner notification services. A cost–benefit analysis. *Arch Intern Med* 1993;153:1225–30.
26. Varghese B, Peterman TA, Holtgrave DR. Cost-effectiveness of counseling and testing and partner notification: a decision analysis. *AIDS* 1999;13:1745–51.

16

Tobacco Prevention and Control

RICHARD A. DAYNARD, MARK A. GOTTLIEB,
ROBERT L. KLINE, EDWARD L. SWEDA, JR.,
AND RONALD M. DAVIS

Tobacco use causes an estimated 400,000 deaths each year in the United States.[1] The annual worldwide toll of mortality from tobacco-attributable disease is about 4 million and is expected to rise to 10 million by 2030.[2] Annually, about 1 million young Americans become regular smokers; for many, their nicotine addiction will be extremely difficult to break, and about half of those who become lifelong smokers will eventually die prematurely from tobacco-related disease. Furthermore, smoking causes about 50,000 deaths each year in the United States among nonsmokers exposed to environmental tobacco smoke (ETS; i.e., passive smoking).[3] Prevention efforts are proceeding on many fronts, some of which do not raise legal issues. Important elements of comprehensive tobacco-control programs include school- and community-based education programs; "counter-advertising" campaigns in the mass media, financed through either tobacco excise taxes or proceeds from the 1997 and 1998 settlements of the state lawsuits against the tobacco companies; and counseling and treatment for tobacco dependence.

Policies that discourage tobacco use and protect nonsmokers from exposure to ETS are also key elements of comprehensive tobacco-control programs. These policies are typically grouped into the categories of price policy (mainly referring to tobacco excise taxation), restrictions on tobacco advertising and promotion, restrictions on smoking in public places and work sites, restrictions on youth access to tobacco, government-mandated health warnings and disclosures on tobacco packaging and advertisements, and tobacco product regulation.[4] Such policies can be adopted through legislation or regulation at the federal, state, and local levels. Important tobacco-control policies also can be promulgated by private entities such as employers, professional sports associations, and health-care organizations (e.g., accreditation bodies such as the Joint Commission on Accreditation of Healthcare Organizations, which requires that hospitals be smoke free as a condition of accreditation). These policies, whether promulgated in the public sector or the private sector, result in the majority of legal disputes and controversies in tobacco control.

LEGAL AUTHORITIES

In this section we review legal authorities that affect tobacco at the federal, state, and local levels. Because litigation has played a prominent role in the interpretation and application of these authorities, and because it forms the legal basis of many new "public policies" (e.g., through the Master Settlement Agreement [MSA]), we also review key developments in tobacco litigation.

Federal Authorities

Considering the amount of harm attributed to tobacco use, tobacco products are under-regulated, particularly at the federal level. In the United States, the Food and Drug Administration (FDA), the Consumer Product Safety Commission, and the Occupational Safety and Health Administration are among the federal agencies that have not successfully regulated tobacco products. In the last half of the 1990s, the FDA sought to regulate the sale and marketing of cigarettes and smokeless tobacco products under the federal Food, Drug, and Cosmetic Act (classifying nicotine as a drug and treating these tobacco products as drug-delivery devices). However, the tobacco industry won a five-to-four Supreme Court victory in May 2000, holding that Congress had not authorized the FDA to assert jurisdiction over tobacco products.[5] Nevertheless, several sources of federal legal authority exist over tobacco products.

The most significant federal statute is the Federal Cigarette Labeling and Advertising Act (FCLAA).[6] Enacted in 1965 in the wake of the first U.S. Surgeon General's *Report on Smoking and Health* (released in 1964) and amended several times, the FCLAA requires one of four rotating warnings to appear on each pack of cigarettes and on all cigarette advertising. It preempts any state or local cigarette warning requirements or advertising restrictions based on smoking and health. In 1971, Congress banned broadcast advertising for cigarettes.[7]

Similarly, the Comprehensive Smokeless Tobacco Education Act of 1986 approached smokeless or "spit" tobacco products by mandating three rotating warnings on packaging and advertisements and banning broadcast advertising for this category of tobacco products.[8] Like the FCLAA, it preempted state and local efforts to restrict advertising or require warnings for smokeless tobacco products. Five rotating warnings are required on cigar packaging for 95% of the U.S. cigar market under consent decrees resulting from Federal Trade Commission actions taken against seven U.S. cigar companies.[9] The only categories of tobacco product left completely unregulated by warning requirements are pipe tobacco and roll-your-own cigarette tobacco.

Two important federal laws address smoking in public places. In 1990, Congress banned smoking on all domestic airline flights of 6 hours or less (and, since then, most airlines have extended the ban voluntarily to include all of their flights within the country, including those to Alaska and Hawaii, lasting more than 6 hours).[10] In addition, the Pro-Children's Act of 1994 prohibits smoking in facilities in which federally funded children's services are regularly or routinely provided.[11]

Another federal legal authority affecting tobacco products is an amendment to the federal Alcohol, Drug Abuse and Mental Health Administration Reorganization Act of 1992, known as the "Synar Amendment."[12] The statute provides for federal substance abuse block grants to states. The Synar Amendment requires each recipient state to enact a state law proscribing the sale of tobacco products to minors or the purchase of tobacco products by minors and to establish a compliance testing and reporting system as a condition of receiving the block grants.

State and Local Authorities

Individual states can use many legislative and regulatory approaches to reduce the prevalence of tobacco use and the harm it causes. The range of options available to a state largely depends on how state legislative, regulatory, and police powers are configured under a state's constitution and various state statutes.

The most notable limitation on state authority to regulate tobacco stems from the FCLAA, the federal law that requires rotating Surgeon General's warnings on every pack of cigarettes sold or advertised. The FCLAA contains a preemption clause that states, "No requirement or prohibition based on smoking and health shall be imposed under State law with respect to the advertising or promotion of any cigarettes the packages of which are labeled in conformity with the provisions of this Act."[13] The FCLAA defines "State" to include political subdivisions of the state. Even though this preemption generally does not affect state action on substantive regulatory areas such as ETS and youth access to tobacco, it profoundly affects state and local measures to restrict cigarette advertising and promotion.

Beyond the restrictions imposed on state action through the preemptive effect of the FCLAA, the primary means of enacting measures to control tobacco at the state level is through legislation. Every state legislature has the power to pass laws to, for example, restrict minors' access to tobacco products, prohibit smoking in public places, and increase tobacco excise taxes. Such legislation also may contain provisions that preempt localities from acting on such matters. Such local preemption is generally counterproductive from a public health standpoint because it prevents localities from passing more rigorous measures.[14,15] State health departments usually have regulatory and enforcement powers that can be applied to tobacco control. In some instances, a state health department may be authorized to promulgate regulations pursuant to particular statutes, such as clean indoor air or tobacco youth-access legislation. In other states, such authority may be reserved to or shared with local health boards at the municipal or county level under a general grant of regulatory authority from state statute related to public health.

The power of municipalities and local boards of health to further the public health varies from state to state. The legal variables include whether the state constitution has a Home Rule provision granting legislative powers to municipalities so that they can enact local tobacco-control measures or whether the state provides statutory authority to local health boards so that they can enact reasonable health regulations to protect the public health. Such constitutional or statutory grants of authority, if available, provide a solid foundation for public health agencies to promulgate regulations implementing a wide range of tobacco-control provisions. On the other hand, state statutes "regulating" smoking in workplaces and restaurants, cigarette vending machines, sales to minors, and other tobacco-control subjects frequently combine weak substantive provisions with clauses preempting local action. Indeed, courts sometimes infer such preemption even in the absence of explicit preemption clauses.

In addition to state legislatures, health departments, and municipal legislation, state attorneys general have some enforcement authority—and, in some cases, regulatory authority—over tobacco. The range of civil and criminal law enforcement powers granted to state attorneys general varies significantly from state to state. Generally, state attorneys general can enforce state laws on unfair and deceptive acts and practices. Such laws may be targeted at tobacco industry marketing and sales activities where appropriate. In some states, the attorney general has rule-making powers.

The attorney general of Massachusetts exercised such powers in 1999 by promulgating regulations restricting outdoor tobacco advertising within 1000 feet of schools and playgrounds.[16] The restrictions were designed to eliminate deception and unfairness in the way cigarettes and smokeless tobacco products were marketed, sold, and distributed to reduce cigarette smoking and smokeless tobacco use by minors. The regulations were not premised on "smoking and health" concerns and therefore were not preempted by the FCLAA, according to the Massachusetts attorney general. On June 28, 2001, the U.S. Supreme Court disagreed with the attorney general's contention and struck down most of the Massachusetts attorney general's regulations.

In all but four states (Mississippi, Florida, Texas, and Minnesota), the state attorneys general have enforcement power stemming from the MSA between 46 states and the major tobacco manufacturers in the United States. [17,18] The remaining four states have separate settlement agreements with tobacco manufacturers that are likewise enforceable by the state attorney general in the court that approved the settlement and consent decree in each state.

Litigation Against the Tobacco Industry

Litigation against the tobacco industry can have several effects. Lawsuits can force tobacco companies to reveal incriminating internal documents, weakening their political power to oppose effective regulation. Lawsuits also increase public discussion about the dangers of tobacco use, as talk shows debate whether people who develop tobacco-caused diseases should be compensated for their own "stupidity" in relying on the industry's assurances that the risks were merely hypothetical. Lawsuits also have the potential to force the industry to change its behavior, either through settlements or "voluntarily" to avoid future punitive damage awards. By forcing the industry to pay even a modest fraction of the medical and personal costs that their products and behavior cause, lawsuits can drive up the price of tobacco products, reducing use particularly among youth. Finally, lawsuits can produce settlements or verdicts that can help fund tobacco-control programs.[19,20]

The most impressive demonstrations of the regulatory power of tobacco litigation are the settlements between all 50 state attorneys general and the tobacco industry. Four states, Mississippi, Florida, Texas, and Minnesota, settled their cases individually during July 1997 through May 1998. The remaining states settled, on terms similar to those of the four individual state settlements, in November 1998, through the MSA. Under the MSA, the states relinquished their claims for reimbursement of tobacco-caused medical costs (past, present, and future) and agreed to provisions that prevented their political subdivisions from bringing such claims. In return, the tobacco companies agreed both to pay money to the states and to change some of their more egregious behavior. In terms of money, the cigarette companies (proportionately to their market shares) agreed to make quarterly payments to each state, in perpetuity, at a rate roughly approximating each state's anticipated tobacco-caused Medicaid costs. A state's payments could have been drastically reduced if the state legislature failed to pass "nonparticipating manufacturer" statutes, which required cigarette manufacturers to either join the MSA or post bonds equal to the financial contributions that would have been required if they had joined; all states have adopted such statutes. Another major adjustment reduces the overall payments when annual national cigarette sales drop.[21] Because a 10% increase in cigarette price reduces overall cigarette consumption by 3% to 5%,[22] the settlement-induced price increases have caused a substantial drop in smoking in the United States. Furthermore, states have used 5% to 8% of payments under the MSA to fund tobacco-control programs.[23]

The MSA's enforceable provisions as applied to the settling defendants, aside from monetary payments to the states, include (*1*) ban on tobacco billboard advertising; (*2*) ban on the use of cartoon characters in tobacco advertising; (*3*) ban on manufacturer advertising, promotion, or marketing activities that have a primary purpose of targeting minors; (*4*) ban on distribution of apparel or merchandise featuring brand names of tobacco products; (*5*) ban on distribution of free cigarette samples to minors (if state law prohibits purchase or possession of tobacco products by minors); (*6*) ban on the sale of packs with fewer than 20 cigarettes; (*7*) modest restrictions on tobacco company lobbying (e.g., prohibiting lobbying against bills that limit youth access to cigarette vending machines or bills that enhance penalties for violating laws restricting youth access to tobacco); and (*8*) maintaining open public access to internal industry "discovery" documents obtained during the state litigation, both through depositories in Minnesota and England and through websites established by the companies (MSA, Sec. III). These promises became part of consent decrees between the states and the settling manufacturers that courts approved in each of the states.

A similar settlement, the Smokeless Tobacco Master Settlement Agreement, was reached at the same time as the MSA between the state attorneys general and the principal purveyor of smokeless tobacco (chewing tobacco and moist snuff), the United States Tobacco Company.

Litigation by or on Behalf of the Tobacco Industry

Beginning in the 1990s, the tobacco industry as a whole, and Philip Morris in particular, embarked on an aggressive campaign of filing lawsuits to thwart the plans and policies of their adversaries. Although the threat of litigation by the industry need not impede strong tobacco-control measures at the state and local levels, it requires that such measures be carefully drafted to avoid successful challenges.

The industry's most spectacular litigation victory was the invalidation of the FDA's assertion of jurisdiction, but there have been others as well. In 1993, several months after the Environmental Protection Agency (EPA) issued a comprehensive report on ETS, the tobacco industry sued the EPA in federal court in Greensboro, North Carolina, even though the EPA had not issued any regulation to limit smoking anywhere. Because no agency action existed to form the basis of a legitimate court challenge, the industry filed a lawsuit with the goal of undermining the scientific case against secondhand smoke at hearings when states and localities across the country considered passing laws limiting or banning smoking in public places. The industry got the ruling it sought in June 1998 from Judge William Osteen in *Flue-Cured Tobacco Cooperative Stabilization Corp. v. EPA.*[24] That ruling, which purported to invalidate a portion of the EPA's report and is under appeal, is analyzed at http://tobacco.neu.edu/tcu/3-1/epa_article.htm.

In 1994, Philip Morris filed its own lawsuit against television network ABC and two of its journalists, Walt Bogdanich and John Martin, for suggesting in a report on the program *Day One* that the industry "spiked" cigarettes with nicotine.[25] The case was settled in August 1995 with a public apology from ABC, which was then republished in a national advertising campaign to blunt criticism from members of Congress and others about the problem of nicotine addiction and cigarettes.

The tobacco industry sued the Commonwealth of Massachusetts in 1996 to block a first-in-the-nation law to require disclosure of ingredients, additives, and nicotine yield ratings by brand for the various companies' cigarettes.[26] A decision invalidating the law is on appeal in the First Circuit Court of Appeals.

In 1999, the industry sued the Massachusetts Attorney General for having adopted regulations banning tobacco advertising within 1000 feet of schools and playgrounds. Despite its public relations efforts to assure the American people that it does not want children to smoke, tobacco interests fought these regulations. The industry sought a declaration that the regulations are invalid because they violate the First Amendment to the U.S. Constitution and that they are preempted by the FCLAA. In *Lorillard Tobacco Co. v. Reilly,*[27] the Supreme Court voted five to four that states' authority to regulate tobacco advertisements was limited by the First Amendment and partially preempted by the FCLAA.

The tobacco industry and its allies have filed numerous lawsuits, and threatened the filing of many others, to fend off legislation that limits smoking in public. These cases generally have tested the powers of local governmental entities. Although they have had mixed success, the potential cost of defending them has often discouraged governmental bodies from taking strong action. For example, R.J. Reynolds Tobacco Co. financed a 1994 lawsuit filed by restaurant owners in Puyallup, Washington. The suit alleged that a recently enacted ordinance requiring restaurants to be smoke free was preempted because state law permitted smoking sections in restaurants and that the city had unlawfully and substantially deprived the plaintiffs of their rights guaranteed by the U.S. Constitution, including the "takings" clause of the Fifth Amendment. Although these arguments seemed dubious, the City Council voted to repeal the ordinance rather than spend the money required to fight the lawsuit.[28]

LEGAL ISSUES AND CONTROVERSIES

Reducing Youth Access to Tobacco

The Synar Amendment

The Synar Amendment to the Alcohol, Drug Abuse, and Mental Health Administration Reorganization Act of 1992 requires states to adopt and enforce laws establishing a minimum age limit for buyers of tobacco products and to show progressive reductions in the availability of tobacco products to minors.[29] The U.S. Department of Health and Human Services (DHHS) is the government agency responsible for a yearly evaluation of its progress. The statute and proposed implementing regulations make the state (rather than municipalities) responsible for ensuring compliance and reporting results to the federal government, but the commentary accompanying the proposed regulations explicitly acknowledges that the state can delegate enforcement efforts "through local governments or private entities." The policy behind the Synar Amendment is to encourage states (by providing financial incentives) to adopt effective tobacco-control measures, including compliance checks. A state's failure to meet these requirements would result in forfeiture of federal block grant funds for substance abuse prevention and treatment.

The threat of forfeiting substance-abuse block grant money is not enough of an incentive for local police officers to enforce youth-access laws that prohibit sale of tobacco to minors. Furthermore, the Synar Amendment is an easy target for the tobacco industry lobby. The tobacco industry vigorously campaigned at the state level to undermine serious enforcement of youth-access laws by successfully lobbying for inclusion of language such as "knowingly" or "intentionally" in the laws prohibiting the sale of tobacco to minors.[30] Such language makes the youth-access laws virtually unenforceable.

Types of restrictions and enforcement

The effectiveness of tobacco-control legislation at the federal and state levels often has been thwarted by the tremendous muscle of the tobacco industry lobby. The success of a tobacco-control program depends on the willingness of local health departments and municipal legislative bodies to adopt effective local tobacco-control measures. One tobacco-control strategy that works best at the local level is municipal licensing of tobacco retailers to control youth access to tobacco products.

In 1993 and 1994, the Institute of Medicine (IOM) conducted an 18-month study on the prevention of nicotine dependence among children and youths.[31] One problem with youth smoking is that teenagers can relatively easily obtain tobacco products. According to a large body of evidence,[32] minors who purchase their own cigarettes are seldom asked for identification to verify their age. Children can also obtain cigarettes easily from vending machines and self-service displays.

In its report, the IOM identified what it considered the essential components of any program to reduce youth access to tobacco. The IOM recommends that states or localities establish a licensing system requiring merchants to obtain a license or a permit to sell tobacco products and revoking or suspending that license if a merchant sells tobacco to minors. The IOM states that "a tobacco retailer licensing program must be the cornerstone of any successful enforcement effort." Nearly every study of youth-access interventions has endorsed this licensing approach, and experience with local licensing and permitting systems has demonstrated the effectiveness of this approach.[33] In 1990, former DHHS Secretary Louis Sullivan, who served in the George H.W. Bush Administration, produced a Model Sale of Tobacco Products to Minor Control Act, which included a provision for licensing tobacco retailers.[34]

The IOM further recommended limiting youth access to tobacco products by (1) banning the sale of tobacco products through self-service displays, a prime source of tobacco products for minors (self-service displays also invite shoplifting); (2) banning the sale of single cigarettes and the free distribution of tobacco products, two sources of tobacco products for adolescents; and (3) banning tobacco vending machines, which younger children rely on as a source for cigarettes.[35]

Because of their limited disposable income, minors are especially susceptible to free sampling. The DHHS has encouraged states and local governments to ban distribution of free tobacco samples because "they inevitably fall into the hands of children and adolescents." In response to this problem, many communities across the country have restricted the distribution of free cigarette samples from areas around schools and other places frequented by minors or have prohibited free samples altogether. Not one of these ordinances and regulations has been challenged in court. Local restriction of free sample distribution does not violate the U.S. Constitution, is within the police power of local government, and is consistent with federal law.

Enforcement mechanisms differ for municipalities and local public health agencies. Specifically, a municipality can enforce a youth-access measure by a simple ticket-and-fine procedure (also known as the "noncriminal disposition" process). A municipality may have to grant its local public health agency a general authority to use the noncriminal disposition process to enforce its regulations. In the absence of such authority, enforcement of public health agency regulations may prove cumbersome.

Municipalities and local public health agencies should first understand what authority they have to enact local measures and ascertain whether state law has preempted any of their authority. With this authority in place, state tobacco-control programs can support cities, towns, and local boards of health in enacting a wide range of youth-access measures. Local regulations can impose tobacco permit licensing schemes and penalties against retailers and their agents for selling to minors. For example, in Massachusetts, cities, towns, and local health agencies are encouraged to pass youth-access regulations that

- Require local merchants to verify by valid government-issued identification that each person purchasing tobacco products is 18 years of age or older
- Require local merchants to place all tobacco products out of the reach of all consumers and in a location accessible only to store personnel
- Establish retailer training requirements and programs
- Conduct periodic unannounced inspections to enforce local laws
- Require local permits regulating the location of vending machines or ban vending machines entirely

Fourth Amendment warrant requirement and compliance checks

To conduct a successful compliance check, public health and other officials need some element of surprise. A formal request to a retailer, by public health officials, to submit to a specific compliance check, for example, would only warn the retailer to carefully check identifications. No enforcement could take place under this arrangement. Thus, local youth-access regulations should emphasize a retailer's general consent to submit to random, unannounced compliance checks. One way to ensure that tobacco retailers give implied consent is to institute a licensing or permitting scheme and condition issuance on consent to compliance checks. This condition is constitutional as long as specific compliance checks are conducted in a reasonable manner.[36]

A basic understanding of search-and-seizure laws helps to ensure smooth compliance checks. The Fourth Amendment to the U.S. Constitution as applied to the states through the Fourteenth Amendment requires that law enforcement officials and their designees obtain a warrant to search private property, even where the property is used for commercial purposes. The warrant rule applies to enforcement of both criminal laws and civil codes, such as health and safety ordinances, violation of which can result in civil penalties. The purpose of the rule is to protect the privacy and security of people against arbitrary intrusions by the government. Failure to obtain a warrant can result in the exclusion of evidence, which often undercuts successful enforcement of criminal and civil penalties. Unless an exception to the warrant requirement applies, critical evidence obtained by a warrantless compliance check could be excluded from a hearing to assess penalties, thereby nullifying formal enforcement. Public health and other officials can obtain a warrant to conduct compliance checks, but alternatives, such as a licensing scheme outlined below, are more efficient. Warrants for administrative searches are issued only if there is "probable cause" to suspect a violation or violations.[37] Accordingly, steps should be taken to ensure that an exception to the warrant requirement applies to compliance checks.

Courts have developed many exceptions to the warrant requirement, two of which are of particular importance for administrative searches. First, a retailer may consent to inspection. Consent may be given immediately before the search or as a condition to obtaining a license to operate a business or market a product. The second exception applies to businesses that operate in "closely regulated commercial activity"; three criteria apply to this exception: (1) governmental interest in the regulatory scheme must be substantial; (2) warrantless searches must be necessary to further the regulatory scheme; and (3) the regulatory scheme must control the time, place, and scope of warrantless searches to limit discretionary enforcement.[38]

Public health officials should take steps to ensure that their regulations or ordinances fulfill the three criteria of the closely regulated commercial activity exception. Tobacco-control laws meet the first criterion of the closely regulated commercial activity exception, which requires a substantial government interest in the regulatory scheme. Local officials have a legitimate governmental interest in developing regulatory schemes for the sale of tobacco products. Compliance checks probably meet the second criterion of the closely regulated commercial activity exception, which requires that warrantless compliance checks further the regulatory scheme. In Massachusetts, the Supreme Judicial Court found that warrantless administrative searches are especially necessary when only a narrow window exists in which to identify a violation.[39] Inspections deter violations if they occur frequently and are unannounced. Similarly, warrantless compliance checks are necessary for the enforcement of tobacco-control laws. To effectively enforce tobacco-control laws, compliance checks must be conducted frequently, and they must be unannounced.

Tobacco-control laws can meet the third criterion of the closely regulated commercial activity exception, which requires that the time, place, and scope of compliance checks reasonably limit the enforcement discretion of the official and his or her designee who conducts the compliance checks. As part of any local tobacco-control law, the manner of enforcement should be defined. Specifically, a regulation or ordinance should state that compliance checks are to be carried out randomly, frequently by certain officials or their designees, and in a certain manner.

Due process requirements

The Due Process Clause of the U.S. Constitution provides two fundamental protections. The first due process protection, frequently referred to as *procedural due process*, requires governmental officials and their agents to follow a fair procedure when enforcing laws. The second, commonly referred to as *substantive due process*, ensures that a law's overall effect on an individual's fundamental rights, such as the right to procreate and the right to marry, is justified or justifiable.

Tobacco-control law involves several due process issues. Procedural due process requires public health and other officials to provide retailers with notice and an administrative hearing before suspending or revoking a permit or license to sell tobacco. Substantive due process may protect an individual's right to smoke in the home, except in limited circumstances. However, the right to smoke is not a protected fundamental right. Therefore, substantive due process does not protect the sale, possession, and use of tobacco products, thereby allowing federal, state, and local regulation of tobacco.

To comply with procedural due process concerns, a licensing or permitting authority must provide notice and an administrative hearing if it revokes or suspends an individual retailer's license or permit to sell tobacco products. Fair notice must be reasonably detailed, accurate, and timely. A reasonably detailed notice must accurately list the charges leveled against the permit or license holder. The adjudicative body should provide additional information about the charges, if the license or permit holder seeks clarification before the hearing. Although verbal notice may fulfill this requirement, issuing a written notice is advisable. Notice must be presented in a timely fashion.

The permit or license holder must have enough time to prepare a defense. If the license or permit holder makes a reasonable request for more time, granting a brief postponement is advisable. The license or permit holder is entitled to disclosure of all evidence that supports revocation or suspension. The licensing or permitting body can conduct its own hearing to revoke or suspend a retailer's license or permit to sell or otherwise distribute tobacco products. In this capacity, the licensing or permitting authority acts as a quasi-judicial entity.

Reducing Exposure to Environmental Tobacco Smoke

From 1992 through 2000, six major reviews of the health effects of ETS concluded that nonsmokers are harmed by such exposure in a variety of ways.[40] These include respiratory effects (acute lower respiratory tract infections in children, including bronchitis and pneumonia; asthma induction and exacerbation in children; chronic respiratory symptoms in children; eye and nasal irritation in adults; and middle ear infection in children); carcinogenic effects (lung cancer and nasal sinus cancer); cardiovascular effects (heart disease mortality; and acute and chronic coronary heart disease morbidity); and developmental effects (impaired fetal growth, low birth weight, or small size for gestational age; sudden infant death syndrome). Responding to concerns raised by the growing body of medical evidence condemning ETS as a threat to human health, government bodies, private businesses, and individuals have taken a variety of actions to limit nonsmokers' exposure to ETS.

Legislation is a common means of minimizing nonsmokers' exposure to ETS. The earliest laws restricting tobacco use (both local and state) were adopted as fire-safety measures. The first modern tobacco-control laws designed to protect nonsmokers from ETS appeared in the early 1970s. In 1975, Minnesota became the first state to pass a comprehensive state Clean Indoor Air Act restricting smoking in public places, restaurants, and public and private workplaces. Although the earliest laws restricting smoking were passed largely at the state level, progress began shifting to the local level by the early 1980s. The specific provisions and scope of these laws vary widely, but, as of December 31, 1999, smoking was restricted in public places in 45 states and the District of Columbia, and 820 local clean indoor air ordinances are now in place.[41]

During the 1980s and early 1990s, many of these laws merely required the designation of nonsmoking areas within rooms in which smoking was permitted, without a requirement for physical barriers or separate ventilation systems. Laws pertaining to restaurants typically required designation of a certain percentage of seats as being in a "no smoking" area; protecting nonsmokers from actual exposure to ETS while they were dining was simply not being accomplished. Recognition of the ongoing nature of the harm for nonsmoking patrons and employees[42,43] led to stronger legislative intervention.

Studies in both workplace and restaurant settings confirm that only policies requiring establishments to be 100% smoke free (rather than requiring only partial restrictions) adequately protect nonsmokers from exposure to ETS.[44] In 1998, California's landmark statewide ban on smoking in restaurants was extended to bars as well. Despite predictions to the contrary, neither the California law nor similar local measures have adversely affected restaurant or bar sales.[45]

The tobacco industry has suggested ventilation equipment as a solution for smoking in public. For example, Philip Morris launched a program called "PM Options" to "help business owners find ways to accommodate all customers and employees comfortably. We understand that the key to success of any accommodation program is the comfort of non-smokers. Ventilation technology can help make this a reality for the hospitality industry."[46,47]

Because smokers can and do eat in smoke-free restaurants as long as they refrain from smoking while there, they are already accommodated. On the contrary, nonsmokers who cannot tolerate a smoke-filled environment do not have access to smoke-filled establishments. What Philip Morris means by "accommodation" is, in effect, to accommodate smoking in these establishments. Significantly, Philip Morris adds the disclaimer that the "programs, resources and information offered by Philip Morris USA do not purport to address health effects attributed to environmental tobacco smoke." In fact, no evidence exists that ventilation and filtration render ETS harmless.

Litigation is one avenue through which policies limiting exposure to ETS have come about. Those who have chosen this route have helped to shape public policy concerning involuntary exposure to ETS by legal claims against cigarette manufacturers, seeking injunctive relief against continuing exposure to ETS using antidiscrimination laws such as the Americans With Disabilities Act (ADA), relying on the principles of the law of nuisance to prevent a neighbor's smoke from seeping into one's apartment or condominium unit or by raising ETS as an issue in the context of a dispute about child custody.[48] For example, the ADA was the basis for a claim by three adults with asthma who sued a major restaurant chain, alleging that they attempted to patronize the restaurants but were forced to leave because of the smoke. A federal judge denied a motion to dismiss the plaintiffs' complaint. After noting that Title III of the ADA was enacted to facilitate disabled persons' access to places of public accommodation, the Court concluded: "Just as a staircase denies access to someone in a wheelchair, tobacco smoke prevents Plaintiffs from dining at Defendants' restaurants."[49] One observer concluded that, to the extent that future jurors more fully understand how harmful ETS is, the more likely plaintiffs are to win ETS-based lawsuits.

In contrast, lawsuits attacking smoke-free policies have contained one or more of the following claims—that smoke-free laws have violated the Equal Protection Clause of the U.S. Constitution, been enacted in a manner that exceeds the authority of the entity that enacted the measure, and violated the separation of powers. These lawsuits have been filed in a variety of states, including New York, Massachusetts, Arizona, Ohio, and Michigan. For example, in *Cookie's Diner v. Columbus Board of Health*, an Ohio court found that city and county boards of health had improperly considered "concerns (such as . . . economics) other than those solely for the protection of public health." Thus, the power of boards to regulate smoking in places open to the public was limited to considerations of "protecting the public health, preventing disease and abating nuisance."[50]

In *Tri-Nel Management, Inc., et al. v. Board of Health of Barnstable, et al.,*[51] a local bar owner in Massachusetts challenged the town of Barnstable's regulation banning smoking in restaurants and bars. The bar owner argued that the board's regulation was "not reasonable because the amount of ETS exposure at restaurants and bars would not be sufficient to cause adverse health effects in general."[51] Unanimously ruling in favor of the board of health, the Massachusetts Supreme Judicial Court (SJC) rejected that argument, noting that "the board has placed in the record four reports interpreting and summarizing scientific studies that identify ETS exposure as a cause of numerous negative health effects."[51] The SJC concluded that the board's regulation is within the standard of reasonableness.[51]

A restaurant owner in Arizona challenged an antismoking measure in Tucson. One of her arguments was that, because the ban did not apply to other establishments such as bars, bowling alleys, or billiard halls, it was unconstitutional.

The Court of Appeals of Arizona, Division Two, Department A, in *City of Tucson v. Grezaffi*,[52] rejected that Equal Protection argument, ruling that absolute "equality and complete conformity of legislative classifications are not constitutionally required."

Tobacco Advertising and Promotion

Regulation of tobacco advertising is governed by the First Amendment to the U.S. Constitution, a federal statute that preempts some tobacco advertising regulations, and the MSA negotiated between the tobacco industry and the state attorneys general. In *Lorillard v. Reilly*,[53] the U.S. Supreme Court set new parameters for analyzing the constitutional and statutory issues.

First Amendment

In First Amendment analysis, advertising is considered in the special category of commercial speech. This area receives less constitutional protection than political or expressive speech because speech aimed at creating business transactions is not considered necessary to the promotion of democracy. Government regulation of political speech receives a high level of scrutiny by courts, but regulation of commercial speech receives a thorough but intermediate level of scrutiny. Constitutionally protected commercial speech may be regulated if the government furthers a substantial interest through a regulation that directly and materially advances that interest in a way that is no more extensive than necessary to achieve that interest.

In *Lorillard*, the U.S. Supreme Court assumed that the tobacco industry's speech was protected and that the government's interest in preventing tobacco-related disease was substantial. The Court further held that a government program restricting tobacco advertising on storefronts directly and materially advanced the government interest in preventing youth from experimenting with tobacco products. The Court relied on extensive scientific data to reach that conclusion but nonetheless held that the regulation was more extensive than necessary and hence invalid. The Court ruled that Massachusetts' attempt to restrict minors' exposure to tobacco advertising interfered with adults' ability to access the information. Particularly troubling to the Court was that the statewide regulation did not take local circumstances into account.

In a small but important victory for public health concerns, the Court upheld the Massachusetts Attorney General's ban on self-service displays of tobacco products. While assuming that the ban raised First Amendment concerns, the Court concluded that restrictions to behind-the-counter sales was an "appropriately narrow means" of advancing the state's "substantial interest in preventing access to tobacco products by minors."

Federal Cigarette Labeling and Advertising Act

In 1964, Congress passed the FCLAA, which required cigarette advertisements and packages to carry government-mandated warning labels. The statute preempts or trumps state and local laws that impose a requirement or prohibition on the basis of smoking and health with respect to advertising or promotion, as mentioned above. In the *Lorillard* case, the U.S. Supreme Court found that the statute preempts all state and local government regulation specifically aimed at tobacco advertising.

Several cities and states had regulated tobacco advertising and asserted a government interest in protecting children from tobacco advertising and preventing children from becoming involved in illegal activities, such as the sale of cigarettes to minors. Some jurisdictions justified the regulations as a zoning ordinance related to the placement of tobacco advertising. The Supreme Court held that Congress had preempted all these state and local laws because at their base were issues concerning the public health.

Master Settlement Agreement and advertising and promotion

Restrictions placed on tobacco advertising have been cited as the most important nonmonetary restriction achieved by the MSA, but they are also extremely complex. The MSA bans "outdoor advertising," which includes billboards and signs in arenas, stadiums, shopping malls, and video arcades. It includes other advertisements placed outdoors and certain advertisements placed inside stores if they remain visible from outside.

Exceptions to this prohibition are significant. A tobacco retailer can place any number of tobacco advertisements anywhere on its property as long as the advertisements are smaller than 14 square feet. This substantially undercuts the restriction described above because the "ban" on outdoor tobacco advertising does not apply to tobacco retail locations—the places most interested in displaying tobacco advertising.

The MSA's advertising restrictions are also subject to an exception for activities at the site of an "adult-only facility." An "adult-only facility" is defined as a restricted area where the operator of the facility ensures, or has a reasonable basis to believe, that no underaged person is present; a bar that limits entry to persons with valid identification probably would qualify. For example, the MSA permits outdoor advertising at the site of a tobacco brand-sponsored event held at an adult-only facility during the event and for 14 days before the event. This includes "Camel nights" at local bars and nightclubs. These events often target young adults by sponsoring events of interest to that age group and are permitted under the MSA clause that allows sponsored concerts in adult-only facilities.

An important achievement of the MSA is the restriction on tobacco advertisements placed on or within private or public vehicles and within transit waiting areas, such as bus stops, taxi stands, train stations, and airports. Tobacco advertising on the tops of taxis and on the sides of buses is no longer allowed.

Before the MSA, the tobacco industry claimed it voluntarily did not target minors with its advertising. The MSA is a legally binding consent decree in which the cigarette manufacturers agree not to target youth. The tobacco companies further agreed "not to take any action the *primary purpose* of which is to initiate, maintain or increase youth smoking" within the settling states (emphasis added).

The MSA provides restrictions on brand name merchandise, including bans on marketing, distributing, offering, selling, or licensing tobacco brand names on shirts, hats, backpacks, and other gear that strongly appeals to children. Tobacco products and tobacco advertisements such as posters are not covered by the merchandising prohibitions. The prohibition also does not apply to the use of coupons by adults to purchase tobacco products, the distribution of merchandise to employees of the participating manufacturers, or merchandise used only within an adult-only facility that is unavailable to the general public.

Under the MSA, the tobacco industry also agreed to prevent distribution of free samples of tobacco products except in adult-only facilities. This restriction does not include marketing practices such as "two-for-one" offers. The MSA prohibits giving anything to underaged persons on the basis of proof-of-purchase or coupons. The coupon and redemption systems will continue, but customers must provide the manufacturer of proof of age to participate.

Special highly complex rules govern tobacco product brand name sponsorships. Generally, the tobacco industry cannot use cigarette brand names to sponsor certain cultural and sporting events, except that each manufacturer may reserve one such brand name sponsorship each year. In addition, brand name sponsorship restrictions do not apply to events held in adult-only facilities.

Under the MSA, a brand name is defined as a "brand name . . . trademark, logo, symbol, motto, selling message, recognizable pattern of colors, or other indicia of product identification" identifiable with a domestic brand of tobacco product. Corporate names are specifically excluded. A brand name sponsorship is "an athletic, musical, artistic, or other social or cultural event" for which a participating manufacturer has paid a fee for the use of the brand name in the name of the event, such as the Winston Cup NASCAR series. It also includes the advertising of the event or an entrant, participant, or team in the event, such as the Winston racing team in NASCAR events.

Several types of brand name sponsorships are completely prohibited. Tobacco companies cannot sponsor (*1*) concerts (except in adult-only facilities); (*2*) events in which the intended audience comprises a significant percentage of youth; (*3*) events in which paid participants or contestants are youth; or (*4*) any athletic event between opposing teams in any football, basketball, baseball, soccer or hockey league.

Each company is allowed only one brand name sponsorship in a 12-month period. A sponsorship is considered a single sponsorship even if it includes many events or locations, such as Virginia Slims tennis tournaments that may be played in many different states throughout the year. Despite the brand name sponsorship limits, events may still be sponsored in the corporate name of the tobacco company as long as the corporate name does not include any domestic brand name of a tobacco product.

These limitations regarding product placement, merchandising, and outdoor advertisements do not apply in the context of brand name sponsorships. For example, outdoor advertising of brand name sponsorships are also allowed at the site of the event for 90 days before the event and 10 days after the conclusion of the event. The result is that cigarette companies can advertise the sponsored event on billboards for 100 days each time an event occurs.

Because third parties, such as retailers and billboard companies, did not sign the document, holding them to the terms of the MSA is difficult. The MSA prohibits tobacco companies from licensing or authorizing third parties to do anything the tobacco companies cannot do under the MSA. In fact, the tobacco companies are obliged to take "commercially reasonable steps" to prevent such action. However, whether a third party allegedly acting on its own may take action forbidden under the MSA is not clear.

Product Regulation and Disclosure

States can undertake a range of untested or cutting-edge regulatory approaches to tobacco products. Such endeavors involve a certain degree of risk because they inevitably invite legal challenges. However, they have the potential to address important public health aspects of the tobacco problem that have not been the subject of federal legislation or regulation. For example, cigarette-caused fires result in nearly 1000 deaths and 3000 injuries each year in the United States. As of April 2002, New York is the only state to have adopted legislation mandating that cigarettes be less incendiary, which becomes effective in 2003. Similar efforts in Massachusetts, Minnesota, California, and Oregon have not yet succeeded.

Although the FDA has enacted most of the drug regulation in the United States, states retain residual power over drugs not regulated by the FDA. Because this applies to tobacco regulation, states have the opportunity to fill the vacuum created by the U.S. Supreme Court's invalidation of the FDA's assertion of jurisdiction over tobacco products in *FDA v. Brown & Williamson Tobacco Corp.*[54] The Court held that, without a direct grant of authority by Congress, FDA regulation of tobacco products as drugs or drug-delivery devices is unavailable. However, a potential parallel regulatory framework exists at the state level. Most states have statutes providing residual powers over drugs not regulated by the FDA. FDA-like regulation of tobacco at the state level could compel disclosure of additional product information to consumers or regulate product design including incendiary characteristics as well as overall toxicity, addictiveness, and lethality.

Massachusetts was the first state to attempt to compel disclosure, by state statute and health regulation, of the identity and weights of additives used in specific brands of tobacco products.[55] The regulation was enjoined on the basis that it amounted to a "taking without compensation," violating the Fifth and Fourteenth Amendments to the U.S. Constitution. As of April 2002, the case is before the U.S. Court of Appeals for the First Circuit. Other than Massachusetts, only Minnesota and Texas have required any reporting of tobacco ingredients.[56] These two states' approaches would not provide basic information such as which ingredients in which quantities are in any particular cigarette brand.

Aside from the Fifth Amendment concerns that stem from the assertion that the ingredients disclosure is a taking of a trade secret, the two affirmative theories most likely to be used to challenge tobacco product regulation at the state level are preemption under the FCLAA and violations of the Commerce Clause of the U.S. Constitution.

PRACTICE CONSIDERATIONS

As discussed above, the law has a huge impact on the ability of public health practitioners to reduce the use of tobacco. Thus, practitioners need to understand how the law can be used to support—or thwart—tobacco control. One reason the law is often a thorn in the side of tobacco-control advocates is that a $40 billion industry is actively engaged in shaping the law to protect its interests—in particular an uninterrupted flow of profit from the sale of tobacco.

Practitioners should heed several "lessons learned" about how the law should be shaped to support the aims of tobacco control. First, tobacco-control legislation should be crafted as strongly and as devoid of loopholes as possible. For example, increasing the tax on tobacco should include a provision that indexes the tax to inflation; otherwise, the tax will lose value over time. One cannot expect to be able to revisit tobacco legislation soon after initial passage to correct problems with the legislation. Similarly, partial bans on tobacco advertising and promotion are generally ineffective because tobacco companies shift marketing expenditures from banned media to media that remain accessible to them.

The language in tobacco-control legislation needs to be scrutinized to search for wording that will emasculate the effectiveness of the legislation. An example noted above is the effort by tobacco interests to include language such as "knowingly" or "intentionally" in laws prohibiting the sale of tobacco to minors (penalties are imposed only on retailers that knowingly sell tobacco to minors).[57]

Tobacco-control legislation needs to be crafted carefully in anticipation of legal challenges by tobacco companies or their allies. The tobacco industry will often challenge in court any legislation that threatens its business, no matter how remote its chances for success. Sometimes the legal challenge will be intended only to delay implementation of the law or to tax the patience and resources of the proponents.

Tobacco companies will often threaten to challenge legislation in court when it is under consideration by a legislative body. The purpose is to frighten legislators from passing a bill or ordinance, over concern about the costs of defending the legislation in court. In anticipation of this tactic, tobacco-control advocates should procure legal support early in the legislative process, including having legal counsel and written legal opinions available.

For several reasons, tobacco-control advocates should recognize that local control over the sale, distribution, and use of tobacco is generally the most effective strategy a tobacco-control program can pursue. First, local legislation is easier to pass than state or federal legislation. In addition, local legislation is adopted at a faster rate. Despite its use of business associations and groups such as the National Smokers' Alliance, the tobacco industry is generally ineffective in defeating or weakening local tobacco-control measures. Second, laws passed at the local level typically are far stronger than laws passed at the state or federal level, both substantively and in terms of enforcement mechanisms established. Local ordinances, bylaws, and health board regulations are usually stronger and more comprehensive than federal and state tobacco-control laws. Third, measures passed at the local level enjoy broad community support. After spending countless hours in town meetings and public hearings, communities are educated in tobacco issues. As a result, local tobacco-control measures gain strong public support. Fourth, compliance rates are higher for local tobacco-control measures, primarily because local enforcement agencies are more accessible and thus more effective than federal and state enforcement agencies. For these reasons, tobacco-control advocates should avoid "deals" offered by tobacco interests or tobacco-friendly politicians that would insert legislative language that would preempt local controls.

EMERGING ISSUES

Legislation and Regulation

At the federal level, legislation has been introduced to provide the FDA with regulatory authority over tobacco products. Strong legislation could enable the FDA not only to reinstate its rules limiting youth access to tobacco and restricting tobacco marketing but also to regulate tobacco product design to reduce toxicity; require effective health warnings through package inserts; and take other steps to reduce the extent of addiction, disease, and death caused by tobacco products. Weak legislation, on the other hand, would limit the FDA's ability to protect both existing smokers and future industry targets, while allowing the companies to say that "we're already regulated so the problem is solved."

At the state level, health advocates will continue their efforts to have tobacco settlement funds appropriated for tobacco-control education and intervention. In some states, advocates may use ballot initiatives to guarantee a fair allocation of settlement funds to tobacco control after failed attempts to accomplish this goal through legislation. Legislation may be introduced in several states requiring disclosure of tobacco product ingredients and smoke components, requiring less incendiary product designs, and, in the continued absence of FDA jurisdiction over tobacco, perhaps requiring design changes to render the products less toxic and addictive. In some states the health departments may already have the authority to impose such requirements.

At the state and local levels, efforts will continue to broaden and strengthen laws restricting smoking in shared airspaces. Cutting-edge issues include restricting smoking in some outdoor public places and prohibiting smoking in vehicles in which children are present. Furthermore, raising the minimum age of sale to 21 years, in parity with alcohol, would be likely to dramatically reduce sales of cigarettes to teenagers.

Litigation Against the Tobacco Industry

The U.S. Department of Justice may settle or win its pending lawsuit against the tobacco industry, which is based on the Racketeer Influenced and Corrupt Organizations Act. Such a settlement or final judgment may restrict various future actions of cigarette manufacturers.

The appeal in the Engle class action case on behalf of ailing or deceased Florida smokers, which so far has resulted in a $145 billion punitive damage verdict and the award of an average of $4 million each in compensatory damages to three of the hundreds of thousands of class members, probably will continue at least through 2003. Favorable appellate court rulings are likely to result in similar cases in other jurisdictions. Other class actions, seeking the cost of medical monitoring for addicted but otherwise healthy smokers, are pending in Louisiana and West Virginia. Other class actions on a variety of theories are pending in California and Illinois state courts and in a New York federal court.

Individual cases on behalf of smokers or their survivors are pending in many states. Multimillion dollar punitive damage verdicts already have been reached in several cases: If these are upheld on appeal, thousands of additional cases will doubtless be filed. The assessed and anticipated liability may exceed even this wealthy industry's ability to pay, which could force one or more companies into bankruptcy reorganization (i.e., "Chapter 11" status). For the companies to continue in business under Chapter 11, rather than being forced to sell their assets, the bankruptcy court needs to conclude that the reorganization plan is "viable" in that the expected liability costs from new sales will not exceed the profits. This could provide an opportunity for the public health community to provide evidence on what would be an appropriate (non-tortious) way to design and market tobacco products.

The tobacco industry may seek Congressional relief from its tobacco liability obligations. Such relief was part of the proposed "Global Settlement" of June 1997 between state attorneys general, private attorneys, and the tobacco industry. Congress did not approve the proposed immunities, leading the industry to jettison the deal. However, pressure from successful tobacco lawsuits may induce the industry to try again, and the public health community needs to be prepared to respond.

Litigation by or on Behalf of the Tobacco Industry

The tobacco industry's goal is to sell as many products as it can. The public health goal is to reduce consumption of tobacco products (at least of the addictive, carcinogenic, and otherwise toxic products on the market) to the greatest extent possible. These goals are fundamentally incompatible. As a result, the tobacco industry will continue to try to thwart effective tobacco-control measures, including threatening and pursuing litigation. This fundamental incompatibility of goals is also the reason that this branch of public health practice is characterized by confrontation with an industry (unlike many other areas of public health), by military metaphors, and frequently by litigation.

ACKNOWLEDGMENTS

We thank Jackie Salcedo, J.D., for her assistance in drafting the section on youth access to tobacco, and Lissy Friedman, J.D., for her assistance with the manuscript.

References

1. Centers for Disease Control and Prevention. Cigarette smoking-attributable mortality and years of potential life lost—United States, 1990. *MMWR* 1993;42:645–9.
2. World Bank. *Curbing the Epidemic: Governments and the Economics of Tobacco Control*. Washington, DC: World Bank, 1999.
3. California Environmental Protection Agency. *Health Effects of Exposure to Environmental Tobacco Smoke*. Sacramento: Office of Environmental Health Hazard Assessment, 1997.
4. Centers for Disease Control and Prevention. *Best Practices for Comprehensive Tobacco Control Programs—August 1999*. Atlanta: CDC, National Center for Chronic Disease Prevention and Health Promotion, Office on Smoking and Health, 1999.

5. *Brown & Williamson Tobacco Co. v. FDA*, 529 U.S. 120 (2000).
6. 15 U.S.C. § 1331 *et seq.*
7. 15 U.S.C. § 1335.
8. 15 U.S.C. § 4401 *et seq.*
9. In the Matter of Swisher Int'l, Inc. Consent Decree dated June 26, 2000; USFTC File No. 0023199.
10. 47 U.S.C. § 41706.
11. Public Law 103-227, § 1041–4.
12. 42 U.S.C. § 300x-26.
13. 15 U.S.C. § 1334b.
14. Siegel M, Carol J, Jordan J, et al. Preemption in tobacco control: review of an emerging public health problem. *JAMA* 1997;278:858–63.
15. Centers for Disease Control and Prevention. Preemptive state tobacco-control laws— United States, 1982–1998. *MMWR* 1999;47:1112–4.
16. 940 Code Mass. Regs. 21.00.
17. Daynard RA. Tobacco liability litigation as a cancer control strategy. *J Natl Cancer Inst* 1988;80:9–13.
18. *Master Settlement Agreement.* Sec. VII Available at http://www.naag.org/tobac/ cigmsa.rtf. Accessed December 6, 2001.
19. Daynard RA. Tobacco litigation: a mid-course review. *Cancer Causes Control* 2001; 12:383–6.
20. National Association of Attorneys General. *Multistate settlement with the tobacco industry.* Available at http://www.tobacco.neu.edu/Extra/multistate_settlement.htm. Accessed October 12, 2001.
21. U.S. Department of Health and Human Services. Economic approaches. *Reducing Tobacco Use: A Report of the Surgeon General.* Atlanta: US Department of Health and Human Services, Public Health Service, CDC, National Center for Chronic Disease Prevention and Health Promotion, Office on Smoking and Health, 2000: pp. 293–370.
22. U.S. Department of Health and Human Services. *Investment in tobacco control: state highlights 2001.* Available at http://www.cdc.gov/tobacco/statehi/statehi_2001.htm. Accessed October 12, 2001.
23. Sweda EL Jr, Daynard RA. Tobacco industry tactics. *Br Med Bull* 1996;52:183–92.
24. *Flue Cured Tobacco Cooperative Stabilization Corp. v. EPA*, 4 F.Supp. 435 (USDC MD NC 1998).
25. *Philip Morris v. American Broadcasting Co., Inc., et al.*, 36 Va. Cir. 1, 1995 Va. Cir. LEXIS 1250 (1995).
26. *Philip Morris, Inc. v. Reilly*, 113 F.Supp. 2d 129 (USDC D Mass. 2000).
27. 121 S.Ct. 2404, 150 L.Ed.2d 532 (2001).
28. Bergman AB. Curtailing youth smoking [editorial]. *Arch Pediatr Adolesc Med* 2001; 155:546–7.
29. 58 *Federal Register* 164: 45156 (August 26, 1993).
30. DiFranza JR, Godshall WT. Tobacco industry efforts hindering enforcement of the ban on tobacco sales to minors: actions speak louder than words. *Tob Control* 1996; 5:127–31.
31. Lynch BS, Bonnie RJ. *Growing Up Tobacco Free: Preventing Nicotine Addiction in Children and Youths.* Washington, DC: National Academy Press, 1994.
32. U.S. Department of Health and Human Services. *Reducing Tobacco Use: A Report of the Surgeon General.* Atlanta: U.S. Department of Health and Human Services,

Public Health Service, CDC, National Center for Chronic Disease Prevention and Health Promotion, Office on Smoking and Health, 2000: pp. 207–8.

33. Office of the Inspector General. *Youth Access to Tobacco*. Washington, DC: U.S. Department of Health and Human Services, December 1992.

34. U.S. Department of Health and Human Services. *Preventing Tobacco Use Among Young People: A Report of the Surgeon General*. Atlanta: U.S. Department of Health and Human Services, Public Health Service, CDC, National Center for Chronic Disease Prevention and Health Promotion, Office on Smoking and Health, 1994.

35. Cummings KM, Sciandra E, Pechacek TF, Orlandi M, Lynn WR. Where teenagers get their cigarettes: a survey of the purchasing habits of 13–16 year olds in 12 US communities. *Tob Control* 1992;1:264–7.

36. *See v. City of Seattle*, 387 U.S. 541, 545–6 (1967).

37. *Camara v. Municipal Court of and City of San Francisco*, 387 U.S. 523, 534–5 (1967).

38. *New York v. Burger*, 428 U.S. 691, 702–3 (1987).

39. *Commonwealth v. Tart*, 408 Mass. 249, 255 (1990).

40. Environmental Protection Agency, 1992; Australian National Health and Medical Research Council, 1997; California Environmental Protection Agency, 1997.

41. United Kingdom Scientific Committee on Tobacco and Health, 1998; World Health Organization, 1999; and US National Toxicology Program in 2000.

42. U.S. Department of Health and Human Services. *Reducing Tobacco Use: A Report of the Surgeon General*. Atlanta: U.S. Department of Health and Human Services, Public Health Service, CDC, National Center for Chronic Disease Prevention and Health Promotion, Office on Smoking and Health, 2000: pp. 16.

43. Siegel M. Involuntary smoking in the restaurant workplace: a review of employee exposure and health effects. *JAMA* 1993;270:490–3.

44. National Cancer Institute. *State and Local Legislative Action to Reduce Tobacco Use: Smoking and Tobacco Control*. Bethesda, MD: National Institutes of Health, 2000; Monograph No. 11.

45. Glantz SA, Smith LRA. The effect of ordinances requiring smoke-free restaurants and bars on revenues: a follow-up. *Am J Public Health* 1997;87:1687–93.

46. Glantz SA, Charlesworth A. Tourism and hotel revenues before and after passage of smoke-free restaurant ordinances. *JAMA* 1999;281:1911–8.

47. Philip Morris USA. *Accommodation: reasonable approaches to public-place smoking*. Available at http://www.philipmorrisusa.com/displaypagewithtopic.asp?id=52. Accessed December 6, 2001.

48. Sweda L. *Summary of Legal Cases Regarding Smoking in the Workplace and Other Places*. 16.2 Tobacco Products Litigation Reporter 4.1-4.79 (2001). Boston: Tobacco Control Resource Center, 2000.

49. *Edwards, et al. v. GDRI, Inc., et al.*, Civil Action No. DKC-97-4327 (USDC D Md. 1999).

50. *Cookie's Diner v. Columbus Board of Health*, 640 N.E.2d 1231, 1241 (Mun. Ct. 1994).

51. *Tri-Nel Management, Inc., et al. v. Board of Health of Barnstable, et al.*, 433 Mass. 217, 741 N.E.2d 37 (2001),

52. *City of Tucson v. Grezaffi*, 23 P.3d 675, 347 Ariz. Adv. Rep. 10 (2001).

53. *Lorillard v. Reilly*, 121 S.Ct. 2404, 150 L.Ed.2d 532 (2001).

54. *FDA v. Brown & Williamson Tobacco Corp.*, 529 U.S. 120 (2000).

55. Sweda EL Jr. Litigation on behalf of victims of exposure to environmental tobacco smoke, the experience from the USA. *Eur J Public Health* 2001;11:201–5.

56. Brigham PA, McGuire A. Progress towards a fire-safe cigarette. *J Public Health Policy* 1995;16:433–8.

57. New York Executive Law sec. 156-c.

58. Mass. Gen. L. Ch. 94, Sec. 307A and 105 Code of Mass. Regs. 660.000.

59. Minn. Stat. Sec. 461.17 (Supp. 1997) and Tex. Health & Safety Code Ann., Secs. 161.251–255 (West Supp. 1998).

60. DiFranza JR, Godshall WT. Tobacco industry efforts hindering enforcement of the ban on tobacco sales to minors: actions speak louder than words. *Tob Control* 1996; 5:127–31.

17

Reproductive Health

BEBE J. ANDERSON AND LYNNE S. WILCOX

The field of reproductive health includes examples of almost every type of public health law. Reproductive health is not a single health exposure or outcome but rather an entire human biologic system. This chapter defines reproductive health broadly, including examples from contraception, abortion, pregnancy, and infertility. (Human immunodeficiency virus [HIV] and sexually transmitted infections, important aspects of reproductive health, are discussed in Chapter 15.) Legal issues in reproductive health include reporting of outcomes (surveillance, vital statistics), program management (who receives and who can provide reproductive health services), insurance coverage (legal mandates for insurance covering contraception or infertility services), government funding of services (Medicaid, Title X), clinic operation (licensing laws), and public health research (human subjects protection and informed consent for pregnant women).

An understanding of reproductive health law requires recognition that both law and medicine have shaped this area. Activities such as sexual behavior, childbearing, and birth control are viewed in most societies as having moral, legal, and cultural implications beyond their health effects, leading to laws intended to control these behaviors. For example, abortion and birth control were subject to state criminal laws that limited access to these services until the mid-1960s, when courts began to find that such laws implicate federal constitutional rights. Thus, several reproductive health law issues implicate constitutionally protected rights, in particular the right to privacy.

In the United States, approximately 6 million pregnancies occur and 4 million live infants are born each year, and approximately 39 million women of childbearing age use some form of birth control. Women who are pregnant receive special attention in state and federal laws. This attention includes ensuring that medical care is available to low-income pregnant women (Title V); monitoring health events, such as maternal deaths (vital statistics reporting); and protecting pregnant women from research risks. Women of reproductive age are subject to a variety of laws, some designed to increase access to reproductive health services and others designed to restrict such access. For example, Title X of the Social Security Act provides family planning services to low-income women, but significant legal restrictions exist at the federal and state levels regarding abortion services or family planning services to minor girls. An estimated 48% of U.S. women aged 15–44 years have had at least one unplanned pregnancy.[1]

Women and couples who use infertility services have other legal concerns, many of which center on the financial cost of advanced infertility techniques. For example, a 1-month cycle of in vitro fertilization (IVF) can cost thousands of dollars but has only one chance in four of resulting in a liveborn infant. This has led to a strong interest among advocates for infertile couples in encouraging legislation that mandates insurance coverage for these services; these mandates have been established in several states. In addition, federal legislation requiring standardized reporting of pregnancy rates by IVF clinics has been passed to provide consumers with standardized data for decision making regarding the use of IVF services.

Thus, the influence of law on reproductive health concerns varies with the outcome of interest and is often affected by the woman's resources. To provide the best reproductive health research and programs, public health practitioners need to be aware of the spectrum of legal influences.

LEGAL AUTHORITIES

Introduction

This section outlines the laws governing reproductive health in the United States, with particular emphasis on the federal Constitution, statutes, regulations, and case law. State law regarding reproductive health is dynamic. Each year, new laws are introduced in state legislatures throughout the country, touching on such issues as provision of abortions, access to contraceptives, and insurance coverage for infertility treatments. Moreover, many state-by-state differences exist in the approach to legislation in this area. Given the number, breadth, and volubility of state regulation in this area, we have not attempted to cite or explain the many laws of individual states.[a] Rather, we have tried to highlight major themes of state regulation in this area to emphasize the need to determine whether a specific state has enacted legislation addressing a particular aspect of reproductive health.

Constitutional Law

Controlling issues under the U.S. Constitution

In contrast to many other areas of public health law, the most important legal authority for reproductive health law issues is the U.S. Constitution. Before 1965, the main sources of law governing reproductive health were state laws, in particular, laws criminalizing the use of contraceptives and prohibiting the performance of abortions.[b] The legal landscape changed dramatically with the U.S. Supreme Court's decision in *Griswold v. Connecticut.*[2]

In *Griswold*, the Supreme Court held that state regulation of the use of contraceptives by married persons invaded "the zone of privacy created by several fundamental constitutional guarantees."[2] The Constitution does not explicitly protect a right to privacy; rather, the Supreme Court has found such a right to be implicit in the Constitution on the basis of the nature of rights explicitly protected by the federal Constitution.[3] Legal restrictions on matters involving reproductive health implicate the constitutional right to privacy because, as the Court has stated, "if the right of privacy means anything, it is the right of the individual, married or single, to be free from unwarranted governmental intrusion into matters so fundamentally affecting a person as the decision whether to bear or beget a child"[4,c] (emphasis omitted). Therefore, state regulation regarding reproductive health must account for the unique, constitutionally protected status accorded decisions regarding pregnancy. Most of the court decisions addressing this right have arisen in the context of abortion; however, the right to privacy is by no means limited to that aspect of reproductive health.[d]

Although the right to privacy under the U.S. Constitution is the primary federal constitutional authority governing the regulation of reproductive health, the constitutional rights to due process and equal protection also are often implicated. To satisfy the requirements of the due process clause of the Fourteenth Amendment, a statute must clearly define the conduct that it prohibits, so a person can avoid engaging in prohibited conduct. In particular, statutes that impose criminal penalties—as many state laws regulating abortion do—and statutes that interfere with constitutionally protected activity are subjected to a higher standard of certainty in their language. Many restrictions on the provision of reproductive health services have been found by federal courts to be unconstitutionally vague and therefore violative of the due process clause of the Fourteenth Amendment.[5] In some of these cases, the statutes' vagueness derives from the use in legislation of terms that have a variety of meanings or no clear meaning to members of the medical community.

Equal protection challenges to restrictions on the provision of reproductive health services focus on the extent to which the laws treat similarly situated persons alike. Federal courts have found some restrictions on the provision of abortion to violate the equal protection clause of the Fourteenth Amendment because they single out abortion providers for requirements that are not imposed on providers of medical procedures involving comparable risks and complexity. Other equal protection challenges have focused on differential treatment of women and of men seeking reproductive health services. Although such claims are frequently raised in challenges to restrictions on, in particular, the provision of abortion, the challenges are usually resolved on other grounds, in particular, vagueness or the right to privacy.

The right to privacy was applied to the abortion context in the landmark decision *Roe v. Wade*,[3] in which the Supreme Court declared that Texas's criminal abortion statutes were unconstitutional. Three years after the *Roe* decision, the Court held that minor women also have a right to privacy, which includes the right to reproductive choice, although the state has broader authority to restrict the exercise of that right in the context of minors.[6]

Since the *Roe* decision, the Supreme Court has repeatedly addressed the constitutionality of various state, and some federal, laws imposing restrictions on the provision of abortions, as the limits and continued vitality of the *Roe* decision have been tested. The most significant post-*Roe* case is *Planned Parenthood v. Casey*.[1]

In *Casey*, a bare majority of the Supreme Court reaffirmed that women have a constitutional right to choose and obtain an abortion without government interference, as it had held in *Roe*. However, the Court altered the analysis to be applied to restrictions on that right. Five members of the Court held that (*1*) before a fetus is viable, a woman has a right to choose to have an abortion and to obtain such an abortion, subject only to state interference that is designed to advance the state's interests in protecting the health of the woman or the potential life of the fetus and that does not constitute an "undue" burden on that right; (*2*) after viability, a state has the power to restrict abortions, provided that the restriction contains exceptions for situations in which a woman's health or life is endangered by continuation of her pregnancy; and (*3*) a state has legitimate interests throughout a pregnancy in protecting both the health of the pregnant woman and the potential life of the fetus.[7] In *Roe*, the Court held that the right to reproductive choice is a fundamental right and the weight to be given the state's interests in regulating abortion depended on the trimester of pregnancy affected. In *Casey*, the trimester approach was replaced with the "undue burden" test: A state regulation violates the right to privacy if it imposes an "undue burden" on that right, meaning that the regulation "has the purpose or effect of placing a substantial obstacle in the path of a woman seeking an abortion of a nonviable fetus."[7]

The Supreme Court has recognized only two purposes that can justify imposing an undue burden on a woman's right to reproductive choice: (1) the state's interest in potential life and (2) the state's interest in protecting maternal health.[7] With respect to the state's interest in potential life, the Court has clearly stated that before viability the state may promote that interest only through means "calculated to inform the woman's free choice, not hinder it."[7]

In its most recent affirmation of the right to reproductive choice, the Court reiterated the requirement that restrictions on the provision of abortions must include an exception for situations in which the woman's health or life will be placed at risk.[8] In that case, the Court found that Nebraska's ban on "partial birth abortions" violated the right to privacy because it lacked such an exception and placed an undue burden on the right by allowing prosecution of physicians for performing the most commonly used procedure for terminating previability second-trimester pregnancies.[8]

Controlling issues under state constitutions

Some restrictions on access to reproductive health services have been challenged on the basis of provisions in state constitutions—in particular in states with constitutions that provide broader protection to privacy rights than the U.S. Constitution.[9] Such challenges also have been brought successfully on the basis of other clauses in state constitutions, in particular, equal protection clauses and privileges and immunities clauses.[10]

Laws and Regulations Related to Program Management

Restrictions on receipt of services

By statute and regulation, many states regulate the provision of contraceptives and other family planning services, including imposing specific informed consent requirements for the receipt of such services. The provision of sterilization services is specifically restricted where federal family planning funds are used: The patient must comply with a specific informed consent procedure; there must be a 30 day gap between provision of informed consent and performance of the procedure; the patient must be over age 21 years; and the patient must be mentally competent.[11] In addition, many states impose specific restrictions on the provision of sterilization.

For minors in most states, access to reproductive health services differs from access to other health care. In general, Anglo-American common law traditionally accorded parents (specifically, fathers) the right to make health-care decisions for their children. However, slightly more than half of the states have altered this ancient doctrine by statutes that specifically authorize a minor to obtain prenatal care and delivery services without parental consent or notification. Half of the states explicitly grant minors the right to consent to contraceptive services without parental involvement. In contrast, many states impose, by statute, limitations on the access of minors to abortion services. Many states have laws requiring that the minor obtain the consent of one or both parents or that the minor or the abortion provider notify one or both parents before an abortion is performed on the minor.

State law provides the primary source of restrictions on the receipt of abortion services. Federal case law interpreting the validity of such statutes under the U.S. Constitution provides the primary controlling law governing such restrictions.

Restrictions on provision of services

A physician's prescription is required for oral contraceptive pills and emergency contraceptive pills in the United States. This requirement serves as a barrier to receipt of emergency contraceptive, which must be obtained promptly after intercourse to be effective.[17] The Food and Drug Administration (FDA) has authority to remove the prescription restriction for a drug and allow it to be distributed over the counter.[12,13]

Some state laws allow certain individuals, facilities, or entities to refuse to participate in the provision of contraceptive supplies or services or abortion services on the basis of moral or religious beliefs.[c] In a few states, such laws have been found to be unconstitutional under either the state or federal constitution as applied to public, "quasi-public," nonsectarian, or nonprofit facilities.[14-16] Some states allow individuals or facilities to deny patients information or counseling about contraceptives, and some actually prohibit state employees or entities or organizations that receive state funds from counseling or referring women for abortion services in some circumstances.

Most states prohibit, by statute, persons other than licensed physicians from performing abortions. Such restrictions have been found to be constitutional under the U.S. Constitution as furthering the state interest of protecting maternal health.[3,17] In a few states, physician assistants can perform abortions under the supervision of a licensed physician, and one state has adopted this as a matter of state constitutional law.

States may not require all second-trimester abortions to be performed in hospitals; such laws violate the U.S. Constitution.[18-20] In almost every state, after a fetus is viable, an abortion can be performed only in accordance with specific statutory requirements.

An increasing number of states have enacted licensing schemes that not only require state licensure of facilities at which abortions are performed but also impose specific requirements regarding staffing, physical plant, administrative procedures, equipment, and other matters. Some of these laws and regulations have been successfully challenged as violating the U.S. Constitution, but others have been upheld by the courts, usually on the basis that they do not create a significant obstacle to women seeking abortions. In addition to the many abortion-specific statutes, several statutory and regulatory schemes governing the provision of medical services apply to abortion providers. Physicians and nurses performing abortion services are required to adhere to the professional and ethical standards contained in the applicable state statutes and regulations governing their professional licensure. Most facilities at which abortions are performed are subject to the federal Clinical Laboratory Improvement Act (CLIA)[21] and to the Occupational Safety and Health Act[22]; local ordinances pertaining to waste disposal; and other local laws, such as fire and building codes and local ordinances, pertaining to building maintenance.

Laws and Regulations Related to Payment for Services

Government funding

Government funding of reproductive health services differs greatly depending on the type of service. Health services related to childbirth—during pregnancy, at birth, and postpartum—are subject to special rules, generally designed to increase the number of women receiving the services, by raising income eligibility levels for pregnant women.

Federal regulations require that state Medicaid programs provide Medicaid-eligible persons with pregnancy-related services, such as prenatal, delivery, and postpartum care and family planning services.[23] Moreover, a woman who was eligible for and received Medicaid coverage for pregnancy-related services during her pregnancy remains eligible for such services during a postpartum period lasting at least 60 days after the birth, even if her financial circumstances change.[23] In response to the changing provision of health care in the United States, many Medicaid programs contract with managed-care providers. To protect women's access to timely and confidential family planning services, Congress has enacted a freedom-of-choice statute, allowing women to go "outside the plan" for family planning services.[24]

Beginning in 1986, in response to concerns about infant mortality, Congress amended the Medicaid laws in an effort to increase the number of pregnant women eligible for prenatal care services and to improve the services they can receive. In particular, Congress created a higher income eligibility limit for pregnant women so that more women would qualify for Medicaid coverage of pregnancy-related services. As a result, by the mid-1990s the Medicaid program paid for almost one third of all births in the United States. In addition, other federal programs—including the Maternal and Child Health program and the Special Supplemental Food Program for Women, Infants, and Children (WIC)— provide funding for aspects of prenatal care. Most states have taken additional steps to increase pregnant women's access to pregnancy-related services, including increasing their Medicaid eligibility levels beyond the minimum levels required by the federal regulations; adopting special administrative rules to make beginning receipt of covered services easier for pregnant women; and increasing the types of pregnancy-related services covered under their Medicaid plans. The strategies used by states to increase the number of women receiving prenatal care have differed, with varying success rates.[25]

Family planning services other than abortion are funded from a variety of public sources, each with its own restrictions. The federal government provides funding for family planning services through four major sources: Title X of the Public Health Services Act and Titles V (the Maternal and Child Health Block Grant), XIX (Medicaid), and XX (the Social Services Block Grant) of the Social Security Act.[26–29] Through the Title X program, the federal government awards grants solely for family planning to service providers—state agencies and private nonprofit agencies—which then can offer such services to uninsured persons at reduced fees and to women in managed-care plans who seek services outside their provider network. Recipients of Title X funds are required to provide not only comprehensive family planning services but also an array of preventive health-care services such as pelvic examinations, Pap tests, breast examinations, screening and treatment for sexually transmitted infections, safer-sex counseling, basic infertility screening, and referrals to specialized health care. Funds under Titles V and XX, which can be used for services including family planning services, are provided only to state government agencies, which may pass the funds on to private agencies. Under the Medicaid program, the federal government reimburses the states for providing services, with family planning services reimbursed at a higher rate than other services. State funds for family planning services come from a variety of sources, including state Medicaid funding.

Minors can obtain federally funded contraceptives confidentially. Title X encourages family participation in federally funded family planning programs; federal courts have invalidated efforts to require notification of a minor's parent on the basis that they violated Title X.[30,31]

Government funding for abortion services is severely restricted. Although the Medicaid program generally provides coverage for medically necessary health care needed by income-eligible persons, medically necessary abortions are not covered. Pursuant to the "Hyde Amendment," state Medicaid plans must cover abortions, and federal reimbursement funds are available for them, only if the procedure is necessary to save a woman's life when her life was endangered by a physical disorder, physical injury, or physical illness or where the woman's pregnancy resulted from rape or incest.[32,f] The U.S. Supreme Court has held that this restriction on coverage of abortions does not violate the federal right to privacy.[33] Nevertheless, some states fund medically necessary abortions on the basis of a state statute or regulation or because ordered to do so by a state court.

Private funding

Private funding for reproductive health services depends on the specific provisions of a given insurance policy or managed-care plan, but some types of coverage are mandated by law. Federal law requires that group health plans, insurance companies, and health-maintenance organizations that offer health coverage for hospital stays in connection with childbirth provide such coverage for mandated minimum periods of time.[34] After most normal vaginal deliveries, a hospital stay of at least 48 hours must be covered for both the woman and her newborn child; after birth by caesarean delivery, a hospital stay of at least 96 hours must be covered.

Legislation has been enacted in some states, and proposed at the federal level, requiring health plans to cover infertility treatments as a benefit in each insurance policy or to make such coverage available for purchase. The details of what the plans must cover—in terms of type of infertility treatments, number of procedures covered, and prerequisites for coverage—vary widely among these state laws. As of 2001, most health plans did not provide any coverage for infertility treatments when not mandated to do so by law.

Beginning in the late 1990s, many states enacted laws requiring that health insurance plans provide partial or comprehensive insurance coverage for reversible methods of contraceptives. Laws in a few states prohibit private insurance coverage for abortion unless the woman pays an extra premium.

Laws and Regulations Related to Public Health Surveillance

The states have the legal responsibility to collect, manage, and compile vital records, a key source of information for many reproductive health issues. States require the registration of all births and deaths. This registration is considered virtually complete in most states and allows a complete enumeration of the numerator (infant deaths) and denominator (infant births) for reporting infant mortality rates. The reporting of maternal deaths is more challenging. While every woman's death is reported, information regarding pregnancy may not appear on the death certificate because of differences in certificate design and definition of maternal death among states. Thus maternal deaths calculated from vital records are generally regarded as underestimates of the true number of deaths. Legal requirements for reporting of fetal deaths also vary from state to state.

Most states gather data on the provision of legal induced abortions. Typically, abortion providers are required by state statute or regulation to provide data to the state health department, state registrar, or state vital statistics officer. Some controversy has arisen about whether induced abortions should be monitored as reportable events comparable with births, deaths, and fetal deaths or as medical procedures comparable with other surgeries.[35] The collection of confidential information about the provision of abortions relates to the state's interest in maternal health and has been found to be constitutional. Noting that "[t]he collection of information with respect to actual patients is a vital element of medical research," the U.S. Supreme Court upheld a requirement that the following information be reported for each abortion performed: identity of the facility and physician performing the abortion; woman's number of prior pregnancies and abortions; gestational age of the aborted fetus; type of abortion procedure; preexisting conditions complicating the pregnancy; medical complications from the abortion; reason the abortion was medically necessary, if applicable; and weight of the aborted fetus.[6,7]

Laws and Regulations Related to Public Health Research and Information

Both the U.S. Department of Health and Human Services (DHHS) and the FDA regulate protection of human subjects in clinical trials. The regulations governing obtaining informed consent require that a woman who is or may become pregnant be informed if the treatment or procedure might involve risks to the fetus or embryo that are currently unforeseeable.[36,37]

The DHHS imposes specific limitations on all research involving pregnant women that it conducts or funds, and these regulations were recently revised. For any research designed to benefit solely the fetus, both the consent of the pregnant woman and the consent of the fetus' father must be obtained, with a few limited exceptions. Only the consent of the pregnant woman must be obtained for research designed to benefit both the pregnant woman and the fetus; research designed to benefit solely the pregnant woman; and research designed to develop important biomedical knowledge but not expected to benefit the individual fetus and woman and presenting no more than minimal risk to the fetus.[38]

The National Center for Health Statistics, part of the DHHS's Centers for Disease Control and Prevention (CDC), conducts national fertility surveys—the National Survey of Family Growth (NSFG)—to gather information about factors contributing to the national birth rate, such as sexual activity, contraceptive use, infertility, fetal loss, expected future births, and the wantedness status of pregnancies and births. Using data collected in the NSFG, researchers have examined such public health issues as adolescent pregnancy, use of family planning services, and maternal and child health.[39]

LEGAL ISSUES AND CONTROVERSIES

Legal Issues Relating to Program Management

Issues related to reproductive health services generally or to services other than abortion

Recent efforts to increase enforcement of statutory rape laws, combined with child abuse reporting laws that require the reporting of statutory rape, may have implications for minors' continued confidential access to all reproductive health services.[40] In recent years, at the federal and state levels, greater attention has been paid to "statutory rape"—meaning consensual sexual activity between a minor and an older person that is criminalized—and part of this attention has focused on revising child abuse reporting laws to require or encourage the reporting of statutory rape.[g] In 1996, Congress amended the Child Abuse Prevention and Treatment and Adoption Reform Act to expand the definition of "sexual abuse" to include, *inter alia*, statutory rape in cases of "caretaker or inter-familial relationships."[41] All states require reporting of child abuse, which includes sexual abuse, to child welfare agencies or law enforcement. Some states specifically include statutory rape as a reportable offense, and in others prosecutors interpret the law as requiring such reporting. Thus, in some states, health-care professionals are statutorily obligated to report instances in which minors have had sexual activity with older or adult partners. In these states, minors needing pregnancy-related health services, treatment for sexually transmitted diseases, or even contraceptives may be deterred from seeking such services for fear that they or their sex partners will be put at risk because of their health-care providers' reporting obligation.

Issues related solely to abortion

Since the criminalization of abortion was barred by the U.S. Supreme Court's decision in *Roe v. Wade*, many states have enacted laws seeking to limit the availability of abortion services. As discussed below, some of these limitations have been found to be unlawful, but many others have successfully withstood legal challenge. Legal barriers to women's access to abortion services have taken many forms but can generally be grouped according to whether they focus on the woman and her decision making or on the manner in which the abortion procedure is provided.

State laws focused on the woman's decision making have required provision of specific information to the woman before performance of the procedure, waiting periods between receipt of such information and performance of the procedure, and/or notice to or consent from the woman's spouse or parent before performance of the procedure. A state may require that an abortion be performed only after the woman has received specified information, which may be scripted by the state and include information unrelated to the medical risks and benefits of the procedure, such as text about and pictures of fetal gestational age and development. The state can impose such requirements even if in doing so it expresses a preference for childbirth over abortion as long as the information is "truthful and not misleading."[7] Moreover, a state may require that a woman wait 24 hours after receiving such information directly from an abortion provider before the procedure is performed, provided that an exception is made for medical emergencies, where delay in terminating the pregnancy would create a serious risk of impairment to the woman's health.[7] In making these rulings, the Supreme Court left open the possibility that the types of restrictions found lawful in the *Casey* case might be found to be an undue burden and therefore unconstitutional on the basis of a different factual record.[7] Since the *Casey* decision, some laws imposing waiting periods and provision of particular information have been challenged, with mixed results.

A state may not require that a woman notify, or receive the consent of, her spouse before she obtains an abortion.[7] However, a state may place greater limits on a minor's ability to exercise the right to seek an abortion than it may place on that of an adult woman. Therefore, a state may require that a minor's parent be notified or give consent before an abortion is performed if the state provides an alternative procedure by which the minor may obtain authorization from a judge to obtain an abortion.[6,42-44] At least with respect to a parental consent requirement, the constitutionally required alternative procedure must satisfy the following four criteria: (*1*) the minor must have the opportunity to obtain court authorization for the abortion if she shows that she is sufficiently mature and informed to make her decision independently of her parents; (*2*) the minor must have the opportunity to obtain court authorization if the court determines an abortion would be in her best interests; (*3*) the procedure must ensure the minor's anonymity; and (*4*) the procedure must be conducted expeditiously so that the minor has an effective opportunity to obtain an abortion.[42]

As mentioned earlier, some state constitutions protect individual rights greater than those provided under the federal constitution. As a result, in some states, restrictions on the provision of abortions to minors have been successfully challenged as violative of state constitutional rights, in particular, rights to privacy and/or equal protection.

States have restricted the manner by which an abortion may be obtained mainly by limiting who may perform an abortion, where an abortion may be performed, when an abortion may be performed, and what specific procedures may be used to perform an abortion. In the late 1990s, many states enacted laws to restrict the abortion procedures used. These "partial birth abortion" bans typically were broadly worded so that they prohibited the performance of most procedures commonly used before fetal viability and generally lacked exceptions to protect women's health. Analyzing the Nebraska "partial birth abortion" statute, the Supreme Court concluded that it imposed an unconstitutional undue burden on a woman's right to terminate her pregnancy before viability by banning the procedure most commonly used for abortions during the second trimester of pregnancy.[8]

Legal Issues Relating to Payment for Services

In the mid-1990s, Congress extensively changed welfare laws, many of which affected reproductive health. As part of the Personal Responsibility and Work Opportunity Reconciliation Act of 1996,[45] Congress repealed the Aid to Families with Dependent Children (AFDC) program and replaced it with the Temporary Assistance for Needy Families (TANF) block grant. TANF recipients are subject to a 5 year limit on benefits and must comply with mandatory work requirements. Women who received cash assistance through AFDC—who were most of the women receiving federal welfare benefits—were automatically enrolled in the Medicaid program, through which they received medical services. With the change to TANF, states were supposed to de-link Medicaid eligibility from receipt of cash assistance to ensure that low-income families with dependent children continued to have access to medical assistance. However, as a result of the changes in welfare laws, many eligible families and children lost their Medicaid benefits, largely because of continued linkage of Medicaid eligibility to cash assistance eligibility, despite different eligibility criteria; improper application of sanctions, such as terminating Medicaid coverage for failure to comply with work requirements; or diversion into a work program before the person was allowed to apply for Medicaid.

Among other changes to welfare laws enacted by Congress during the mid-1990s were provisions intended to reduce out-of-wedlock childbearing. Those changes included creation of an "illegitimacy bonus" to reward states for reduction in their rates of out-of-wedlock births. State efforts to achieve that goal included programs and policies intended to increase the use of contraceptives among low-income women and other measures to prevent teen pregnancies.

In recent years, a trend requiring health insurance plans to provide contraceptive coverage has emerged, with many bills enacted at the state level and many more introduced. A continuing controversy with respect to such laws has been the extent to which religion-owned or -affiliated health plans or employers will be subject to such requirements. Some states have enacted contraceptive insurance coverage laws without any such exemptions, whereas others have included exemptions limited to organizations that are operated for religious purposes, and still others have exemptions that cover any organization affiliated with a religious organization that objects to coverage of contraceptives on religious grounds.

The federal government's restrictions on Medicaid reimbursement for abortion services do not limit the extent to which states may cover such services. States remain free to include—and where mandated by state law, must include—reimbursement for abortion services denied federal funding.[33] Several states have chosen by statute to provide broader coverage for abortions than required by the federal Medicaid regulations—some covering all medically necessary abortions, others covering abortions performed because of fetal anomalies. In almost half of the 50 states, denial of funding for medically necessary abortions has been challenged on state constitutional grounds; in most of those states, state courts have ordered that the state provide such funding.[46-52]

Restrictions on the provision of abortion that increase the costs of the procedure may amount to an unconstitutional undue burden.[7] The Supreme Court has not specified how great a cost increase must be to violate the right to privacy; this issue is frequently raised in opposition to licensing requirements that make the provision of abortions more costly for providers and their patients. Laws that impose delays on the provision of abortion are sometimes challenged on the grounds that they increase the cost associated with obtaining an abortion and thus, particularly for low-income women, may impose a substantial obstacle in the path of women seeking abortion.

Legal Issues Relating to Public Health Research and Information

Historically, women often were excluded from human subject research and clinical trials to avoid risk of harming a developing fetus. A 1977 FDA guideline specifically excluded women of childbearing potential from participating in early studies of drugs. As a result of such exclusions, knowledge about the risks for or efficacy of a particular treatment or drug for women generally and pregnant women in particular often was unavailable. In recent years, the federal government has adopted policies and guidelines to encourage inclusion of women of childbearing potential in research study populations and in all phases of clinical drug development. As a result, more women are being included in clinical studies, although data are not always collected in a manner allowing for sex analysis. The inclusion of women of childbearing potential is required only in studies of life-threatening conditions.

Studies involving pregnant women have special restrictions, as discussed above, meant to ensure that such studies are conducted ethically. However, such restrictions may make pregnant women less likely to be included as research subjects. In addition, some of the specific restrictions recently adopted by DHHS are likely to be controversial, such as the requirement that the consent of the father be obtained for any research designed to benefit solely the fetus, even where the risk to the fetus is minimal.[38,h]

Legal Issues Relating to Individual Health Behaviors

In recent years, law enforcement personnel, judges, and elected officials in the United States punished women for conduct during pregnancy that might harm the developing fetus, particularly drug or alcohol use. Using existing laws, local prosecutors have charged pregnant substance abusers with such crimes as child abuse, child neglect, delivery or distribution (through the umbilical cord) of an unlawful substance to a minor, contributing to the delinquency of a minor, and assault with a deadly weapon (i.e., cocaine). In almost every state in which women have contested such charges, courts have rejected the charges or reversed imposed penalties, finding that using these criminal statutes to punish women for their conduct during pregnancy is without a legal basis or is unconstitutional. In doing so, some courts have noted that prosecuting pregnant women for their conduct during pregnancy is counterproductive because it may discourage them from seeking health care during pregnancy.[53]

Many states have modified their civil child protection laws to cover situations in which a child is born dependent on, tests positive for, or has been harmed by an illegal drug or alcohol consumption, either by defining "child neglect" to include these situations or by requiring reporting of such births to child welfare authorities. In some states, efforts have been undertaken to civilly commit pregnant women to protect their fetuses from potential harm; a few states have laws specifically authorizing civil commitment or detention of women who use a controlled substance or abuse alcohol during pregnancy.

PRACTICE CONSIDERATIONS

The public health practice aspects of laws related to reproductive health are broad and highlight the challenges of balancing contrasting concerns: state versus federal responsibilities; medical privacy versus accurate data; legislation of mandates versus the scientific evidence to support such mandates; concerns about new clinical issues versus the resources required to regulate those issues; and many others. Space limitations prohibit a comprehensive discussion, but the following examples illustrate common public health aspects of state and federal regulation of reproductive health issues.

Pregnancy

Maternal health is a rediscovered issue in the public health arena.[54] After years of focusing on infant mortality, public health professionals have recognized that little hope exists for additional reductions in rates of preterm delivery and other adverse newborn outcomes unless the health of pregnant women is examined. Thus, support for maternal mortality review committees has revived. These committees were prevalent in the mid-twentieth century but faded into oblivion during the last decades of the century. Two major reasons for their decline included the 100-fold decrease in maternal deaths from 1900 to 1980 [54] and the substantial risk for litigation when a young woman died during childbirth, which discouraged reviewers from gathering details of the factors that might have contributed to her death.

Several states have established or re-established maternal review committees. In 2001, the American College of Obstetricians and Gynecologists collaborated with the CDC in assessing the legal issues facing these committees, including questions about anonymity, confidentiality, and legal protection from liability. Statutes differ among states in addressing the protection of review committee members from civil liability and protecting the confidentiality of information collected during the review process.[55] In most states, a formally organized review committee and the data it collects are protected from civil liability or disclosure.

Birth Control

During the past few years, Congress and several state legislatures have debated mandatory insurance coverage for contraceptive benefits for women, and legislation has been passed to support mandatory coverage. Some argue that access to contraception coverage is a women's rights issue, noting, for example, that access to Viagra for men should be balanced by access to contraception for women.[i] Others believe that contraceptive insurance coverage will improve health outcomes for women and infants.

Is lack of benefits coverage for contraceptive methods an important barrier to preventing unplanned pregnancies? The highest rates of live-born infants resulting from unintended pregnancies occur among low income women,[56] who are least likely to hold jobs that provide mandated coverage. Unintended pregnancy remains high in the United States but is lowest among well-educated white women, who are most likely to benefit from insurance coverage. The public health impact of these changes in coverage remains to be seen.

Abortion

Reporting of legally induced abortions illustrates a combination of mandatory state regulations and voluntary state reporting to a federal agency. Forty-four U.S. reporting areas collect abortion data as required by state statute or regulation. Every hospital, Medicare facility, or licensed clinician in required areas must report each induced abortion performed to the central department of health by a standardized form for that reporting area. The time period for filing reports after legal induced abortions varies widely by state.[57]

Since 1969, the CDC has documented the number and characteristics of abortions to monitor unintended pregnancies and to help identify preventable causes of complications and deaths associated with abortions.[58] States provide summary data to the CDC that contains no personal identifying information. The CDC compiles these state reports into a national report that describes the characteristics of women obtaining abortions across the country. However, each state faces unique challenges in obtaining this information. For example, some states report abortions according to the state in which the procedure occurred; some report according to the resident state of the woman obtaining the procedure; and some report by both.[58] These multiple approaches make the states with the greatest need for family planning services or other approaches to reducing unintended pregnancies difficult to identify.

Infertility Services

CDC reporting of pregnancy rates in U.S. assisted reproductive technology (ART) clinics is one of the few examples of mandated nationwide reporting to a federal public health agency. The Fertility Clinic Success Rate and Certification Act (FCSRCA),[59] passed in 1992, described the CDC's role: collect data from all ART clinics in the country; report pregnancy success rates for each ART clinic; and develop a model certification program for embryo laboratories. FCSRCA defines ART as procedures that involve handling of oocytes and sperm in establishing pregnancy; the definition does not include the use of artificial insemination or fertility drugs alone. Other federal responsibilities in this field include the role of the FDA, which oversees the handling of human tissues, including gametes and embryos. In addition, CLIA[21] provides for additional oversight of laboratory quality control by the Health Care Financing Administration (now called the Centers for Medicare and Medicaid Services). However, the United States does not have substantial earmarked public funds to support ART oversight or regulation, such as has been available in several other countries.[60]

The CDC produces annual reports describing both clinic-specific and summary national data on pregnancy rates in ART. In addition, the CDC has produced several specific reports that provide the scientific bases on which policies could be built. For example, reports of the interaction between number of embryos transferred and risk of multiple gestations,[61,62,j] reports of the risk for donor eggs in multiple gestations, and reports of low-birth-weight and monozygotic twinning among infants resulting from ART all offer information on health risks related to these services. These reports could potentially provide the basis for regulation of ART clinical sites or practice.

EMERGING ISSUES

Assisted Reproductive Technology

Assisted reproductive technology is rapidly evolving and gaining increased use, but legal responses to the new technology have been slow. Older techniques have become the subject of specific regulation; for example, some states have laws regarding the donation of sperm for artificial insemination, and many states have statutes regarding surrogacy arrangements. Most of the legal response in the United States to the use of ART has been through individual court cases in which principles of law not specific to the ART context were applied. Many commentators have noted a need for legislative and regulatory activity to guide the resolution of existing issues and new issues that arise as technologic advances continue. Future court cases may address whether efforts to regulate ART clash with the constitutional right to procreate, first recognized by the Supreme Court in 1942.[63] At the start of the twenty-first century, advances in techniques of IVF, cloning, and sex and genetic selection techniques for embryos had gained the attention of researchers, public health practitioners, and the general public, but specific legislative, regulatory, and case law responses to the issues raised by use of those techniques were largely undeveloped.

In vitro fertilization routinely involves the creation of extra embryos, which subsequently are frozen and stored for possible future use by the couple in case implantation of the first embryo is unsuccessful or the couple wants more children later. The medical success of this technique has led to legal disputes over control or use of the stored embryos when couples divorce or die or their intentions change. To resolve such disputes, courts often focus on the enforceability of the contract governing disposition of any unused embryos, but application of contract law principles is complicated by the issue of whether stored embryos are property, persons, or something in between.[64,65] A few states have enacted laws specifically relating to agreements for the disposition of stored embryos.

In contrast to the United States, some other countries have enacted legislation to address issues raised by ART. For example, Great Britain, Canada, and the State of Victoria in Australia established commissions of experts and scholars to study ART and recommend legislation governing it. Britain passed the Human Fertilization and Embryology Act in 1990, which regulates IVF and some other infertility treatments through a licensing scheme and requires, *inter alia*, that IVF participants be counseled, provide written consent for disposition of embryos, and enter into an agreement for the disposition of embryos in the case of death, divorce, or change in circumstances.[66] In 1984, the State of Victoria in Australia enacted the Infertility (Medical Procedures) Act, which imposes, *inter alia*, counseling, consent, and disclosure requirements for IVF.[67] The States of South Australia and Western Australia have enacted legislation requiring licensing of providers of IVF.[68]

Medical Abortion

Considerable attention has focused on the use of medical, rather than surgical, techniques for inducing abortion since the FDA began reviewing, and ultimately approved, the use of mifepristone (i.e., RU-486) as an abortifacient in the United States. The availability of mifepristone had been expected to increase women's access to abortions, mainly because additional health-care providers might offer this nonsurgical type of abortion service. However, the extent to which access increases may be limited by the array of state laws restricting the provision of abortions. Most state laws regulating "abortion" do not limit their scope to surgical abortions or to post first-trimester abortions, and therefore providers of medical abortions will be subject to such laws. In some situations, lawsuits may be brought challenging the application to medical abortions of laws that were enacted to regulate the provision of surgical abortions. In particular, such laws might be challenged successfully on the grounds that they impose significant burdens on the provision of such abortions, they do not serve the state's interest in maternal health by making the provision of medical abortions safer, or they violate equal protection rights of abortion providers or their patients.[69,70]

Physician-only laws, which limit who can perform an abortion, may conflict with some states' practice acts, which grant nonphysician practitioners authority to dispense drugs, thus creating uncertainty about whether certain nonphysicians can perform medical abortions in those states. Health-care personnel providing medical abortions may have to comply with laws that single out facilities at which abortions are performed for special requirements not imposed on other physicians' offices or outpatient clinics. Although some of those laws are limited to facilities at which surgical abortions only or second- or third-trimester abortions only are performed, in other states such requirements are not so limited and in some cases even apply to private physicians' offices. Similarly, laws requiring parental consent or notice, waiting periods, or provision to the patient of specific information will apply to medical abortions. Laws relating to examination and/or disposal of fetal tissue might in some states be interpreted as applying to medical abortions, possibly making it necessary for patients to collect and deliver to their physician the expelled fetal tissue.[69,70]

CONCLUSION

The law governing reproductive health issues will continue to change in the United States, at both the federal and state levels. Technologic advances relating to reproduction will challenge the legal system. Issues of reproductive health surveillance and research will be affected by evolving regulations regarding human subjects' protection. Public interest in reproductive health services will remain high because of the moral and cultural implications. Inevitably, issues in reproductive health will see new laws and new litigation, accompanied by extensive public dialogue.

Notes

[a] Given the extensive legislative activity surrounding reproductive health issues, each year the National Abortion and Reproductive Rights Action League (NARAL) and NARAL Foundation publish a state-by-state review of laws governing abortion and reproductive rights. See, for example, NARAL & NARAL Foundation. *Who Decides? A State-by-State Review of Abortion and Reproductive Rights*. Washington, DC: NARAL Foundation & NARAL, 2001. Summaries of the laws of specific states and citations to those laws can be found in this publication.

[b] Generally, states began criminalizing abortion by statute in the mid-nineteenth century; before that, abortion in most states was legal, at least before "quickening" of the fetus—the point of recognizable movement by the fetus in utero. By the end of the 1950s, a large majority of states banned abortion except when necessary to preserve the life of the mother. See *Roe v. Wade*, 410 U.S. 113, 132–41 (1973).

[c] In *Eisenstadt*, the U.S. Supreme Court held that unmarried persons had a right to use contraceptives under the federal constitution. *Eisenstadt v. Baird*, 405 U.S. 438 (1972).

[d] For example, a federal district court found that the right to privacy encompasses the right of a woman to become pregnant by artificial insemination. See *Cameron v. Board of Education*, 795 F. Supp. 228, 237 (S.D. Ohio 1991).

[e] The laws granting exemptions to "facilities" or "entities" are premised on the questionable fiction that facilities or entities have moral or religious beliefs. Moreover, few of these laws limit the exemption to religious institutions, and fewer still are limited to institutions engaged solely in religious activities.

[f] The Hyde Amendment is a rider added annually to the DHHS appropriations bill. Although each year it limits coverage for medically necessary abortions, in certain prior years it has excluded coverage in circumstances of rape or incest and has included coverage where a woman's life was endangered by a mental condition, as well as by a physical condition.

[g] States differ in the extent to which they criminalize consensual sexual activity by a minor. For example, in some states, the severity of the offense depends on the age of the minor's sex partner, whereas other states criminalize sexual activity with a minor irrespective of the age of the sex partner. Compare, for example, Ca. Pen. Code § 261.5 (severity of offense varies depending on whether minor is under 18 or under 16 and on whether partner is over 18, over 21, or within 3 years of the minor's age) with Wis. Stat. § 948.02 (anyone having sexual contact or intercourse with person under age 13 is guilty of a Class B felony and anyone having sexual contact or intercourse with a person under age 16 is guilty of a Class BC felony).

ʰ Some fetal protection policies are vulnerable to legal challenge on the grounds that they constitute sex discrimination. Title VII, 42 U.S.C. § 2000e-2(a)(1), prohibits discrimination on the basis of sex in employment, and the Pregnancy Discrimination Act, 42 U.S.C. § 2000e(k), specifically requires that women affected by pregnancy, childbirth, or related medical conditions be treated the same for all employment-related purposes "as others not so affected but similar in their ability or inability to work." In *International Union, UAW v. Johnson Controls*, 499 U.S. 187 (1991), the U.S. Supreme Court held that an employer's sex-specific fetal protection policy violated Title VII, as amended by the Pregnancy Discrimination Act. The Court found that the employers' policy of excluding women with childbearing capacity from jobs where they would be exposed to lead at levels that could endanger a developing fetus constituted impermissible sex discrimination.

ⁱ In December 2000, the U.S. Equal Employment Opportunity Commission found that two employers' failure to cover the expenses of prescription contraceptives to the same extent that they covered the expenses of other prescription drugs and devices used to prevent other medical conditions constituted a violation of Title VII of the Civil Rights Act of 1964, as amended by the Pregnancy Discrimination Act, 42 U.S.C. 2000e *et seq.* See also *Erickson v. Bartell Drug Co*, 141 F. Supp. 2d 1266 (W.D. Wash. 2001) (finding that exclusion of prescription contraceptives from health insurance benefits violated Title VII), appeal filed, No. 01–35870 (9th Cir. Sept. 13, 2001).

ʲ A few countries, including Austria, Germany, and Switzerland, have passed laws limiting how many eggs can be fertilized outside of the body or limiting the number of embryos that can be transferred at one time into a woman's uterus.

References

1. Henshaw S. Unintended pregnancy in the United States. *Fam Plan Perspect* 1998; 30:24–9, 46.
2. *Griswold v. Connecticut*, 381 U.S. 479 (1965).
3. *Roe v. Wade*, 410 U.S. 113 (1973).
4. *Eisenstadt v. Baird*, 405 U.S. 438 (1972).
5. *Colautti v. Franklin*, 439 U.S. 379 (1979) (finding viability determination requirement and standard of care provision unconstitutionally vague).
6. *Planned Parenthood of Central Missouri v. Danforth*, 428 U.S. 52 (1976).
7. *Planned Parenthood v. Casey*, 505 U.S. 833 (1992).
8. *Stenberg v. Carhart*, 530 U.S. 914 (2000).
9. *American Academy of Pediatrics v. Lungren*, 940 P.2d 797, 828–9 (Cal. 1997) (finding that parental consent law violated privacy rights of minors under California constitution); *In re T.W.*, 551 So.2d 1186 (Fla. 1989) (same, under Florida constitution).
10. *Planned Parenthood of Central New Jersey v. Farmer*, 762 A.2d 620 (N.J. 2000) (finding that parental notice law violated equal protection rights under New Jersey constitution).
11. 42 C.F.R. § 50.203.
12. Grimes DA, Raymond EG, Jones BS. Emergency contraception over-the-counter: the medical and legal imperatives. *Obstet Gynecol* 2001;98:151–5.
13. 21 U.S.C. § 353(b)(3).
14. *Hodgson v. Lawson*, 542 F.2d 1350 (8th Cir. 1976) (finding that public hospital must

make its existing facilities available for performance of abortions).

15. *Valley Hospital Association v. Mat-Su Coalition for Choice*, 948 P.2d 963 (Alaska 1997) (finding that quasi-public hospital's policy prohibiting performance of most abortions violated state constitutional right to privacy).

16. *Doe v. Bridgeton Hospital Association*, 366 A.2d 641 (N.J. 1976) (finding that quasi-public hospital cannot refuse to permit facilities to be used to perform first trimester elective abortions).

17. *Mazurek v. Armstrong*, 520 U.S. 968 (1997).

18. *City of Akron v. Akron Center for Reproductive Health*, 462 U.S. 416, 431–9 (1983).

19. *Planned Parenthood v. Ashcroft*, 462 U.S. 476, 481–2 (1983).

20. *Reproductive Services v. Keating*, 35 F. Supp. 2d 1332 (N.D. Okla. 1998).

21. 42 U.S.C. § 263a *et seq.* (2001) (Clinical Laboratory Improvement Act).

22. 29 U.S.C. § 651 *et seq.* (2001) (Occupational Safety and Health Act).

23. 42 C.F.R. § 440.210.

24. 42 U.S.C. § 1396a(a)(23)(B).

25. U.S. General Accounting Office. States used Medicaid to improve access and services. In: *Medicaid Prenatal Care: States Improve Access and Enhance Services, but Face New Challenges.* Washington, DC: U.S. General Accounting Office, Health, Education, and Human Services Division, 1994; pp. 12–41.

26. 42 U.S.C. § 300 *et seq.* (Title X).

27. 42 U.S.C. § 701 *et seq.* (Maternal and Child Health Block Grant).

28. 42 U.S.C. § 1396 *et seq.* (Medicaid).

29. 42 U.S.C. § 1397 *et seq.* (Social Services Block Grant).

30. *New York v. Heckler*, 719 F.2d 1191 (2d Cir. 1983).

31. *Planned Parenthood v. Heckler*, 712 F.2d 650 (D.C. Cir. 1983).

32. Public Law No. 106-554, Title V, §§ 508–9, 114 Stat. 2763.

33. *Harris v. McRae*, 448 U.S. 297 (1980).

34. 29 U.S.C. § 1185(a) (1996).

35. Saul R. Abortion reporting in the United States: an examination of the federal-state partnership. *Fam Plan Perspect* 1998;30:244–7.

36. 21 C.F.R. § 50.25(b)(1).

37. 45 C.F.R. § 46.116(b)(1).

38. 45 C.F.R. § 46.201 *et seq.*

39. Mosher WD, Bachrach CA. Understanding U.S. fertility: continuity and change in the National Survey of Family Growth, 1988–1995. *Fam Plan Perspect* 1996;28:4 12.

40. English A, Teare C. Symposium statutory rape realities: scholarship and practice article: statutory rape enforcement and child abuse reporting: effects on health care access for adolescents. *DePaul Law Rev* 2001;50:827–64.

41. 42 U.S.C. § 1506g(4)(B).

42. *Bellotti v. Baird*, 443 U.S. 622, 643 (1979) (plurality opinion) (*Bellotti II*).

43. *Lambert v. Wicklund*, 520 U.S. 292, 295 (1997) (reaffirming requirements for bypass articulated in *Bellotti II*).

44. *Hodgson v. Minnesota*, 497 U.S. 417 (1990).

45. Public Law No. 104-193, 110 Stat. 2105.

46. *Comm. to Defend Reproductive Rights v. Myers*, 625 P.2d 779 (Cal. 1981).

47. *Moe v. Secretary of Administration & Finance*, 417 N.E.2d 387 (Mass. 1981).

48. *Women of Minnesota v. Gomez*, 542 N.W.2d 17 (Minn. 1995).

49. *Right to Choose v. Byrne*, 450 A.2d 925 (N.J. 1982).

50. *New Mexico Right to Choose/NARAL v. Johnson*, 975 P.2d 841 (N.M. 1998).

51. *Doe v. Dep't of Soc. Servs.*, 487 N.W.2d 166 (Mich. 1992).

52. *Fischer v. Dept. of Public Welfare*, 502 A.2d 114 (Pa. 1985).

53. *State v. Ashley*, 701 So.2d 338 (Fla. 1997).

54. CDC. Achievements in public health, 1900–1999: healthier mothers and babies. *MMWR* 1999;48:849–58.

55. American College of Obstetricians and Gynecologists. State review provisions. In: Berg C, Danel I, Atrash H, Zane S, Bartlett L, eds. *Strategies to Reduce Pregnancy-related Deaths: from Identification and Review to Action.* Atlanta: U.S. Department of Health and Human Services, CDC, 2001: pp (Appendix D) 1–36.

56. Abma JC, Chandra A, Mosher WD, Peterson LS, Piccinino LJ. Fertility, family planning, and women's health. New data from the 1995 National Survey of Family Growth. National Center for Health Statistics. *Vital Health Stat* 1997;23(19).

57. Koonin LM. Reporting of medical (nonsurgical) abortions: information for providers. (Appendix). Am J Obstet Gynecol (Suppl) 2000;183:S24–5.

58. Koonin LM, Strauss LT, Chrisman CE, Parker WY. Abortion surveillance—United States, 1997. *MMWR* 2000;49(No. SS-11).

59. 42 U.S.C. § 263a-1 *et seq.*

60. Jones HW, Cohen J, eds. IFFS Surveillance '98: an international surveillance of issues dealing with assisted reproductive technology. *Fertil Steril* 1999;71 (Suppl 2).

61. Schieve LA, Peterson HB, Meikle SF, et al. Live-birth rates and multiple birth risk using in vitro fertilization. *JAMA* 1999;282:1832–8.

62. Schieve LA, Meikle SF, Peterson HB, Jeng G, Burnett NM, Wilcox LS. Does assisted hatching pose a risk for monozygotic twinning in pregnancies conceived through in vitro fertilization? *Fertil Steril* 2000; 74:288–94.

63. *Skinner v. Oklahoma*, 316 U.S. 535 (1942) (finding that Oklahoma's Habitual Criminal Sterilization Act interferes with fundamental right to procreate).

64. *Davis v. Davis*, 842 S.W.2d 588 (Tenn. 1992) (resolving dispute in divorce proceeding over custody of frozen embryos).

65. *Kass v. Kass*, 696 N.E.2d 174 (N.Y. 1998) (requiring compliance with terms of agreement for disposition of frozen embryos).

66. Human Fertilisation and Embryology Act (1990) (UK).

67. Infertility Treatment Act (1995) (Austl. [Victoria]).

68. Reproductive Technology Act (1988) (South Austl.); Human Reproductive Technology Act (1991) (Western Austl.).

69. Jones BS, Heller S. Providing medical abortion: legal issues of relevance to providers. *J Am Med Womens Assoc* 2000(3 Suppl);55:145–50.

70. Borgmann CE, Jones BS. Legal issues in the provision of medical abortions. *Am J Obstet Gynecol* 2000;183 (2 Suppl):S84–S94.

18

Environmental Health and Protection

PAUL A. LOCKE, HENRY FALK, CHRIS S. KOCHTITZKY,
AND CHRISTINE P. BUMP

This chapter provides a context for the practice of environmental health law. It is meant as both a road map for the practitioner and an introduction to some of the ways in which environmental health problems can be approached. Although the vast range of environmental health law is difficult to condense, we can give practitioners a flavor of how the tools available to practitioners developed and where environmental health and protection law may be going. Ultimately, the reader must protect environmental health by selecting from among, and employing, the legal tools presented here. Because of the complexity and scope of the law, the modern environmental health practitioner is faced simultaneously with an extensive group of legal tools and a changing landscape in which to apply them.

The major federal laws associated with environmental health and protection (Table 18–1) are broad and heterogeneous, reflecting the diversity of activities that defines environmental health. As we use it in this chapter, the term *environmental health* "comprises those aspects of human health, including quality of life, that are determined by interactions with physical, chemical, biological and social factors in the environment. It also refers to the theory and practice of assessing, correcting, controlling and preventing those factors in the environment that may adversely affect the health of present and future generations." [1]

In addition to these federal authorities, state laws and municipal or local

TABLE 18–1. Major Federal Environmental Protection Laws

FEDERAL LAW	SUMMARY OF INTENT AND PROVISIONS
Clean Air Act (CAA)	The CAA protects human health and the environment from outdoor air pollution. It requires the EPA to establish minimum national standards for air quality and assigns primary responsibility to the states to ensure compliance with these standards. Areas not meeting the standards, referred to as "nonattainment areas," are required to implement pollution-control measures. The CAA establishes federal standards for mobile sources of air pollution, for sources of 188 hazardous air pollutants, and for the emissions that cause acid rain. It establishes a comprehensive permitting system for all major sources of air pollution. It also addresses the prevention of pollution in areas with clean air.
Federal Water Pollution Control Act (CWA)	The CWA is the principal law addressing prevention of pollution of surface waters. Originally enacted in 1948, it was totally revised by amendments in 1972 and 1987. The 1972 amendments required all municipal and industrial wastewater to be treated before discharge into waterways, increased federal assistance for municipal treatment plant construction, and strengthened and streamlined enforcement. Before the 1987 amendments, however, programs under the CWA were primarily directed at point source pollution, wastes discharged from discrete and identifiable sources, such as pipes and other outfalls. Little attention had been given to nonpoint source pollution (storm water runoff from agricultural lands, forests, construction sites, and urban areas). The 1987 amendments directed states to develop and implement nonpoint pollution-management programs. Federal assistance was authorized to support control activities.
Comprehensive Environmental Response, Compensation, and Liability Act (CERCLA) and the Superfund Amendment and Reauthorization Act (SARA)	CERCLA and SARA established a fee-maintained fund to clean up abandoned hazardous waste sites. CERCLA authorizes the federal government to respond to spills and other releases of hazardous substances, as well as leaking hazardous waste dumps. Hazardous substances are identified under the SDWA, the CWA, CAA, and the TSCA or are designated by the EPA. Response is also authorized for releases of "pollutants or contaminants," which are broadly defined to include anything that can threaten the health of "any organism." Most nuclear materials and petroleum are excluded. CERCLA also established the Agency for Toxic Substances and Disease Registry (ATSDR) with mandates to (1) establish a National Exposure and Disease Registry, (2) create an inventory of health information on toxic substances, (3) create a list of closed and restricted-access sites, (4) assist in toxic substance emergencies, and (5) determine the relation between toxic substance exposures and illnesses. SARA added responsibilities in health assessment, toxicology, and medical education.

(continued)

TABLE 18–1—Continued

FEDERAL LAW	SUMMARY OF INTENT AND PROVISIONS
Emergency Planning and Community Right-to-Know Act (EPCRA)	EPCRA requires industrial reporting of toxic releases and planning to respond to chemical emergencies. EPCRA established state commissions and local committees to implement procedures for coping with releases of hazardous chemicals and mandated annual reporting on environmental releases of such chemicals by facilities that manufacture or use them in significant amounts.
Federal Insecticide, Fungicide, and Rodenticide Act (FIFRA)	FIFRA governs pesticide products and their use. FIFRA requires the EPA to regulate the sale and use of pesticides in the United States through registration and labeling. It directs the EPA to restrict use of pesticides to prevent unreasonable adverse effects on people and the environment, taking into account the costs and benefits of various uses. FIFRA prohibits the sale of any pesticide in the United States unless it is registered and labeled indicating approved uses and restrictions. The EPA registers each pesticide for each use. In addition, FIFRA requires the EPA to reregister older pesticides based on new data and scientific discoveries. Establishments that manufacture or sell pesticide products must register with the EPA, and managers of these facilities are required to keep records and allow inspections by the EPA or state regulatory staff.
Food Quality Protection Act (FQPA)	The FQPA amends both the FFDCA and the FIFRA. It requires the re-registration of all pesticides used in the United States to account for new scientific understanding and to provide adequate protection for particularly sensitive populations such as children and pregnant women. Specifically, (1) it requires recognition that people can have concurrent exposure to many different chemicals (before this, each pesticide was regulated in isolation, as if exposure occurred only one chemical at a time); (2) it recognizes that exposure can occur from many sources or pathways including pets, lawns, soil, carpets, and even house dust; and (3) it includes provisions to protect children, who may be more vulnerable to the effects of environmental pollutants such as pesticides, and excludes cost–benefit analysis from the regulatory decision-making process.
National Environment Policy Act (NEPA)	The NEPA requires the EPA to review environmental impact statements. The basic purposes of the NEPA are to (1) declare a national policy to encourage harmony between humans and the environment; (2) promote efforts that will prevent or eliminate damage to the environment and biosphere and stimulate the health and welfare of humans; (3) enrich the understanding of the ecologic systems and natural resources important to the United States; and (4) establish the White House Council on Environmental Quality.

(continued)

TABLE 18–1. Major Federal Environmental Protection Laws—Continued

FEDERAL LAW	SUMMARY OF INTENT AND PROVISIONS
Oil Pollution Act (OPA)	The OPA streamlined and strengthened the EPA's ability to prevent and respond to catastrophic oil spills. A trust fund financed by a tax on oil is available to clean up spills when the responsible party is incapable or unwilling to do so. The OPA requires oil storage facilities and vessels to submit to the federal government plans detailing how they will respond to large discharges. It also requires the development of Area Contingency Plans to prepare and plan for oil spill response on a regional scale.
Pollution Prevention Act (PPA)	The PPA states that it is the policy of the United States that "pollution should be prevented or reduced at the source whenever feasible; pollution that cannot be prevented should be recycled in an environmentally safe manner, whenever feasible; pollution that cannot be prevented or recycled should be treated in an environmentally safe manner whenever feasible; and disposal or other release into the environment should be employed only as a last resort and should be conducted in an environmentally safe manner." The PPA focused industry, government, and public attention on reducing the amount of pollution produced in the United States through source reduction.
Residential Lead-Based Paint Hazard Reduction Act	This Act directs the Department of Housing and Urban Development and the EPA to require disclosure of information on lead-based paint hazards before the sale or lease of most housing built before 1978. This ensures that purchasers and renters of housing built before 1978 receive the information necessary to protect themselves from lead-based paint hazards but does not require any testing or removal of lead-based paint by sellers or landlords.
Safe Drinking Water Act (SDWA)	The SDWA is the key federal law for protecting public drinking water systems from contamination. First enacted in 1974 and substantively amended in 1986 and 1996, the SDWA establishes standards and treatment requirements for drinking water, controls underground injection of wastes that might contaminate water supplies, and protects ground water. The SDWA established the current federal–state arrangement in which states may be delegated primary implementation and enforcement authority for the drinking water program. The state-administered Public Water Supply Supervision program remains the basic program for regulating the nation's public water systems. In 1996 Congress substantially revised the SDWA. Among other things, flexibility was added to its standard setting provisions, the EPA was required to conduct cost–benefit analyses for most new standards, consumer information requirements were expanded, provisions to improve small system compliance and protect source waters were added, and a State Revolving Loan Fund to help finance needed projects was created.

(continued)

TABLE 18–1—Continued

FEDERAL LAW	SUMMARY OF INTENT AND PROVISIONS
Solid Waste Disposal Act (SWDA), Resource Conservation and Recovery Act (RCRA), and Hazardous and Solid Waste Amendments (HSWA)	Federal solid waste law has gone through four major phases. The SWDA focused on research, demonstrations, and training. The RCRA refocused on concern with the reclamation of energy and materials from solid waste. It authorized grants for demonstrating new resource recovery technology and required annual reports from the EPA on means of promoting recycling and reducing the generation of waste. In a third phase, the federal government began a more active regulatory role, embodied in the RCRA. The RCRA instituted the first federal permit program for hazardous waste and prohibited open dumps. In a fourth phase (HSWA), the federal government attempted to prevent future clean-up problems by prohibiting land disposal of untreated hazardous wastes, setting liner and leachate collection requirements for land disposal facilities, setting deadlines for closure of facilities not meeting standards, and establishing a corrective action program. The ATSDR was directed to work with the EPA to (*1*) identify new hazardous wastes to be regulated, (*2*) conduct health assessments at RCRA sites, and (*3*) consider petitions for health assessments from the public or states.
Toxic Substances Control Act (TSCA)	The TSCA regulates the testing of chemicals and their use. The EPA may require manufacturers and processors of chemicals to conduct and report the results of tests to determine the effects of potentially dangerous chemicals on living things. Based on test results and other information, the EPA may regulate the manufacture, importation, processing, distribution, use, and/or disposal of any chemical that presents an unreasonable risk of injury to human health or the environment. A variety of regulatory tools are available to the EPA under the TSCA, ranging in severity from a total ban on production, import, and use to a requirement that a product bears a warning label at the point of sale.

ordinances could contain useful tools for environmental health practitioners. A detailed discussion of these authorities is beyond the scope of this chapter. However, the major common law theories on which they are based are outlined in Table 18–2.

LEGAL AUTHORITIES

Federal and State Authorities

The legal authorities available to environmental health practitioners are broad and extensive. They are based largely in state police powers and the Interstate

TABLE 18–2. Overview of State Police and Plenary Power Common Law Actions

TYPE OF ACTION	DESCRIPTION
Negligence	Negligence is the failure to do something that a reasonable person, guided by the considerations that normally regulate human affairs, would do or the doing of something that a reasonable person would not do. To succeed in bringing a negligence claim, the plaintiff must prove (*1*) that the party responsible for toxic material had a duty to either warn others about the risks associated with the toxic materials under the particular circumstances or to take precautions to prevent injury to others; (*2*) that the party responsible for toxic material breached that duty; (*3*) that the toxic material was the proximate cause of the plaintiff's injury; and (*4*) that damages, if collected, can remedy the injury. Breach of duty has been found for an insecticide manufacturer failing to warn users that the product was lethal* and for the corporate owner of a toxic waste cite failing to prevent the release of toxic materials.†
Negligence per se	If the injured party in a negligence action seeks to prove violation of a statutory or regulatory standard, the action is one of negligence per se. To prevail in a negligence per se claim, the plaintiff must show that (*1*) the plaintiff is a member of the class of individuals that the legislative provision in question is designed to protect from a particular type of harm and (*2*) the plaintiff suffered the particular type of harm contemplated by the legislative provision.‡
Strict liability	Parties who carry on "abnormally dangerous" activities that harm persons or land are held strictly liable for the damage or injuries caused by their activities, regardless of the level of care taken to prevent such injuries. The court, not the jury, determines whether an activity is abnormally dangerous. Crop dusting,§ operating hazardous waste facilities,¶ and generating nuclear power** have all been determined to be abnormally dangerous activities. The Restatement (Second) of Torts § 520 sets out six factors to determine whether an activity is abnormally dangerous: (*1*) the existence of a high degree of risk to the person or land of others; (*2*) the likelihood that the harm resulting from the activity will be great; (*3*) the inability to eliminate the risk through reasonable care; (*4*) the extent to which the activity is not a manner of common usage; (*5*) the inappropriateness of the activity related to where it is carried on; and (*6*) the extent to which the value of the activity outweighs its dangerousness.

(continued)

TABLE 18–2—Continued

TYPE OF ACTION	DESCRIPTION
Trespass	Trespass occurs when an actual intrusion occurs onto, above, or below land where the plaintiff has an interest when this intrusion is intentional, reckless, negligent, or the result of ultra-hazardous activity.†† Trespass was found when a defendant's production of aluminum caused fluoride particles to escape onto the plaintiff's farmland, rendering it unusable for grazing.‡‡
Nuisance	Nuisance is the nontrespassory invasion of another's interest in the private use and enjoyment of land.§§ Nuisance has been found for contamination of neighboring groundwater by leaking gasoline storage tanks.¶¶ Nuisance and trespass actions are complementary, and in environmental tort cases the line distinguishing them is blurred.***
Fraud	Fraud is claimed when the defendant knowingly conceals the dangerous nature of the toxic substance and suffered an injury from exposure to it. Fraud was found when an employee was permanently disabled after using a chemical product that his employer claimed was not harmful.†††
Breach of warranty and misrepresentation	Breach of warranty and misrepresentation are causes of action based on a seller's express or implied representation of their product on which the consumer justifiably relied.‡‡‡ Misrepresentation was found when a seller of a gasoline station stated, when asked, that the station had no problems; in reality, a 2000 gallon spill had occurred 5 years earlier.§§§ In breach of warranty and misrepresentation cases, the plaintiff must prove that the misrepresented fact caused the alleged injury.

*Hubbard-Hall Chem. Co v. Silverman, 340 F 402 (1st Cir. 1965).
†Ewell v. Petro Processors of La., Inc, 364 So 2d 604 (LA. Ct. App. 1978).
‡Gerrard, § 33.01(1)(a).
§Langan v. Valicopters, Inc, 567 P 2d 218 (Wash. 1977). The court imposed strict liability against an aerial pesticide sprayer for damages to organic crops.
¶Sterling v. Veliscol Chem. Corp, 855 F 2d 1188 (6th Cir. 1988). The court imposed strict liability to recover for personal injuries and property to residents living near a chemical waste burial site.
**Silkwood v. Kerr-McGee Corp, 464 U.S. 238 (1984). The court imposed strict liability for radiation injuries stemming from the operation of a nuclear power plant.
††Restatement (Second) of Torts, Chapter 7.
‡‡Martin v. Reynolds Metals Co, 342 P 2d (Or. 1959).
§§Restatement (Second) of Torts, § 821D.
¶¶Exxon Corp. v Yarema, 516 A 2d 990 (Md. App. 1986).
***Gerrard, § 33.01(1)(c).
†††Berkley v. American Cyanamid Co, 799 F 2d 1489 (5th Cir. 1985).
‡‡‡Gerrard, § 33.01[1][e].
§§§Damon v. Sun Co, 87 F 3d 1467 (1st Cir. 1996).

Commerce Clause, the authority ceded to the federal government by the states in the U.S. Constitution. The Interstate Commerce Clause, the scope of which was expanded greatly during the New Deal years,[2] is the basis for almost all modern federal environmental laws.[2]

This section summarizes the legal authorities in four tables. The first table (Table 18–1) describes the major federal environmental protection laws. The second table (Table 18–2) contains an overview of common law actions available under the police or plenary powers of most states. These authorities underlie the actions that state and local governments can exercise, even in the absence of federal law and regulation. Table 18–3 describes the major federal public health laws that have environmental authorities. Table 18–4 illustrates the range of media-based approaches contained in federal law and indicates some of the laws and agencies that are associated with controlling certain compounds or classes of compounds.

Overview of state police and plenary power common law actions

Many cases brought against environmental polluters contain claims based on tort law and theory. Environmental tort suits can seek recovery for personal injury as well as for property damage. Historically, recovery has been allowed only for actual physical injury. More recently, plaintiffs have been able to collect for the enhanced risk for future disease, fear of contracting a disease, and damage to one's immune system.[3] Environmental tort actions generally allege that exposure to a toxic substance has caused the plaintiff's injury. Common law causes of action for tort include negligence, negligence per se, strict liability, nuisance, trespass, fraud, and breach of warranty and misrepresentation (§ 33.01[1]).[3] Negligence is the most frequently pleaded claim, followed by strict liability. Table 18–2 contains a fuller explanation of these tort actions.

Overview of the major federal environmental protection laws

The environmental health authorities of the U.S. Environmental Protection Agency (EPA) derive primarily from 13 major environmental statutes that have been enacted or amended over the past 30 years. The multiplicity of federal environmental laws contrasts sharply with federal public health law, which has evolved over the past 250 years and is captured in three main pieces of legislation. Table 18–3 summarizes the components of the major federal public health laws today.

As the substantial number of environmental and public health statutes suggest (Tables 18–1 and 18–3), the process of federal regulation in these areas is complex and fragmented. To demonstrate the complexity of the administration of these regulatory processes, Table 18–4 cross-references some of the major federal regulations of specific chemical groups by individual media. The six separate chemical groups, separated into six separate media, are regulated by four

TABLE 18–3. Major Federal Public Health Laws

FEDERAL LAW	SUMMARY OF INTENT AND PROVISIONS
Federal Food, Drug and Cosmetic Act (FFDCA)	The FFDCA is the basic U.S. food and drug law. It ensures that foods are pure and wholesome, safe to eat, and produced under sanitary conditions; that drugs and devices are safe and effective for their intended uses; and that cosmetics are safe and use appropriate ingredients.
Occupational Safety and Health Act (OSHA)	The OSHA requires safe and healthful conditions for working people by authorizing enforcement of the standards developed under the OSHA and by assisting and encouraging the states in ensuring safe and healthful working conditions. The goal was to ensure that employers provide their workers a place of employment free from recognized hazards to safety and health, such as exposure to toxic chemicals, excessive noise levels, mechanical dangers, heat or cold stress, or unsanitary conditions. Standards set under the OSHA regarding toxic materials or harmful physical agents are based on levels that most adequately ensure that no employees will suffer material impairment of health or functional capacity even if such employees have regular exposure to the hazard dealt with for their entire working life. Whenever practicable, the standard promulgated shall be expressed in terms of objective criteria.
Public Health Service (PHS) Act	The Public Health Service (PHS) was established in July 1798. Subsequent legislation has vastly broadened its scope. The PHS Act of 1944 consolidated and revised all legislation relating to the PHS. Its legal responsibilities have been broadened and expanded many times since 1944. Currently, the PHS *(1)* coordinates with the states to set and implement national health policy; *(2)* generates and upholds cooperative international health-related agreements, policies, and programs; *(3)* conducts medical and biomedical research; *(4)* sponsors and administers programs for the development of health resources and the prevention and control of diseases; *(5)* provides resources and expertise to the states and other public and private institutions in the planning, direction, and delivery of physical, environmental, and mental health-care services; and *(6)* enforces laws to ensure the safety and efficacy of drugs and protect against impure and unsafe foods, cosmetics, medical devices, and radiation-producing projects. Today, the vast majority of activities at the CDC, FDA, HRSA, IHS, and NIH are conducted under the auspices of the PHS Act.

TABLE 18–4. Federal Regulations of Chemical Groups by Media

	CAA*	CWA	SDWA	TSCA	RCRA	CERCLA	SARA	EPCRA	FIFRA	FFDCA†	FQPA	RLHRA‡	OSHA¶
Metals, air	✓												✓
Metals, water		✓	✓										
Metals, land					✓	✓	✓	✓					
Metals, household				✓						✓			
Metals, food										✓	✓	✓	
Pesticides, air	✓												
Pesticides, water		✓	✓										
Pesticides, land					✓	✓	✓	✓					
Pesticides, crops									✓		✓		
Pesticides, household									✓	✓	✓		
Pesticides, food										✓	✓		
Phthalates, air	✓												✓
Phthalates, water		✓	✓										
Phthalates, land					✓	✓	✓	✓		✓			
Phthalates, food											✓		

Dioxins/furans, air	✓											
Dioxins/furans, water		✓										
Dioxins/furans, land			✓									
Dioxins/furans, food									✓			
PAHs, air	✓											
PAHs, water		✓	✓									
PAHs, land			✓		✓	✓	✓					
PAHs, household								✓				
PAHs, food											✓	
PCBs, air	✓											
PCBs, water		✓	✓									
PCBs, land			✓	✓	✓	✓						
PCBs, food									✓			✓

*EPA.

†EPA/FDA.

‡HUD.

¶OSHA.

separate agencies using 13 individual laws. On the whole, these tables demonstrate that federal environmental protection and health authorities and tools are not easily boiled down or pigeon-holed.

Litigation

Litigation by government agencies

Litigation is an important tool for environmental health practitioners. Federal environmental laws provide authorities for administering agencies to sue parties that are out of compliance with their permits or are otherwise running afoul of the law. All the major federal environmental statutes contain such provisions. For example, the Clean Air Act (CAA) authorizes the EPA to issue administrative compliance and penalty orders and seek injunctions and civil and criminal penalties (42 U.S.C. § 7413). The Toxic Substances Control Act (TSCA) provides for civil and criminal penalties and states that substances produced in violation of the Act can be seized (15 U.S.C. §§ 2614, 2615, 2616, and 2617). The Federal Water Pollution Control Act (CWA) states that the EPA can issue compliance orders, bring civil actions, and assess administrative, civil, and judicial penalties against violators (33 U.S.C. § 1319). In addition to the ability to seek penalties, issue compliance orders, and bring civil and criminal actions, some environmental statutes provide agencies with the ability to take immediate action in the event of an imminent and substantial endangerment (see 33 U.S.C. § 1319[c]).

State environmental health practitioners can often take advantage of these federal authorities because federal environmental protection programs are frequently delegated to states.[4] In certain cases, if a state has not begun an action against a violator, the federal government may step in (33 U.S.C. § 1319[a]). State laws may also contain authorities for independent state actions; and traditional common law remedies, such as public nuisance, may also be available (Table 18–2).

In contrast to federal environmental laws, the major federal public health law (the Public Health Service Act) does not provide extensive options for enforcement. Even though certain actions are authorized (such as quarantine [42 U.S.C. § 264–272]), few, if any, authorities seem to be available to bring civil and criminal enforcement actions or seek damages.

Citizen suits

Federal environmental statutes contain provisions that allow citizens to bring civil suits against those who violate environmental statutes, including federal agencies, if they fail to fulfill their statutory mandates.[a] These authorities empower citizens to act as private "attorneys general" to force compliance with the law. For example, under the Resource Conservation and Recovery Act (RCRA), a citizen can begin a civil action against any person, including the United States (e.g., the EPA) or any other government agency for violations of RCRA permits, regulations, or other requirements. Anyone may begin a civil suit against any person who is contributing, or has contributed to, past or present handling, storage, treatment, transportation, or disposal of hazardous or solid waste that may imminently and substantially endanger health and the environment (see 42 U.S.C. § 6972[a][1][A] and [B]). Citizen groups have successfully used the citizen suit provisions of the CWA to collect penalties from companies for non-compliance with (and exceedences to) their National Pollutant Discharge Elimination System permits.[4,b] Citizen groups have also sued the EPA and other federal agencies for failure to comply with environmental laws (§ 4.3).[4]

LEGAL ISSUES AND CONTROVERSIES

Historical Underpinnings

History of federal environmental law and regulation

Current U.S. environmental law and regulation is a relatively recent development that has been concerned primarily with standard setting, monitoring and oversight, and enforcement.[5] In their present form, environmental laws and regulations have existed since the creation of the EPA in 1970. Before the EPA, federal efforts regarding the environment fell into two categories. Most environmental or ecosystem protection efforts were handled by the Department of the Interior and the Department of Agriculture (USDA) and their predecessors, and most environmental/human health protection efforts were handled by the Department of Health, Education, and Welfare (DHEW) and its predecessors.[6]

The EPA was created to consolidate into one agency a variety of federal research, monitoring, standard-setting and enforcement activities to ensure integrated environmental protection.[7] In his letter to Congress calling for the creation of the new agency,[8] President Richard Nixon recognized this country's need for a unified, comprehensive, environmental protection effort[8]:

The Government's environmentally-related activities have grown up piecemeal over the years. . . . Our national government today is not structured to make a coordinated attack on the pollutants which debase the air we breathe, the water we drink, and the land that grows our food. Indeed, the present governmental structure for dealing with environmental pollution often defies effective and concerted action. . . . [D]espite its complexity, for pollution control purposes the environment must be perceived as a single, interrelated system. Present assignments of departmental responsibilities do not reflect this interrelatedness.

Programs from the Department of Interior (including the Federal Water Quality Administration and all pesticide research efforts), the DHEW (the National Air Pollution Control Administration, the Bureau of Solid Waste Management, the Bureau of Water Hygiene, the Bureau of Radiological Health, and certain programs from the Food and Drug Administration), the Atomic Energy Commission and the Federal Radiation Council, and the USDA were brought together to form the new comprehensive environmental agency, the EPA.

Given its creators' clear intent, the new agency would be designed to be a unified, comprehensive, and interconnected organization that addressed the environment as a whole and regulated human interaction with the environment in the same way.[8] This was, however, not how the new agency and its regulatory efforts developed. Instead of turning away from the historical trend of regulating human interactions with the environment in a medium-by-medium, piecemeal fashion, Congress and the White House methodically established one environmental program after another that focused on only one environmental area. In 1970, Congress substantially amended the CAA.[9] In 1972, it passed the Federal Environmental Pesticide Control Act, which substantially amended the Federal Insecticide, Fungicide and Rodenticide Act (FIFRA).[10] This was followed closely by substantial amendments to the Safe Drinking Water Act in 1974, the Toxic Substance Control Act in 1976, and the Federal Water Pollution Control Act in 1977. In the 1980s the Comprehensive Environmental Response, Compensation, and Liability Act of 1980 (CERCLA or "Superfund") was enacted, and the Hazardous and Solid Waste Amendments of 1984 were added to the list of focused pieces of environmental legislation.[11,12] Superfund was amended in 1986; the original 20-page Act was expanded by over 200 pages of new or changed provisions.[13] These program-specific and highly detailed amendments continued through the 1990s as Congress passed significant legislation altering the Safe Drinking Water Act (see Public Law 104-182, August 6, 1996, 110 Stat. 1614 *et seq.*), the Federal Food, Drug and Cosmetic Act, and FIFRA (see Public Law 104-170, August 3, 1996, 110 Stat. 1489 *et seq.*, commonly referred to as the Food Quality Protection Act of 1996 [FQPA]).

The historical forces that operated at this time were considerable and somewhat explain why the federal environmental protection system evolved as a series of interconnected media-based programs instead of as an organic whole. After World War II, the new chemical, plastics, and petroleum industries were creating new highly visible forms of pollution that were affecting people and ecosystems on much larger geographic scales than previously. As the scope of pollution became less local and more national, the lack of uniformity in state and local environmental laws became glaringly apparent.[6] In addition, starting in the late 1960s and continuing into the 1970s and 1980s, several events related to the environment garnered national attention—for example, Rachel Carson's publication of *Silent Spring;* the banning of DDT in 1972; the declared public health emergency at Love Canal, New York, in 1978; and the public health advisory issued by the Centers for Disease Control (now the Centers for Disease Control and Prevention) (CDC) for Times Beach, Missouri, in 1982. These and other events created pressure on Congress and the EPA to quickly address the problem at hand, which led to the 13 separate major environmental laws that exist today (Table 18–1). In the end, some of the same flaws that led to the creation of the EPA as a unified federal environmental regulatory agency still exist, despite the best intentions of those who created the EPA. In 1988, the EPA published a historical analysis of its regulatory efforts, which concluded that "ideal preconditions for a more coherent and successful future seem today as elusive as they have always been: EPA's laws are still reauthorized and amended one at a time in a manner inimical to cross-media and unified-field ecological thinking."[6]

Despite its fragmented nature, the present federal environmental system has several notable strengths that have resulted in a cleaner, healthier, and less polluted environment.[14] First, federal environmental protection laws contain a variety of tools for environmental health practitioners. Thus environmental health professionals can take advantage of the information, expertise, and enforcement authorities that the major federal environmental laws create. Second, the national system of regulations is more or less uniform, thereby discouraging all polluting industries from locating in one municipality, state, or region. Finally, the environmental law system is participatory and multitiered. It creates federal authorities that states can use and contains extensive opportunities for citizen and stakeholder involvement.

History of federal public health law and regulation

In July 1798, President John Adams signed into law a bill creating the Marine Hospital Service, now known as the United States Public Health Service (PHS). By the end of the nineteenth century the scope of activities of the Marine Hospital Service began to expand to include the control of infectious diseases. Responsibility for quarantine was originally a function of the states rather than the federal government, but an 1877 yellow fever epidemic that spread quickly from New Orleans up the Mississippi River clearly indicated that infectious diseases (like industrial pollution) do not respect state borders. The epidemic resulted in passage of the National Quarantine Act of 1878, which conferred quarantine authority on the Marine Hospital Service. The Service continued to expand its public health activities as the nation entered the twentieth century. [15]

A 1902 law increased cooperation between federal and state public health authorities and cemented the cooperative approach that is often considered emblematic of the federal and state public health relationship. The PHS was charged with convening a conference of state health authorities at least on an annual basis. Beginning at this same time, environmental health and sanitation became even more central to the work of the PHS when it was asked to investigate a typhoid fever outbreak in Yakima County, Washington, and traced the source of the disease to badly managed human waste disposal practices. The resulting rural sanitation efforts were applied to other areas of the country and helped to encourage establishment of county health departments.[15] In 1912, the PHS was given federal legislative authority to investigate the diseases of humans and conditions influencing the propagation and spread thereof, including sanitation and sewage and the pollution either directly or indirectly of the navigable streams and lakes of the United States. All types of illness, whatever their cause (including environmental pollution), now came within the purview of the PHS.[15] One of the last major overhauls of the public health law came in 1944 when the Public Health Service Act codified on an integrated basis all the authorities of the PHS and strengthened the administrative authority of the Surgeon General.[15]

In contrast to environmental protection, Congress has created an organic statute for public health and its environmental components. Beginning in this postwar period, important investigations began on the hazards of exposure to radiation and toxic chemicals in various industrial settings and on lung disease in miners and granite cutters. The PHS also became more actively involved in studies of water pollution during this time. In addition, the CDC was established, with a mission to control infectious disease. The CDC's mission eventually grew to include the control and prevention of chronic disease and the study and improvement of occupational and environmental health.[15]

Although the history of federal public health law, including environmental public health law, is longer than that of environmental law, it is not without gaps. The shortcomings of federal public health law came into focus in the 1950s and 1960s as the federal health bureaucracy tried to address problems associated with pollution. One of the original reasons for moving the environmental programs from the DHEW to the EPA was the belief that the public health model was not effectively addressing the emerging environmental health problems.

The federal public health system has a long and distinguished history. Originally, its focus on infectious diseases provided a unifying foundation on which later efforts were built aimed at controlling chronic diseases. Because the public health model is traditionally cooperative rather than adversarial and relies on developing and nurturing partnerships, it was not effective during the 1960s and 1970s in tackling the escalating pollution from industrialization. Nevertheless, the public health system has several important strengths. First, because it is cooperative, it can bring together local, state, and national groups to solve problems. Second, because it is evidence based and intervention focused, it can forge solutions to environmental problems, which can result in measurable progress. Third, it is a unified system. The Public Health Service Act pulled together almost all public health authorities, so a central legal repository exists for public health authorities. Unlike the EPA, the PHS has a unified organic statute under which it can function.

Cooperative Federalism: Seeking the Appropriate State–Federal Balance

The environmental health programs in the United States, especially the regulatory programs administered by the EPA, are based on the idea of cooperative federalism. Under cooperative federalism, Congress regulates, offering states the choice of either establishing regulatory programs and schemes that reflect federal standards or having federal standards that preempt state law.[2] In addition, when Congress enacts laws that occupy a field such as environmental law, states are forbidden to regulate in a way that impedes the federal scheme or place an undue burden on interstate commerce.[2]

In the field of environmental health law, the respective roles of the state and federal governments have waxed and waned. In the 1960s and before, it was generally thought that the federal role in environmental protection and enforcement should be minimal. This view changed substantially during the 1970s and 1980s, with expansion of the federal laws and regulatory authorities. During the 1990s and the beginning of the twenty-first century, the state–federal relationship is again undergoing re-evaluation, and once again there is talk of "de-evolution" of authority back to the states. Throughout the 1990s, the U.S. Supreme Court supported the de-evolution of domestic programs to the states and reigned in Congress' power to enact protective laws.[16]

As responsibilities of environmental health regulatory programs have been devolved to the states, state responsibility in pollution control increased significantly. During 1981–1984, "the delegation of environmental programs to the states doubled from 33 percent to 66 percent of all eligible programs."[6] The Environmental Council of the States reported that as of 2000 "more than 75% of the total number of the major delegable environmental programs[d] have been delegated or assumed by the states."[17,d] Eligible provisions of the CAA have been delegated to 42 states, the CWA to 34 states, the RCRA to 37 states, and the FIFRA to 39 states.[17] This increase in state responsibility appears not to have been adequately covered by federal funds. From 1986 through 1996, state spending on the environment increased 140%, while EPA funding to the states decreased 17%.[17] In fiscal year 1996, the states collectively spent $12.5 billion on environmental protection, while the EPA provided $2.5 billion of its total $6.5 billion budget to the states.[17]

In addition to their partnership with the federal government in setting standards and enforcing federal regulation, states have actively enforced and administered state environmental laws such as facility siting and property transfer laws.[18] Every states does, in fact, have detailed laws regulating air pollution, water pollution, waste disposal, and resource management. Many state laws are modeled after federal legislation. Fifteen states[e] have adopted state environmental policy acts (SEPAs) that are either identical to or closely resemble the National Environmental Policy Act (NEPA).[19] California's and New York's SEPAs are considered more stringent than the NEPA in several ways. They define terms left undefined in the NEPA and require the state to consider additional environmental effects not included in the NEPA impact statement.[19] States continue to "differ significantly in their programs, rules, regulations, and in their capacities for effective implementation."[20] Several states have enacted innovative laws or established novel programs. California is widely recognized for its Proposition 65,[21] which established stringent drinking water standards and warnings to the public about harmful and potentially harmful substances. New Jersey's Environmental Cleanup Responsibility Act.[22] and Massachusetts' regulation of toxic substances.[23,f] exceed federal standards, as do Arizona's, Wisconsin's, and Connecticut's groundwater protection regulations.[24–26] Michigan, Pennsylvania, Rhode Island, and Illinois are among states that have declared a clean environment to be a state constitutional right,[27–30] and Michigan's Citizen Suit Act requires state courts to review any private or agency action that adversely affects the environment.[27]

The federal environmental health infrastructure put into place in the 1970s and 1980s was a broadly supported "response to perceived inadequacies with [state] law and the frustration with the failure of decentralized approaches to environmental protection."[32] The problems of transboundary pollution and the possibility of a "race to the bottom" among states has been effectively addressed by a centralized federal regulatory authority. Uniform federal regulations also improve national efficiency. Under the CAA, the federal government defines, monitors, and enforces emission standards for newly manufactured automobiles. Allowing 50 different state standards for automobile manufacturers would be extremely inefficient.[33]

In most environmental regulatory schemes, the states are "junior-partners in the federal–state regulatory enterprise."[33] Nevertheless, states have retained the right to formulate state policy in addition to and beyond that established by federal authorities. Federal oversight of state programs has actually raised the standards of many states,[34] and in some instances (such as the establishment of state environmental protection acts and the improvement of pollution standards) federal regulations have served as a catalyst for advancing more aggressive state action and the expansion of state programs.

The federal–state relationship is complicated and delicate. Federal standards have provided a consistent level of nationwide environmental quality and have tremendously reduced pollution. However, because states vary significantly in climate, terrain, sources of pollution, economic conditions, and preferences for environmental protection, state flexibility and enforcement are crucial. For practitioners, this cooperative federalism brings both good and bad news. The good news is that many legal tools are available in both federal and state arenas to improve environmental health. The bad news is that the optimum use of such tools is rarely obvious.

Making Preventive Decisions in an Uncertain Scientific Climate

Environmental health laws often have goals that are aspirational and difficult to achieve.[g] However, because almost all environmental health laws seek to protect public health and welfare, action is usually necessary before a complete picture about an environmental hazard has emerged. Many decisions regarding environmental health are made using less than optimal data. Although the need for environmental health laws and regulations to be preventive is widely recognized, the public and regulated entities often have difficulty accepting the uncertainty that accompanies decision making that incorporates data gaps.

A technique called *risk assessment* is commonly used to justify regulations and standards. In a risk assessment, science and data are analyzed to obtain a measure of the potential individual and population harms that could occur through exposure to a substance.[35] Risk assessment is generally a four-part process that begins with a hazard identification. In a hazard identification, a determination is made as to whether exposure to a compound or agent should be of concern. After the hazard identification, a dose–response analysis occurs in which toxicologic data are compiled to create a dose–response curve (or margin of exposure) that links exposure with harm. Dose–response analysis is complicated because toxicology or human epidemiology data, if available, are nearly always available only for doses far above environmental levels. Next, an exposure assessment is conducted; it analyzes information about the scope, nature, route, and duration of the exposure to the agent in question. Finally, the hazard, dose–response, and exposure information are integrated into a risk characterization, which generally describes the potential population and individual risks. For carcinogens, this risk is most commonly expressed probabilistically—that is, a one-in-one-million chance of contracting cancer. For compounds that are not carcinogens, risks are often described by comparing the exposure or dose level with a theoretical reference dose that should not be exceeded.

The preparation of a risk assessment requires much professional judgment. If data are not available, default assumptions or inferences that are public health protective are frequently used. For example, without specific knowledge, adults are often assumed to drink an average of 2 liters of water per day.[36] These assumptions can be controversial.[h] The information obtained in a risk assessment is used by a risk manager, who is often a government employee, to make decisions about how to manage environmental risks. This risk manager combines the information contained in the assessment with social, cultural, and political factors.

In contrast to risk assessment, disease and exposure surveillances are the traditional tools of public health. This philosophy is clearly evident in *Healthy People 2010,*[37] which guides national efforts to set a health agenda and chart health improvement. For example, *Healthy People 2010* sets a series of goals related to environmental exposures or diseases associated with environmental exposure, such as asthma. These goals are generally community based and measurable, and the *Healthy People 2010* protocol calls for regularly updating progress toward reaching its goals. The *Healthy People 2010* goals are not regulatory.[i]

Environmental health practitioners should become familiar with risk assessment and risk management and understand their roles in, and impact on, environmental health regulation. In addition, environmental health law practitioners should recognize that risk assessment and risk management are processes that employ as much art as science. They should not shy away from asking hard questions about how such analyses were carried out, especially about default assumptions, inferences, data sources, and analysis techniques. Several federal and state agencies, including the EPA, have published guidance manuals explaining how these assessments are meant to be carried out.[38] Environmental health law practitioners should also be familiar with how the Department of Health and Human Services sets its environmental health goals and measures them through the *Healthy People 2010* process. It employs traditional public health tools to set objectives and work toward them.

PRACTICE CONSIDERATIONS

Tools for Environmental Health Protection

A multitude of approaches can be taken to advance environmental health and protection. For example, to reduce harmful releases from a facility, authorities can specify the allowable amount to be released (in a permit such as a discharge permit allowed under the CWA) or specify technologic approaches that will ultimately limit releases (as in the CAA's approach to hazardous air pollutants) or penalize the facility by imposing liability for damages from specified releases (as in Superfund). Traditional public health tools, such as surveillance of hazardous conditions (i.e., childhood lead poisoning) and cooperative approaches (such as grants to states to support environmental health programs), also are available. Using these tools, a state public health department can begin or improve an asthma surveillance program or start or increase environmental health information and outreach efforts to citizens. The complexity of environmental health protection is substantial because these different approaches can be mixed in many ways. In addition, multiple actors, including the federal government, state governments, and citizens, all could be tackling the same problem using different tools.

The Office of Technology Assessment[39] identified 12 types of environmental protection tools, divided into three broad categories: single-source tools, multi-source tools, and tools that do not directly limit pollution. Single-source tools, often described as "command-and-control" tools, have been most extensively used. They can (*1*) ban or limit production or use of a product, (*2*) specify the technology for how a product can be made or how pollution can be controlled, (*3*) set standards on the basis of potential harm from exposure for the reduction of releases, or (*4*) set standards on the basis of what a desirable or best technology might achieve. Almost every environmental statute relies to some degree on "command-and-control" approaches.

Multisource tools allow individual facilities or multiple entities the option to vary or even trade emission limits so that a collective protection limit is met, even if limits are exceeded at individual facilities. These tools provide greater flexibility in meeting standards than single-source tools. Finally, a variety of tools exist that do not specify release limits but rely on "carrots and sticks" to either encourage environmental protection through subsidies or technical assistance or discourage releases by requiring public disclosure, payment of fees, or imposition of liability. These tools take various forms, including civil penalties and criminal sanctions, as well as public disclosure of information about pollution. (Most traditional public health tools fall into this category.)

Applying Environmental Health Protection Tools

The environmental health tools used by public health agencies and the environmental protection tools used by environmental agencies complement each other and are rarely mutually exclusive. Nevertheless, they are infrequently found in the same federal environmental statute. The CAA, for example, does not primarily utilize public health tools. On the other hand, CERCLA contains tools that embody both the environmental health and environmental protection traditions. CERCLA created a new public health agency, the Agency for Toxic Substances and Disease Registry (ATSDR), to carry out many of its environmental health functions. Each of these statutes is discussed in some detail to illustrate this point.

The Clean Air Act

The clearly stated purpose of the CAA is "to protect and enhance the quality of the Nation's air resources so as to promote the public health and welfare" (42 U.S.C. § 7401[b][1]). Even from this most cursory review of the key titles in the Act, regulatory provisions clearly dominate and were considerably strengthened from earlier iterations of the CAA that Congress considered insufficiently protective of public health (§ 3.2).[4] As amended by the CAA Amendments of 1990, the CAA contains almost the full range of environmental protection tools to achieve its stated goals. It established National Ambient Air Quality Standards (pollution levels that states are required to meet by preparing and enforcing implementation plans); created a program for reducing emissions from mobile sources (by requiring the EPA to set standards for emissions levels from vehicles); established a methodology for reducing toxic air pollutants (by setting technology-based standards); and sought to reduce acid rain deposition through an allowance program for electric utilities. In addition to these major provisions, additional sections exist that create research programs, including environmental health research.[j]

The CAA outlines a limited role for federal public health authorities. Even in areas where public health could be expected to lead, the statute indicates that PHS agencies are to play a secondary role. Subsection 103(d) of the Act (42 U.S.C. § 7403[d]) illustrates Congress' approach. This subsection, "Research, investigation, training, and other activities," specifically calls for environmental health research. The EPA Administrator, in consultation with the Secretary of the DHHS, is ordered to conduct a research program on the short-and long-term effects of air pollutants and prepare environmental health assessments for hazardous air pollutants. The subsection also creates an Interagency Task Force, which includes several PHS agencies, such as the ATSDR and the National Institute of Environmental Health Sciences. However, the statutory language indicates that the EPA is expected to control this research agenda. The CAA thus creates an opportunity to bolster environmental health research but does not seem to give PHS agencies a leadership role in its design and implementation.

The balance in the CAA is overwhelmingly weighted toward traditional regulatory tools. Additional (or more effective) surveillance of respiratory disease, a role for state health departments in respiratory health education in communities, additional involvement of health agencies at any number of points in the regulatory process, or application of other environmental health tools would most likely be helpful in achieving the public health goals of the CAA. However, the CAA does not contain these tools.[k]

Superfund

Superfund, enacted in 1980, was amended extensively in 1986 by the Superfund Amendments and Reauthorization Act. Its main goal is to protect public health by cleaning up inactive or abandoned sites at which hazardous substances are being released. The "Superfund" name comes from the funding mechanism created by a tax imposed on the petroleum, chemical, and other industries. It assigns liability and apportions responsibility for the cost of cleaning up the sites among classes of persons (e.g., individuals, state and federal government entities, and corporations) deemed to have been responsible for these releases. Environmental protection tools play an important role in making CERCLA effective. CERCLA also uses significant environmental health tools.

Among its features, CERCLA created a National Priorities List (a method for establishing clean-up priorities among the thousands of sites in the country at which hazardous substances are found), a National Contingency Plan (guidance for conducting more immediate response actions when necessary), and a detailed remedial process for evaluating and cleaning up the sites (see 42 U.S.C. § 9605[a]).

Many of the most important tools of CERCLA relate to its liability and enforcement provisions. Strict, and joint and several liability, which can result in one or several significant polluters at a site being responsible for all clean-up costs even though many parties may have contributed to the pollution, is the centerpiece of CERCLA's environmental protection scheme (42 U.S.C. § 9601.) Additional provisions relate to identification of potentially responsible parties, e.g., information requests (42 U.S.C. § 9603), cost recovery actions that the government or a private party can bring to recoup its clean-up expenses (42 U.S.C. § 9607), the abatement of imminent and substantial hazards to public health (42 U.S.C. §§ 9604[a] and 9606), administrative orders issued by the federal government to compel private parties to undertake response actions (42 U.S.C. § 9606), penalties for failure to comply (42 U.S.C. § 9609), and citizen lawsuit provisions (42 U.S.C. § 9659).

CERCLA also contains significant health-related provisions that use classic environmental health tools. When enacted, CERCLA established a new agency within the PHS known as the ATSDR.[40] In cooperation with the EPA and other PHS agencies, the ATSDR has the responsibility to "effectuate and implement the health related authorities" of Superfund (42 U.S.C. § 9604[I][1]). Among other things, the ATSDR conducts public health assessments at all National Priorities List sites, maintains national registries of persons exposed to toxic substances and of illnesses and diseases, develops toxicology profiles for each substance on a hazardous substance priority list, and conducts epidemiologic or other health studies and health surveillance and health education programs when appropriate (42 U.S.C. §§ 9604[i][1] and [2]). CERCLA also created a mechanism whereby the ATSDR provides extensive public health review, evaluation, and feedback on environmental sampling, monitoring, and remediation to the EPA. In addition, CERCLA authorized a substantial basic research program at NIEHS, along with worker training and education programs (42 U.S.C. § 9604[i][1] to [18]).

CERCLA marries a nonregulatory, newly created public health agency (ATSDR) with a regulatory agency (EPA). In practice, this resulted in extensive opportunities for collaboration and coordination among public health and environmental agencies to fulfill the mandates of a major environmental protection statute. Environmental health practitioners should consider the potential for such partnerships in other critical situations that arise in the practice of environmental law.

EMERGING ISSUES

Environmental Health Aspects of Chemical, Biologic, and Radiologic Terrorism

The September 11, 2001, terrorist attacks on New York City and Washington, DC, and the dissemination of anthrax through the US postal system brought into focus some of the gaps in our public health systems' preparedness for responding to terrorism. Public health responsibilities during and after such events must be performed expeditiously and coordinated effectively. All terrorist actions will have environmental health consequences and will require a sustained environmental health presence. Appropriate environmental health response—including air and water monitoring, disease tracking, laboratory analysis of samples, and protection of the health and safety of responders—is vital. Although federal and state statutory authority exists to provide integrated and rapid action in certain cases, more effective environmental health response planning and a fuller assessment of the gaps in authority, leadership, and workforce are needed.

Environmental surveillance and monitoring; case ascertainment; environmental sampling in air, water, and other media; and provision of potable water and clean-up of toxic releases are just some of the tasks that will challenge environmental health responders in the event of other terrorist attacks. Environmental health law practitioners are also likely to face the following issues:

- Lack of clarity about unusual legal enforcement powers during terrorist events
- Operation under completely different chain of command and legal authority structure when a response plan is implemented
- Unusual instances of public health professional liability
- Lack of clarity regarding the availability to the public of the information collected (security vs. right to know)
- Need to use nontraditional and less-than-optimal surveillance methodologies and analyses to make decisions because of the breakdown of public health information systems

Each of these challenges requires public health and legal practitioners to take several steps to respond to the new complexities. First and foremost, public health laws will have to be revisited and revised to address these previously unimaginable situations. Second, public health and legal practitioners will need to collaborate more closely to plan joint action and to coordinate activities before and during emergencies so that a better understanding of roles, responsibilities, and authorities within the unique circumstances emerges.

National Health Tracking

Environmental protection tools provide considerable information about pollutants in the environment. Unfortunately, limited data are available concerning exposures and the distribution of diseases and their relation to the environment. As a result, our public health system is working without even the most basic information about chronic diseases and environmental health factors. In addition, our system of environmental protection has no good way of evaluating whether it is improving public health and reducing disease.

The Pew Environmental Health Commission (PEHC), a blue ribbon panel of policy and scientific experts from industry, government, and academia, described this situation as a national "environmental health gap."[1] It concluded that information about trends in health conditions potentially related to the environment is largely unavailable.[1] Furthermore, the tracking systems that do exist at state and local levels are a patchwork. No agreed-on minimum standards exist, and almost no synchronization exists in the collection, analysis, and dissemination of the information.

Environmental health tracking for pollutants is crucial because hazards often can be removed or contained before they cause harm. Although such monitoring would be valuable, it is not sufficient by itself. Tracking actual exposures to hazards in the environment is frequently the missing link between public health efforts to evaluate a risk and the ability to respond to a health threat from that risk in a specific community. Thus, improving national efforts to track population exposures to contaminants and providing this information to local public health officers is essential.

To fill this environmental health gap, the PEHC offered the following recommendation[1]:

Create a federally supported Nationwide Health Tracking Network with the appropriate privacy protections that informs consumers, communities, public health practitioners, researchers, and policy makers on chronic diseases and related environmental hazards and population exposures. This will provide the capacity to better understand, respond to and prevent chronic disease in this country. (p. 10)

By creating a national system that links disease endpoints with potential environmental exposures, the environmental health and environmental protection traditions would be effectively joined. This national health tracking system would provide environmental health practitioners with information that could be used to more effectively plan and target resources, as well as discover emerging disease and exposure trends. Ultimately, a national health tracking network has the potential to greatly assist in achieving the goal that underlies almost every environmental law—protection of public health and welfare.

Notes

ᵃ See, for example 42 U.S.C. § 7604; 33 U.S.C. § 1365(a); 42 U.S.C § 6972(a)(1)(A).
ᵇ An illustrative case is *Sierra Club v. Simkins Industries, Inc.*, 847 F.2d 1109, cert. denied, 491 U.S. 904 (1989).
ᶜ The U.S. Supreme Court ruled that the Gun-Free School Zones Act exceeded Congress' right to regulate interstate commerce and was therefore unconstitutional.
ᵈ Many federal statutes provide that states can administer and enforce their own programs in lieu of the federal program. Generally, states cannot implement programs if the EPA finds that the state program is not equivalent to the federal program, is not consistent with the federal program, or does not provide adequate enforcement. See, for example, 42 U.S.C § 6929 (RCRA); and 33 U.S.C. § 1342(b) and (c)(1) (CWA permit program for pollution discharges).
ᵉ California, Connecticut, Georgia, Hawaii, Indiana, Maryland, Massachusetts, Minnesota, Montana, New York, North Carolina, South Dakota, Virginia, West Virginia, Washington, and Wisconsin.
ᶠ The Massachusetts Toxics Use Reduction Act reduces industrial use of toxins through mandatory planning approaches. At least 12 other states have toxic use reduction laws, McElfish note 8.1.
ᵍ For example, the CWA states that "it is the national goal that the discharge of pollutants . . . shall be eliminated by 1985" (see 33 U.S.C. § 1251[a][1]). This goal has not yet been met.
ʰ One of the more controversial and public health protective assumptions is the assumption that the dose–response curve associated with carcinogenicity is linear. According to the proposed EPA cancer risk guidelines, linear extrapolation "is generally conservative of public health, in the absence of information about the extent of human variability in sensitivity of effects. For linear extrapolation, a straight line is drawn from the point of departure to the origin0—zero dose, zero response." EPA. "Proposed Cancer Risk Assessment Guidelnes." 61 *Federal Register.*
ⁱ Consider goal 8-1, which aims to reduce the population exposed to air above the EPA's health-based standard for hazardous air pollutants. The Department of Health and Human Services will undoubtedly use surveillance data for this analysis.
ʲ See, for example, 42 U.S.C. § 7404 (research relating to fuels and vehicles) and 42 U.S.C. § 7403(d) (environmental health effects research).
ᵏ It is feasible that, as this chapter suggests, public health agencies could use authorities such as those contained in the Public Health Service Act to conduct these functions. We make this point here only to show that the CAA does not embrace them.
ˡ For example, as *America's Environmental Health Gap*[1] points out, endocrine and metabolic disorders such as diabetes, and neurologic conditions such as migraines and multiple sclerosis, increased approximately 20% during 1986–1995. For most of the country, asthma is not systematically tracked, even though this disease has reached epidemic proportions (pp. 8–9).

References

1. Pew Environmental Health Commission. *America's Environmental Health Gap: Why the Country Needs A Nationwide Health Tracking Network* (Technical Report). Baltimore: Pew Environmental Health Commission, September 2000, p. 86.
2. Gostin LO. *Public Health Law: Power, Duty, Restraint.* Berkeley: University of California Press, 2000 p. 40.
3. Gerrard MB, ed. *Environmental Law Practice Guide: State and Federal Law.* New York: Matthew Bender, LEXIS Publishing, 1992, 2001: § 33.01(2).
4. Rodgers WH, Jr. *Environmental Law* 2nd ed. St. Paul, MN: West Publishing Company, 1994 [with 1995 pocket part], Section 4.2.
5. EPA. Agency overview. In: *EPA Organization and Functions Manual.* Available at http://www.epa.gov/history/org/origins/overview.htm. Accessed September 15, 2001.
6. Lewis J. Looking backward: a historical perspective on environmental regulations. *EPA J* 1988 (March). Available at http://www.epa.gov/history/topics/regulate/01.htm. Accessed January 7, 2002.
7. President's Advisory Council on Executive Organization. Memo for the President [Nixon]. April 29, 1970. Available at: http://www.epa.gov/history/org/origins/ash.htm. Accessed September 15, 2001.
8. Special Message from the President to Congress about Reorganization Plans to Establish the Environmental; Protection Agency and the National Oceanic and Atmospheric Administration, July 9, 1970 [online] Available at http://www.epa.gov/history/org/origins/reorg.htm. Last updated, May 1, 2000.
9. Public Law 91-604, December 31, 1970, 84 Stat. 1676 *et seq.*
10. Public Law 92-516 (7 U.S.C. §§ 136 *et seq.*), October 21, 1972, 86 Stat. 973.
11. Public Law 96-510 (42 U.S.C § 9601 *et seq.*), December 11, 1980, 94 Stat. 2767 (Superfund).
12. Public Law 98-616 (42 USC § 6921[d]), November. 8, 1984, 98 Stat. 3221 (1984 RCRA amendments).
13. Public Law 99-499, October 17, 1986, 100 Stat. 1777.
14. Campbell Mohn C, Breen B, William Futrell J, eds. Chemicals In: 17 *Sustainable Environmental Law.* St. Paul, MN: West Publishing Company, 1993: p. 1352.
15. Parascandola JL. Public Health Service. In: Kurian GT, ed. *A Historical Guide to the U.S. Government.* New York: Oxford University Press, 1998: pp. 487–93.
16. *United States v. Lopez,* 514 U.S. 549 (1995).
17. The Environmental Council of the States. *Home Page.* Available at http://www.ecos.org. Accessed January 7, 2002.
18. Campbell-Mohn C, Been B, Futtrell WJ, eds. Chemicals. *Sustainable Environmental Law.* St. Paul, MN: West Publishing Company 1993: § 17.2(8)(2) and § 17.2(B)(1).
19. Mandelker DR. State environmental policy acts. In: *NEPA. Law and Litigation.* 2nd ed. St. Paul, MN: West Publishing Company Release 9, August 2000: § 12.01, 12-2.
20. Kraft ME. *Environmental Policy and Politics: Towards the 21st Century.* New York: Harper Collins College Publishers, 1996: p. 103.
21. Cal. Health & Safety Code § 25249.1 *et seq.*
22. N.J. Stat. Ann. § 13.1K-6 *et seq.*
23. Massachusetts Toxics Use Reduction Act (TURA), Mass. Gen. L. Ch. 21[1], § 1-23 (1989).
24. Ariz. Rev. Stat. Ann. § 49-201 *et seq.*
25. Wis Stat. Ann. § 1600.001 *et seq.*

26. Conn. Gen. Stat. Ch. 446K, § 22a-416 *et seq.*
27. Skillern FF. *Environmental Protection Deskbook.* 2nd ed. New York: McGraw Hill, Inc., 1995: p. 705.
28. Michigan Constitution, Article IV, § 52 (1983).
29. Pennsylvania Constitution, Article I, § 27 (West Purdon 1994).
30. Rhode Island Constitution, Article I, § 17 (Michie 1987).
31. Michigan Stat. Ann. § 14.528 (204) (1989 & Supp. 1994).
32. Percival RV. Regulatory evolution and the future of environmental policy. In: *University of Chicago Legal Forum.* Chicago: University of Chicago, 1997: pp. 159–98.
33. Dwyer JP. The role of state law in an era of federal preemption: lesson from environmental regulation. *Law Contemp Prob* 1997;60:203–30.
34. McElfish J, Novick SM, Stever DW, Mellon MG, Fogarty JPC, Stewart SL. State environmental laws and programs. In: Novick SM, Stever DW, Mellon MG Fogarty JPC, Stewart SL eds. *Law of Environmental Protection*, vol. 1. St. Paul, MN: West Publishing Company, 1987, Release 17, 3/97, § 6.02(3), 6.18.
35. National Research Council. *Risk Assessment in the Federal Government: Managing the Process.* Washington, DC: National Academy Press, 1983.
36. Environmental Protection Agency. *Exposure Factors Handbook.* Volume I: General Factors. Update to Exposure Factors Handbook. Office of Research and Development, National Center for Environmental Assessment, U.S. Environmental Protection Agency: 3-1. Publication no. EPA/600/P-95/002Fa, August 1997. Available at http://www.epa.gov/NCEA/pdfs/efh/sect3.PDF. Accessed December 15, 2001.
37. U.S. Department of Health and Human Services. *Healthy People 2010.* Available at http://www.health.gov/healthypeople/document/. Accessed January 4, 2002.
38. Environmental Protection Agency. *Proposed Guidelines for Carcinogen Risk Assessment (April 23, 1996).* Office of Research and Development, National Center for Environmental Assessment, U.S. Environmental Protection Agency. *Federal Register* 61(79):17960–8011. Publication No. EPA/600/P-92/003C April 1996. Available at http://www.epa.gov/NCEA/raf/pdfs/propcra_1996.pdf. Accessed January 7, 2002.
39. U.S. Office of Technology Assessment, *Environmental Policy Tools: A User's Guide.* OTA-ENV-634. Washington, DC: U.S Government Printing Office, September 1995.
40. Public Law 96-510, § 104(i)(1)–(5), 94 Stat. 2778.

19

Injury Prevention and the Law

STEPHEN P. TERET AND TOM CHRISTOFFEL

During the twentieth century, the relative significance of injuries increased as other causes of mortality and morbidity declined. Today in the United States, about 150,000 injury-related deaths and 70 million nonfatal injuries occur each year. Injury ranks third among all causes of death and is the second most costly health problem in the U.S. About one third of U.S. injury-related deaths are motor-vehicle related, one third involve other unintentional injuries, and one third involve homicides and suicides.[1,2]

Historically, injuries were given scant attention as a public health issue. Not until the second half of the twentieth century did a scientific understanding of injury etiology and prevention begin to emerge. A key conceptual insight was that the agent involved in injury is *energy* and that injury involves the transfer of energy to human tissues in amounts and at rates that change the cellular structure, tissues, blood vessels, and other body structures. The fact that energy transfers can be controlled to reduce the likelihood and severity of injury gave birth to the modern field of injury prevention. Kinetic, electrical, and thermal energy are generated during travel, work, play, and the performance of life's many other activities. Energy can be transferred to the human body when a car crashes, lightening strikes, or scalding water spills. If the energy is transferred to the human body in small enough amounts, the body can accommodate it without suffering injury; if the energy is transferred in large amounts and the body is not otherwise protected, injury will occur.

Transfers of energy often can be managed by the use of energy-attenuating devices, such as air bags or other items that diffuse the energy. For example, a fall from a height might not injure a person who lands on a soft, large surface, which spreads the decelerative kinetic energy over time and space. However, a fall from the same height in which the person lands on a hard and pointed surface probably will result in damage because the same forces of deceleration were concentrated in time and area. Research pioneers measured energy transfers to humans in car crashes, assaults, falls, and other events and, even more importantly, developed and put in place protection for humans through restraints, barriers, and cushions (e.g., seatbelts, bullet-proof vests, and air bags), leading to enhanced safety for the public.

Injuries are not distributed evenly throughout the population. The descriptive epidemiology of injuries reveals that young people, males, elderly, and the poor are at elevated risk, and, because injuries disproportionately affect children and adolescents, many years of potential and productive life are regularly lost to trauma. In fact, in the United States, injuries steal more years of potential life than does heart disease or cancer. The cost of injuries to our society, whether measured in human suffering or in dollars, remains unacceptable.[3]

The major categories of injury include motor vehicle–related injuries, intentional violence (especially firearm-related violence), drowning, poisoning, fires and burns, suffocation, and falls. Of these, motor vehicle–related injuries and violence take the greatest number of lives, and, for this reason, many of this chapter's examples of how the law addresses injuries are from the fields of motor vehicle–related and violence-related injury prevention. Another method of categorizing injuries is whether they are work related. Although this categorization significantly affects how the law will deal with preventing the effects of the injuries, the etiologies of the injuries are often the same, whether they occur at work or elsewhere. Of emerging consideration to the field of injury prevention are iatrogenic, or medically related, injuries, which traditionally have not been counted in the 150,000 annual injury-related deaths. Medical injuries could add almost another 100,000 victims to the toll of injuries.

William Haddon conceptualized the prevention of injury as involving the following 10 strategies.[4]

- Prevent the creation of the hazard.
- Reduce the amount of the hazard.
- Prevent the release of a hazard that already exists.
- Modify the rate or spatial distribution of the hazard.
- Separate, in time or space, the hazard from that which is to be protected.
- Separate the hazard from that which is to be protected by a material barrier.

- Modify relevant basic qualities of the hazard.
- Make what is to be protected more resistant to damage from the hazard.
- Begin to counter the damage already done by the hazard.
- Stabilize, repair, and rehabilitate the object of the damage.

Many of these strategies are most effectively accomplished through the intervention of law. In using law to deal with any public health problem, governments and agencies at multiple levels can employ several different approaches. First, they can fund public health programs, such as screening and surveillance efforts, health education, and a wide variety of preventive services. In each of these cases government provides public services that can often be voluntarily accepted or rejected, such as home-safety audits. Alternatively, governments can employ statutory controls. Injury-prevention statutes can take the form of specific requirements, such as mandatory seatbelt-use laws or zoning ordinances requiring installation of fire sprinklers, or they can consist of broad regulatory programs, as with the federal Occupational Safety and Health Act or the National Traffic and Motor Vehicle Safety Act.

In enacting statutory laws, legislative bodies can pursue several different conceptual approaches. Statutory commands may govern the behavior of an individual for the protection of that individual or another, or the law may govern the design of environments and products to decrease the risk for injury. Statutory commands can be phrased either to require or to prohibit actions. Table 19–1

TABLE 19–1. Intent of Laws that Prevent Injuries Related to Use of Two Products, by Injury Factors

PRODUCT/FACTOR	INTENT OF LAW
Motor Vehicles	
Humans (people)	Prohibit drag racing; require seatbelt use
Vehicle/agent (things)	Prohibit speedometers that register >80 mph; require air bags
Environment (places)	Prohibit rigid barriers within specified distance of roadway; require break-away sign posts
Firearms	
Humans (people)	Prohibit discharge within city limits; require storage in locked compartments
Vehicle/agent (things)	Prohibit plastic handguns; require safety mechanisms
Environment (places)	Prohibit firearms in certain places (e.g., airports, bars, courtrooms, schools); require bulletproof partitions in late-night convenience stores

provides examples of how injury-prevention laws can be directed at the human factors of individual behavior (people); at products (things)—such as vehicles or other agents associated with injuries; or at environmental conditions (places).

Most of Haddon's strategies for reducing injury, particularly those involving the pre injury and injury phases, call for mandatory counter measures that have the force of law to support them. Law plays an important role in the implementation of such approaches, whether, for example, in the form of a ban on the manufacturing or sale of plastic handguns (e.g., preventing the hazard in the first place) or the requirement of child proof caps on medicines and household cleaners (e.g., creating a material barrier separating the hazard from that which needs to be protected).

In short, legal strategies for injury prevention offer an assortment of options, as is illustrated by efforts to reduce firearm injuries. Of the more interventionist approaches to firearm legislation (i.e., those that go beyond the establishment of educational and training programs), one can distinguish between laws that control the availability of guns (or some particular types of guns) and laws that control the use of guns. Baker, Teret, and Dietz developed a categorization of existing gun-control laws by focusing on the different stages in the life history of a gun.[5] These commentators noted that prevention measures can be implemented at the time the gun is designed, manufactured, sold or transferred, possessed by the potential user, or used.

Most persons who work in the injury prevention field favor the use of any and all strategies that could diminish the incidence and severity of injuries. However, they also understand that strategies that provide automatic protection tend to be more effective. In other words, asking people to try to drive more safely is a necessary part of injury prevention, but designing cars so that, in the event of a crash, the likelihood of serious injury is reduced is probably even more effective.[6] Thus, society has enacted laws both for the purpose of requiring people to drive safely and for compelling car manufacturers to provide safe vehicles.

LEGAL AUTHORITIES

The prevention of injuries is intertwined with legislation, regulation, and litigation. Injury-prevention laws can be traced at least to the Code of Hammurabi, which included strict building safety requirements.[7] In the field of injury control, the challenge traditionally has not been one of scientific discovery of the detailed etiology of injuries, as in disease control. Most injury etiology is readily apparent: A vehicle strikes a pedestrian, a dropped cigarette ignites a house fire, or a trigger is pulled on a gun. The challenge for preventing these and many other types of injuries is to modify risky behaviors, environments, and products, and here the law has played a leading role. Specific legislation, regulation, and litigation have been devised to reduce the risk for and severity of injury by controlling the behaviors of individuals and corporations, requiring safer environments and products and effectively responding to trauma-producing events. Table 19–2, reprinted with modifications from a text for practitioners entitled *Injury Prevention and Public Health*,[8] lists some of the milestones in the development of injury-prevention laws in the United States. Here we provide examples to highlight the principal legal authorities that help protect the public against injury.

Motorcycle injuries exemplify the ease of discerning the cause of an injury but the difficulty of controlling the occurrence of the injury through the use of law.[9] As has long been known, operating a motorcycle is a risky activity. The death rate to motorcyclists, particularly from head injury, is high relative to that from other forms of transportation. Use of a motorcycle helmet also has long been known to significantly reduce the risk for fatal head injury. Helmet use can be increased by the passage of mandatory motorcycle helmet laws. Because the use or nonuse of a helmet is a highly visible and public behavior, when states pass and enforce helmet use laws, the helmet use vastly increases and death rates to motorcyclists drop. Yet, despite the success of mandatory motorcycle helmet laws, states have a long history of passing, repealing, and repassing such laws, with bitter debate over the propriety of such laws. The laws are condemned by some as paternalistic deprivations of highly valued personal freedoms, and the laws are lauded by others as cost-effective injury prevention strategies needed to control a financial burden borne by society as a whole rather than restricted to the motorcyclists themselves. Thus, with head injuries to motorcyclists, the etiology of the injury and a method for its prevention are readily apparent, but the legal and social forces involved in preventing these injuries are subject to substantial debate.

Public health in the United States has traditionally possessed an extensive legal armamentarium, including legal authority to isolate or quarantine; abate nuisances and obtain other injunctive relief; impose penal sanctions; establish permit and license requirements; and seize, embargo, or ban dangerous items. The basis for such legal intervention is clear. U.S. courts have been willing to uphold compulsory public health measures with respect to not only communicable diseases but also health problems where contagion is not involved, such as mandating fluoride in public drinking water or requiring vision and hearing tests for school children. Where clear risk for disease or injury has been identified and where relevant public health expertise supports the proposed response, government has been afforded extensive authority to intervene to protect the public's health.[10]

As with all public health law, the authority to protect the health and safety of the public, and to prevent injury, is found most clearly in the police powers that are reserved to the states. Thus, much of injury prevention law is created

TABLE 19–2. Milestones in Injury Prevention Law

YEAR	MILESTONE
1966	**Congress establishes National Highway Traffic Safety Bureau.** Congress, in 1966, passed the National Traffic and Motor Vehicle Safety Act (15 U.S.C. 1381 *et seq.*), which established the National Highway Traffic Safety Administration (originally called the National Highway Safety Bureau), which promulgates safety standards for motor vehicles
1968	**Court decides *Larsen v. General Motors*** (391 F.2d 495). The Eighth Circuit Federal Court of Appeals held that auto makers must anticipate that their products will be involved in crashes and must design their products to minimize injuries that will occur in the foreseeable crashes. The Court found that the manufacturers have a duty "to provide a means of safe transportation or as safe as is reasonably possible under the present state of the art"
1968	**Congress passes Gun Control Act.** Following the assassinations of President John F. Kennedy, Dr. Martin Luther King, Jr., and Robert F. Kennedy, Congress passed the Gun Control Act (18 U.S.C. Ch. 44), which, among other provisions, banned the importation of small, cheap handguns known as "Saturday Night Specials"
1970	**Congress passes the Occupational Safety and Health Act** (29 U.S.C. 651 *et seq.*). To ensure as far as possible safe and healthful working conditions to every working man and woman in the United States, this Act established the Occupational Safety and Health Administration in the Labor Department
1972	**Congress enacts the Consumer Product Safety Act** (15 U.S.C. 2051 *et seq.*) **and Others**. This Act addressed the risk for injury posed to the U.S. public by dangerous or defective consumer products. The Act established the Consumer Product Safety Agency, which administers the Flammable Fabrics Act (15 U.S.C. 1191, *et seq.*), the Federal Hazardous Substances Act (15 U.S.C. 1261 *et seq.*), and the Poison Prevention Packaging Act (15 U.S.C. 1471 *et seq.*)
1973	**Congress enacts the Emergency Medical Services Systems Act** (Public Law 93–154). On November 16, 1973, Congress passed the EMSSA as an amendment (a new Title XII) to the Public Health Service Act. The EMSSA provided that the federal government could award grants and enter into contracts regarding planning, establishment, expansion, personnel training, and research of and for emergency medical services at the local level within states. In addition, the Act promulgated guidelines for emergency medical services systems, including those related to training, communications, access, facilities, and public information and access. A modern analog now appears at 42 U.S.C.S. § 300d *et seq.* (2001)

(continued)

TABLE 19–2—Continued

YEAR	MILESTONE
1974	**Congress passes the Child Abuse and Prevention and Treatment Act** (Public Law 93–247). Enacted January 31, 1974, this law provided for the establishment of the National Center on Child Abuse and Neglect to analyze and perform research on child abuse and neglect; serve as a clearinghouse for programs on the prevention, identification, and treatment of child abuse and neglect; and provide national training and technical assistance. It authorized the Secretary of Health, Education, and Welfare to award grants and enter into contracts to facilitate the performance of those functions
1978	**Tennessee becomes first state to enact a child passenger safety law.** The law that was initially passed in Tennessee contained a provision based on an amendment to the bill at the time the legislature was debating it. This amendment, later known as the "child crusher" amendment, permitted an adult to hold a small child on the adult's lap. Because of the danger presented by this provision, the Tennessee law was later amended to delete this exception to the rule that children must be restrained in devices designed to protect them
1984	**First lawsuit heard against car manufacturer for failure to provide an air bag.** *Burgess v. Ford Motor Co.* was tried in Alabama. It involved a young woman who, as a front-seat occupant of a Ford vehicle, was seriously injured in a frontal collision. The lawsuit alleged that Ford was negligent in its failure to provide an air bag in the car. Ten days into the trial of this lawsuit, Ford settled the case for $1.8 million
1985	**All states have child passenger safety laws.** In a short time from Tennessee's adoption of the first such law, all states and the District of Columbia adopted laws, with varying provisions, to require that all young children be restrained in devices designed to protect them in car crashes. Gaps in coverage of these laws, however, resulted in a call for more uniform and inclusive laws (see Teret SP, Jones AS, Williams AF, Wells JK. Child restraint laws: an analysis of gaps in coverage. *Am J Public Health* 1986;76: 31–4)
1987	**California enacts first legislation requiring helmets for child bicycle passengers aged ≤4 years.** California Vehicle Code § 21212 (2001) requires that all persons aged <18 years wear "a properly fitted and fastened bicycle helmet that meets [ANSI standards or others]. This requirement also applies to a person who rides upon a bicycle while in a restraining seat that is attached to the bicycle or in a trailer towed by the bicycle." Violations are punishable by $25 fines, for which parents or legal guardians are jointly and severally liable with their children

(continued)

TABLE 19–2. Milestones in Injury Prevention Law—Continued

YEAR	MILESTONE
1988	**Congress enacts the Child Abuse Prevention, Adoption and Family Services Act (Public Law 100–294)**. Enacted on April 25, 1998, this Act amended the Child Abuse Prevention and Treatment Act (Title I), the Child Abuse Prevention and Treatment and Adoption Reform Act of 1978 (Title II), and the Family Violence Prevention and Services Act (Title III). The three Acts were extended to provide continuing grants, data gathering, and technical assistance in these areas by the federal government. Related legislation can be found generally in Title 42 of the U.S.C.
1990	**Howard County, Maryland, adopts law requiring children aged ≤16 years to wear bicycle helmets**. After a classmate was killed when his bicycle was struck by a car, middle-school students in Howard County, Maryland, researched the epidemiology of bicycle-related injuries and then lobbied the county government to pass the first law in the nation requiring teenagers to wear bicycle helmets.
1993	**Congress passes the Handgun Violence Prevention Act (Brady Law)** (Public Law 103–159). After years of lobbying following the attempted assassination of President Ronald Reagan and the serious head injury to Press Secretary James Brady, Congress passed a law amending the Gun Control Act (18 U.S.C. 921 *et seq.*) calling for background checks of people buying guns from gun dealers
1997	**E coding mandated in 23 states.** "E coding"—the cause-of-injury coding for external injuries, specifying both the mechanism of injury and the intent—of death certificates is crucial to generating data for injury-prevention programs. By 1997, these states had adopted mandatory E coding: Arizona (1989), Rhode Island (1989), Washington (1989), California (1990), New York (1990), Vermont (1990), Delaware (1992), Connecticut (1993), Maryland (1993), Missouri (1993), Pennsylvania (1993), Virginia (1993), Massachusetts (1994), Nebraska (1994), New Jersey (1994), South Carolina (1994), Wisconsin (1994), Kentucky (1995), New Hampshire (1995), Tennessee (1995), Utah (1995), Florida (1997), and Georgia (1997)
1997	**Using consumer protection authority, Massachusetts becomes the first state to mandate child-resistant safety mechanisms on handguns.** Massachusetts Attorney General Scott Harshbarger required, by regulation, that handguns sold in Massachusetts have certain safety devices (Mass. Regs. Code Title 940, Section 16.00) These regulations were tested in court and upheld (*American Shooting Sports Council v. Attorney General*, 711 N.E. 2d 899 [Mass. 1999]), and some of the regulations were adopted as statutory law by the Massachusetts legislature

Source: Modified from Christoffel and Gallagher.[8]

by state legislatures, and the breadth of such laws is enormous. We previously have made reference to the many types of state laws that are designed to reduce the risk of injury,[11] including, for example:

- Driving rules governing the conduct of the driver, such as acquisition of a license, driving curfews for younger drivers, use of seatbelts and child restraints, adherence to speed limits, criminalization of driving while intoxicated, and mandates for motorcycle helmet use
- Laws governing the condition of motor vehicles, such as requirements for mandatory inspections
- Penal laws prohibiting assaultive and abusive behaviors
- Laws regulating the acquisition, carrying, and use of guns
- Regulation of the sale, possession, and use of other dangerous products such as poisons, explosives, drugs, and alcohol
- Building codes that regulate the design and function of structures
- Fire-safety laws governing the use of flammable products

This list underscores that the many laws and regulations bearing on injury prevention operate outside the purview of public health agencies.

Often, a state will delegate some of its police power to the localities within the state, thereby allowing the localities to address specific injury risks germane to them, such as requiring protective measures for windows to prevent children from falling from a city's high-rise buildings or fencing to guard swimming pools. However, for political considerations and other reasons, states may specifically preempt localities from enacting safety laws. For example, most states proscribe local legislative initiatives to control access to firearms.[12] States also create administrative agencies that can promulgate safety regulations, such as in the area of occupational safety. The safety of devices, such as elevators or sprinkler systems in buildings, can be regulated through administrative agencies at the state or local level.

Although the federal government does not possess the police powers of the states, it does regulate safety, principally through its governance of interstate commerce and its ability to control taxing and spending. Most consumer products have some connection with interstate commerce, and Congress has created agencies to control the safety of these products. For example, the Consumer Product Safety Commission (CPSC) has the authority to regulate the design of many household items. Strong debate exists within the safety community and among the product manufacturers as to whether the federal safety agencies adequately protect the public, but at least in theory the law provides a mechanism by which the risk of serious injury can and should be reduced. Similarly, the National Highway Traffic Safety Administration has extensive authority to promulgate safety standards for motor vehicles.

As with many areas of law, injury-prevention laws—although varied and numerous—are not enacted in any systematic manner. Many injury-prevention statutes date back decades; others are relatively new government initiatives. Unfortunately, these laws have generally been enacted in such an unplanned, uncoordinated fashion that, overall, they constitute an unsystematic statutory hodgepodge. Rarely, if ever, are they codified into a coherent whole.

LEGAL ISSUES AND CONTROVERSIES

Injury prevention has long relied on laws, and the nation's courts generally have upheld such laws. As with public health laws regarding infectious disease, public health and safety authorities have an extensive and well-established legal armamentarium.

Law can be an effective tool for reducing the toll of injury. However, injury prevention also involves powerful economic and political interests. By requiring safer environments and products, injury-prevention laws can affect the profits of individual companies and of entire industries (e.g., by requiring air bags in automobiles). Thus, the substantial power of business interests over government policy in the United States sometimes accounts for difficulty in enacting and enforcing injury prevention laws. Industry possesses immense political power and controls critical information needed to tailor public policy.

Efforts to pass legislation or regulation to reduce risks for injury often meet opposition from individuals or from industry in the form of one or more of the following three objections. First, such a law or regulation would be unconstitutional. Second, the law or regulation would not effectively reduce the rate or severity of injuries. Third, although the law or regulation might be constitutional and might even be effective, it should not be enacted for social, political, or economic reasons.

Of these objections, the issue of constitutionality probably can be addressed most straightforwardly because a substantial body of precedent has been developed over the years that has ruled on the constitutionality of injury-prevention laws. Many injury-prevention laws that have been challenged as depriving affected individuals of their constitutional rights have been upheld by courts as reasonable exercises of the government's police powers to protect the public.[11] Thus, laws that control the conduct of an individual for the protection of another person, such as speeding laws or laws proscribing assaultive behavior, are readily recognized as valid. Laws that govern a person's conduct for the principal benefit of that same person's safety have undergone a different type of scrutiny. Some of these laws have been upheld because the individual being protected is a member of a vulnerable class, such as children, for which the government has assumed a paternalistic role. Other laws have been upheld on the basis that, although the law protects the individual whose own behavior is being governed, it also protects the financial well-being of society.

For example, in *Simon v. Sargent,*[13] a federal District Court considered the argument of a motorcyclist that a mandatory helmet law was unconstitutional because it unduly interfered with a matter of concern that was personal to the motorcyclist and without consequences to the general public. The court disagreed with the motorcyclist, stating that, "From the moment of injury, society picks the person up off the highway; delivers him to a municipal hospital and municipal doctors; provides him with unemployment compensation if, after recovery, he cannot replace his lost job, and, if the injury causes permanent disability, may assume the responsibility for him and his family's continued subsistence. We do not understand a state of mind that permits (the motorcyclist) to think that only he himself is concerned." Similarly, courts have ruled that seatbelt laws do not violate any constitutionally protected rights of vehicle drivers and occupants.[14]

A more specific example of a constitutional objection is that pertaining to some laws that limit availability to guns. For this issue, some individuals and groups have argued that the Second Amendment to the U.S. Constitution makes illegal laws such as those that ban certain types of firearms (e.g., Saturday Night Special handguns or assault weapons). However, except for one case decided in October 2001 by the U.S. Court of Appeals for the Fifth Circuit Court,[15] federal and state courts have consistently upheld the constitutionality of such laws,[16] ruling that the Second Amendment confers a collective right related to state militias rather than an individual right allowing persons to own whatever guns they want.

Although other alleged constitutional rights have been argued in efforts to invalidate statutes designed to prevent injuries, the validity of the laws usually has been upheld. For example, in *Queenside Hills Realty Co., Inc. v. Saxl, Commissioner of Housing and Buildings of the City of New York,*[17] a law requiring sprinkler systems in multiple dwellings was challenged on the basis that due process was violated in requiring expensive modifications to a building that had been constructed in compliance with previous laws. The U.S. Supreme Court recognized that the "police power is one of the least limitable of government powers," and the Court declined to invalidate the statute.

Sometimes police practices, rather than statutes, have been objected to on the basis of alleged constitutional violations. For example, the use of highway sobriety checkpoints at which police stop vehicles has been alleged to be an illegal seizure, in violation of the Fourth Amendment to the U.S. Constitution. In *Michigan Department of State Police v. Sitz,*[18] the U.S. Supreme Court recognized that states have an interest in eradicating the drunken driving problem and that, although stopping a vehicle is a seizure of sorts, such practice is warranted by the need to address the compelling problem of alcohol-related injuries on the highways.

Because the police powers for the protection of the public were reserved to the states in the U.S. Constitution, the federal government does not base its injury-prevention legislation efforts on the police powers. Instead, acts of Congress that affect injury prevention usually are based on the interstate commerce powers of the federal government and on the federal power to tax and spend. For example, when the CPSC regulates a product, the authority to regulate is premised on that product being in interstate commerce. Sometimes this has been questioned in the courts, as in *United States of America v. One Hazardous Product Consisting of a Refuse Bin.*[19] In this case, the CPSC's standards for safer refuse bin design to protect against the known hazard of injuries to children from bins that tip over were challenged on the basis that the bins were not in interstate commerce—the bins in question remained at their locations and were emptied by the refuse-removal companies that owned the bins and had placed them at their customers' premises. However, the legality of the regulation was upheld.

In using its tax and spend powers, the federal government has influenced states to pass injury-prevention laws. For example, by either withholding or granting federal funds such as highway safety funds, contingent on the actions of a state, the federal government has been able to influence states' passage of speed-limit laws, drinking-age laws, and others.[20]

Another legal issue that arises when state legislatures consider bills, including those that address the incidence of injuries, is whether the legislature is preempted from acting. Generally, if the federal government has fully covered an issue by the federal legislation or regulation or if Congress has declared that states should not pass laws on a particular subject on which Congress has acted, then the states are barred from legislating in this area. Such is the case with many aspects of motor-vehicle design. For example, by passing the National Traffic and Motor Vehicle Safety Act of 1966 and by promulgating Federal Motor Vehicle Safety Standards, Congress and the National Highway Traffic Safety Administration preempted states from passing laws about vehicle design. Sometimes federal regulation will expressly be deemed to provide only minimum standards, however, and the way will be clear for states to enact stricter standards, as with many consumer products.

Somewhat similar to the preemption principle as applicable to the relationship between the federal and state governments is the relationship between state and local governments: States sometimes will preempt their localities from passing certain laws. For example, in the mid-1980s, the National Rifle Association (NRA) declared as one of its foremost legislative priorities the passage of state preemption laws regarding gun control. This was a political decision by the NRA that would allow it to contest its issues in 50 state legislatures (plus Congress) instead of innumerable city councils. Subsequently, more than half the states in the nation passed preemption laws for firearms, thus disallowing local governments (such as highly populated cities with elevated rates of gun violence) from legislatively addressing their gun violence problem in the manner they deemed best.[12]

The courts that decided the cases discussed in this section took an expansive view of the Constitutional role of government. This was typical at the time of these decisions. More recently, trends within the judiciary, including judicial concern regarding government regulation on behalf of the public's well being, have made legal prediction less certain.

In addition to questioning the validity of a proposed law, opponents of injury-prevention legislation and regulation also frequently question the law's potential effectiveness. However, evaluative literature on injury prevention laws has demonstrated the effectiveness of many of the laws.[11] Laws that address the design of built environments and products and laws that address public behaviors will be among the most effective. In contrast, laws that address private behaviors, such as the conduct of an individual within his or her own home, will be difficult to enforce and therefore are at risk of being less effective.[6]

The third type of objection to injury-prevention laws is that they are too costly, either from a purely economic standpoint or in terms of individual autonomy and/or sociopolitical values, even though they may be constitutional and demonstrably effective. However, these are political rather than legal or epidemiologic questions. They are legitimate issues for open public debate, but they sometimes may be put forward in the absence of objectively conducted evaluation. Instead, certain techniques (e.g., cost–benefit analysis or risk assessment) may be used to fashion government policy, even though they may disproportionately emphasize easily monitized costs (such as implementation costs to industry) relative to public benefits (such as the financial and emotional burdens violence imposes on the friends and families of victims).

PRACTICE CONSIDERATIONS

Improved Use of Law in Preventing Injuries

For the public health or injury-prevention practitioner, the enactment, implementation, and enforcement of laws seems a logical approach to lowering the incidence and severity of injuries of all types. For example, the risk for childhood drowning can be affected by pool fencing laws; the risk for dog bites can be affected by leash laws; the risk for gunshot wounds can be affected by laws governing the design of handguns; and the risk for tap water scalds can be affected by housing codes. How the practitioner can maximize the effectiveness of the law in preventing injuries is, in part, a function of the constraints placed on the practitioner by law and politics.

Some practitioners, particularly those employed by government bodies, will be restricted in lobbying for the enactment of laws. Also, practitioners whose salaries are paid by funds from foundations will experience some limitations in lobbying for legislation. However, not all lobbying is proscribed,[21] and not all legislative-oriented activities constitute lobbying. This is a technical area of the law, a full description of which is beyond the scope of this chapter, but literature exists to help practitioners determine the legal extent of their efforts. Much can be done to objectively educate legislators and regulators about the foreseeable effects of proposed laws on the basis of what has already been done in evaluating existing laws.

An area deserving further attention is the implementation of injury-prevention laws. Often, to achieve its desired effect, a law will require action on the part of officials. For example, seatbelt-use laws will be fully effective only if law enforcement officials are willing to enforce them. Child access prevention laws regarding gun storage in the home may be of limited effect if prosecutors understandably choose not to bring charges against the already bereaved parents of an injured child. In a domestic dispute, weapons may not be seized if a department has not instructed its officers about the proper methods of such seizures. Administrative programs, such as the Occupational Safety and Health Administration, will be rendered ineffective if inadequately funded and staffed. Injury-prevention practitioners can become involved in implementing laws and in studying how inadequate or inappropriate implementation can thwart the intent of a law.

Tort Litigation

Notwithstanding the existence of laws and regulations designed to reduce the risk for injury, many people have argued that the conduct and products of manufacturers still present too high a risk for avoidable injury. Therefore, injury prevention practitioners, including safety advocates, have turned to litigation as a tool for protecting the public. In 1968, a successful lawsuit brought against General Motors[22] for its failure to mitigate injuries to a motorist by designing a "crashworthy" car established the responsibility of manufacturers to foresee the human damage that could occur with the use of their products and to do what is reasonable to prevent that damage. Both before and since then, lawsuits have been brought against the makers of injurious products. These lawsuits have had particular significance when, because of political influence, the safety of the product has failed to come under legislative or regulatory control. For example, litigation against car makers for failure to provide air bags in their vehicles helped make this lifesaving device available,[23] and litigation against gun makers has helped to stimulate the redesign of handguns.[24]

Preemption also can affect tort litigation. For example, the U.S. Supreme Court has ruled that, because motor-vehicle occupant safety was governed by the federal motor-vehicle safety standards, a state court could not impose liability on a car manufacturer for failure to provide an air bag, in that such a ruling would be tantamount to a state's regulation of an area preempted by the federal government.[25]

EMERGING ISSUES

Perhaps more than ever before, the future of injury-prevention law depends on evolving political tensions in the United States and elsewhere. For example, some commentators have suggested that in the United States during the 1990s, under presidential administrations of both major U.S. political parties, the funding and political support eroded for meaningful intervention to reduce injuries associated with motor vehicles, other consumer products, and in the occupational setting.

One of the most threatening issues on the injury-prevention legal horizon is international, reflecting the fact that national governments may become secondary players in the public policy arena. The critical concern is the move to use "free-trade agreements" to negate federal, state, and local public health laws, including injury-prevention laws. For example, national governments have ceded substantial power to nonelected entities, such as the World Trade Organization. The treaty agreements establishing these entities are based on a laissez-faire economic approach that defines limits on trade—even limits of meritorious purpose—as impermissible restraints on trade.

Under this approach, efforts to use law to manage emerging public problems can be dampened. Thus, the impact of a statutory restriction, such as a limit on a known carcinogen, even though it may have overwhelming scientific and popular support, may be diminished or even nullified. A recent example involves truck-safety standards and the North American Free Trade Agreement (NAFTA). A NAFTA panel ruled that the United States must allow commercial trucks from Mexico to have full access to all U.S. highways, regardless of any and all federal and state highway safety standards. The United States is subject to financial trade sanctions if the panel is not obeyed. A U.S. Department of Transportation/General Accounting Office study found that more than one third of trucks from Mexico that were inspected as they attempted to enter a narrow commercial border zone in the United States suffered from serious safety violations. The United States was able to inspect less than 1% of such vehicles. Under the NAFTA rule, trucks from Mexico will be free to travel throughout the United States and will presumably do so in even greater numbers. The U.S. Congress moved to stop this application of the NAFTA agreement, but the administration was prepared to veto such legislation. In many instances, however, Congress has refrained from intervening when public health laws have been disallowed under NAFTA and other trade agreements.[26,27]

CONCLUSION

Law has played an important and well-accepted role in the area of injury prevention. The role of public health and safety professionals must be to identify injury problems for which the law can provide solutions, use appropriate and objective scientific methods to characterize such problems, and help garner public support sufficient to permit the passage of appropriate laws. The law can continue to be one of the most effective tools in reducing the incidence and severity of injuries in the United States.

References

1. Committee on Injury Prevention and Control, Institute of Medicine. In: Bonnie RJ, Fulco CE, Liverman CT, eds. *Reducing the Burden of Injury: Advancing Prevention and Treatment.* Washington, DC: National Academy Press, 1999.
2. Fingerhut LA, Warner M. *Injury Chartbook in Health, United States, 1996–97.* Hyattsville, MD: CDC, National Center for Health Statistics, 1997.
3. Robertson LS. *Injury Epidemiology.* New York: Oxford University Press, 1992.
4. Haddon W Jr. Energy damage and the ten countermeasure strategies. *J Trauma* 1973; 13:321–31.
5. Baker SP, Teret SP, Dietz PE. Firearms and the public health. *J Public Health Policy* 1980;1:224–9.
6. Institute of Medicine, Committee on Trauma Research. *Injury in America: A Continuing Public Health Problem.* Washington, DC: National Academy Press, 1985.
7. Johns CHW. *Babylonian and Assyrian Laws, Contracts and Letters, 1904* [facsimile edition]. New York: The Legal Classics Library (Gryphon Editions), 1987. Available at http://www.commonlaw.com/Hammurabi.html. Accessed November 16, 2001.
8. Christoffel T, Gallagher SS. *Injury Prevention and Public Health: Practical Knowledge, Skills, and Strategies.* Gaithersburg, MD: Aspen Publishers, Inc., 1999.
9. Teret SP, Gaare R. The law and the public's health. In: Gaare R, ed. *BioLaw.* Frederick, MD: University Publications of America, 1986.
10. Gostin LO. *Public Health Law: Power, Duty, Restraint.* Berkeley: University of California Press, 2000.
11. Christoffel T, Teret SP. *Protecting the Public: Legal Issues in Injury Prevention.* New York: Oxford University Press, 1993.
12. Teret SP, DeFrancesco S, Bailey LA. Gun deaths and home rule: a case for local regulation of a local public health problem. *Am J Prev Med* 1993;9(Suppl 1):44–6.
13. *Simon v. Sargent*, 346 F. Supp. 277, 279 (D Mass.) Aff'd., 409 U.S. 1020 (1972).
14. *State v. Hartog*, 440 N.W. 2d 852 (Iowa 1989), cert. denied, 493 U.S. 1005 (1989), rehearing denied, 493 U.S. 1095 (1990).
15. *United States of America v. Emerson*, 5th Cir., No. 99-10331, decided October 16, 2001.
16. Vernick JS, Teret SP. Firearms and health: the right to be armed with accurate information about the Second Amendment. *Am J Public Health* 1993;83:1773–7.
17. 328 U.S. 80 (1946)
18. 496 U.S. 444 (1990).
19. 487 F.Supp. 581 (1980)
20. *South Dakota v. Dole*, 483 U.S. 203 (1987)

21. Vernick JS. Lobbying and advocacy for the public's health: what are the limits for nonprofit organizations? *Am J Public Health* 1999;89:1425–9.
22. *Larsen v. General Motors Corporation*, 391 F.2d 495 (8th Cir., 1968).
23. Teret SP. Litigating for the public's health. *Am J Public Health* 1986;76:1027–9.
24. Vernick JS, Teret SP. A public health approach to regulating firearms as consumer products. *Univ Pennsylvania Law Rev* 2000;148:1193–211.
25. *Geier v. American Honda Motor Co.*, 529 U.S. 861 (2000).
26. Gamboa S. White House issues 2nd veto threat. *Associated Press*, July 19, 2001. Available at http://www.trucksafety.org/ap0701.html. Accessed November 16, 2001
27. Congress passes strict safety rules. *Public Citizen News*. September/October 2001.

20

Occupational Safety and Health Law

GARY RISCHITELLI

This chapter focuses primarily on the statutory and administrative legal systems that regulate occupational safety and health in the United States. Important judicial interpretations of the law governing occupational safety and health are also briefly reviewed. The practice of occupational health and the unique aspects of workers' compensation systems are not discussed except as they relate to the legal structure protecting worker health and safety.

HISTORY

The impact of occupational and environmental exposures on the health of individuals and communities has been recognized since antiquity. Hippocrates (4th century BC), a physician of ancient Greece now revered as the "father of medicine," recognized the impact of occupation and the environment on the health of individuals and communities. One of his treatises, "On Airs, Waters, and Places," described the relation between disease and location, climate, water, food, housing, and work.[1]

Occupational risks associated with specific jobs or industrial processes were also recognized and catalogued as medical knowledge was refined and recorded. Agricola (1494–1555) observed the breathlessness and early mortality among miners in Carpathia in his book *De Re Metallica*. He also recognized the social

416

and economic impacts of occupational illness and injury, describing women who had married seven times because of the premature demise of their husbands who worked in the mines.[2]

Occupational medicine began to evolve as both a medical specialty and an essential component of primary medical care. Bernardino Ramazzini (1633–1714), the father of modern occupational medicine, published *De Morbis Artificum Diatriba* in 1714, the first comprehensive textbook of disease and occupation. He introduced the concept of the occupational history as part of the medical evaluation of all individuals, exhorting his students and colleagues to ask patients, "What is your occupation?"

The growing concern and occasional public outrage over the working conditions during the Industrial Revolution stimulated governments to begin to establish laws regarding worker health and safety. In Britain, Sir Thomas Legge was appointed the first Medical Inspector of Factories in 1898, a position he used effectively to improve working conditions.[2] In response to the known hazards of the early industrial economy, these early attempts at protecting working men and women and regulating child labor focused primarily on accidental injuries, with far less emphasis on exposure-related diseases. This emphasis on accidental injury remains to some degree even in the occupational safety and workers' compensation laws of today.

Similarly, on the west side of the Atlantic Ocean, Dr. Alice Hamilton, the first female faculty member at Harvard Medical School, was a champion for American workers' health and safety. Her autobiographical text, *Exploring the Dangerous Trades*, was first published in 1925 and remains a classic in occupational health literature.[3] Hamilton drew public and scientific attention to the burden of illness and injury among American workers in the early twentieth century.

Initial attempts at regulating workplace safety in the United States were at the state level. Massachusetts passed the first law governing worker safety in 1877. By 1900, most other heavily industrialized states had passed some type of worker safety law covering at least some specific workplace hazards. These early attempts at regulation typically lacked sufficient resources for effective enforcement, and the increasing mechanization and pace of work only increased the danger of the industrial workplace.[4]

Early federal involvement in worker safety focused on workers in highly dangerous occupations or on those with a clear connection to interstate commerce, such as merchant seamen, railroad workers, and miners. A federal Office of Industrial Hygiene and Sanitation was established in the U.S. Public Health Service that, along with the U.S. Bureau of Labor Standards created as part of the New Deal government in 1934, studied several recognized occupational hazards.

Passage of the Walsh-Healy Public Contracts Act in 1936 marked the beginning of a more active involvement of the federal government in regulating work-place safety. The Act required the Department of Labor to ensure that federal contractors met minimum health and safety standards.

Like many legislative interventions, federal preemption of occupational health and safety regulation followed public outrage after a tragic disaster. Although 14,000 workers were killed and over 2 million were injured annually during the late 1960s, a widely publicized fatal mine explosion in West Virginia ultimately spurred the passage of the Federal Coal Mine Health and Safety Act of 1969.[5] This was the forerunner of a more general occupational health and safety act 1 year later.

Although President Lyndon Johnson had proposed a comprehensive occupational health and safety program to Congress in 1968, the bill never reached the House or Senate floor. President Nixon continued the effort, and, after considerable conflict and compromise, the Occupational Safety and Health Act of 1970 (OSHA) was passed by the 91st Congress and signed into law on December 29, 1970.

Now, at the start of the twenty-first century, the world is experiencing an explosion of rapidly evolving technologies. Workers face a vast array of chemical, physical, and biologic exposures, the health implications of which are poorly understood. In addition, many of the occupational diseases of antiquity, such as silicosis and lead poisoning, continue to persist. Protecting the health of workers and their communities remains a public health priority.

DIMENSIONS OF THE PROBLEM

Although accurate estimates of the burden of occupational injury and disease are difficult to obtain, nearly 430,000 new nonfatal occupational illnesses were recorded in 1997.[6] Estimates of work-related fatal illnesses are much more difficult to obtain because diseases are often multifactorial and may have long latencies. An estimated 50% of occupational illnesses are undiagnosed because workers and their physicians fail to recognize the occupational association. Most physicians in the United States receive limited or no training in occupational health and usually fail to ask about occupational and environmental exposures during the medical history. Even physicians trained in occupational medicine often have difficulty assessing the possible contribution of occupation and environment to disease. Difficulty abounds because over 70,000 chemicals are in use, of which only about 10,000 to 12,000 have undergone even basic toxicity assessments.

The National Institute for Occupational Safety and Health (NIOSH) has identified the top 10 contemporary occupational illnesses[7] and has established a National Occupational Research Agenda (NORA)[8] to establish priorities for research and prevention. NIOSH has estimated that 1.2 million American workers are exposed to silica, resulting in 250 deaths each year from silicosis, and that 1200 workers die each year from asbestosis.[9] Unfortunately, today's workers appear to face the risk of the occupational diseases of both the future and the past.

Occupational injuries represent a much larger and more visible burden on the nation's health and productivity. Approximately, 5.7 million work-related injuries leading to 3.6 million hospital emergency visits occurred in 1997. These injuries include strains and sprains (799,000), back injuries (472,000), bruises and contusions (166,000), lacerations (134,000), fractures (119,000), burns (30,000), amputations (10,850), and deaths (5915 in 2000).[6,10] Approximately 2 million persons are disabled as a result of these injuries, leading to 200 million lost workdays and approximately $25 billion in costs per year. In the United States, 17 workers are killed in fatal occupational accidents every day. The frequency and cost of these injuries are a significant drain on the national economy in addition to the tragic burden on workers and their families.

VARIETY OF RESPONSIBILITIES AT LOCAL, STATE, AND FEDERAL LEVELS

Occupational health has become an increasingly specialized area and has lost many of its traditional connections with public health agencies and practitioners. Many of the early occupational health practitioners were sanitarians, some of whom became the founders of modern industrial hygiene. Today, many industrial hygienists, occupational health nurses, and occupational physicians continue to be trained in schools of public health but usually pursue a specialized curriculum, which focuses on the recognition, evaluation, control, and treatment of health hazards in industry and the environment. Occupational health and safety practitioners may also come from other disciplines such as engineering, environmental science, chemistry, physics, and psychology.

Prevention activities such as education, consultation, and regulatory enforcement have been largely delegated to separate occupational safety and health agencies at federal, state, and local levels distinct from the traditional public health authorities. This has further widened the professional gulf between occupational safety and health personnel and their public health colleagues.

LEGAL AUTHORITIES

Federal authority over safety and health issues in the workplace largely arises from the Commerce Clause of the U.S. Constitution, which grants Congress the power "to regulate commerce . . . among the States."[11] The Commerce Clause has been construed broadly to allow Congress to pass laws that regulate a wide range of activities that directly or indirectly affect interstate commerce, including the health and safety of workers.

Congress delegated much of this regulatory authority for the work environment to federal administrative agencies, primarily the Occupational Safety and Health Administration (OSHA), through the Occupational Safety and Health Act (OSHAct) of 1970.[12] The Act established OSHA and NIOSH, the two major federal agencies concerned with worker health and safety. OSHA has authority under the Act to promulgate regulations (standards) and conduct inspections to carry out the Act's main purpose, which is "to assure so far as possible every working man and woman in the Nation safe and healthful working conditions . . ." NIOSH houses the scientific, engineering, and health research activities contemplated by the OSHAct. Instead of the U.S. Department of Labor, NIOSH is located in the Department of Health and Human Services (DHHS) to reflect its mission of improving workplace health and safety through research, prevention, education, and training. It is now part of the Centers for Disease Control and Prevention (CDC).

Under the "supremacy clause" of the Constitution, Congress can pass laws that preempt, or even prohibit, state laws that address the subject matter of federal legislation.[13] The OSHAct has such a clause that effectively preempts state regulation of workplace safety, except where federal OSHA has delegated authority to a state-run OSHA program. State-run programs are required to provide standards that are at least as protective as federal standards. States, however, are also prevented from establishing standards that are significantly more burdensome lest they run afoul of the interstate commerce clause, another area of exclusive federal preemption.

Federal OSHA has jurisdiction over workplace safety and health issues in all states that do not operate their own OSHA-approved programs. In fact, any occupational safety and health issues regulated by a state that does not have an OSHA-approved program are preempted by OSHA jurisdiction if OSHA has a standard addressing the hazard or issue.

The OSHAct

In general, the OSHAct covers all private employers and their employees in the 50 states, the District of Columbia, Puerto Rico, and all other territories under federal government jurisdiction. Coverage is provided either directly by the federal OSHA or through an OSHA-approved state-based job safety and health program. States with OSHA-approved job safety and health programs must set standards that are at least as effective as the equivalent federal standard and most state-plan states simply adopt standards identical to the federal standards.

As defined by the Act, an employer is any "person engaged in a business affecting commerce who has employees, but does not include the United States or any state or political subdivision of a State." Therefore, the Act applies to all employers and employees in manufacturing, construction, transportation, agriculture, health care, retail, and private education. The OSHAct includes secular employees of religious groups and nonprofit organizations.

Section 3(5) of the Act specifically excluded employees of state and local governments (unless they are in one of the states with OSHA-approved state safety and health programs). Section 4(b)(1) of the Act excluded working conditions regulated by other federal agencies under other federal statutes. The Department of Labor, as a matter of policy, has also excluded self-employed persons, farms that employ only immediate members of the farmer's family, and domestic households where an individual has been hired to perform household tasks such cooking, cleaning, or child care.[14]

The Act assigns to OSHA two principal functions: setting safety and health standards and conducting workplace inspections to enforce compliance with the standards. OSHA standards may address working conditions, equipment, processes, or outcomes. Safety standards include regulations designed to prevent falls, electrocutions, fires, explosions, cave-ins, and machine and vehicle accidents and injuries. Health standards regulate exposures to a variety of chemical, physical, and biologic health hazards through engineering controls, use of personal protective equipment (e.g., respirators, ear protection), and work practices. The standards may require employers to meet environmental or engineering specifications, use specific technologies or practices, or simply set targets that employers must meet using whatever means are practical or feasible. Employers bear the responsibility to become aware of and understand the standards applicable to their industry, to reduce or eliminate work hazards to the extent possible, and to comply with the standards.

Where OSHA does not have a specific standard for a hazardous exposure or condition, employers are still responsible for complying with the "general duty" clause of the OSHAct. The general duty clause—Section 5(a)(1)—states that each employer "shall furnish . . . a place of employment which is free from recognized hazards that are causing or are likely to cause death or serious physical harm to his employees." Employers, therefore, have an affirmative duty to identify and remove hazards that pose a probable danger to employee health and safety even if no specific OSHA standard addresses that risk. Employees also have a duty under the Act to "comply with occupational safety and health standards and all rules, regulations, and orders issued pursuant to this act."

OSHA was authorized under Sec. 8(a) of the OSHAct to conduct workplace inspections to identify hazards and enforce safety and health standards. Every establishment covered by the Act is subject to inspection. Similarly, states with their own occupational safety and health programs are authorized to conduct inspections using state compliance officers.

Employees are granted several important rights by the Act. Among them are the right to (1) file a confidential complaint with OSHA about the safety and health conditions in their workplace, (2) contest the time period granted by

OSHA for correcting violations, and (3) accompany OSHA workplace inspections. Employees who exercise their rights are protected against employer retaliation. Employees must notify OSHA of the alleged reprisal; if OSHA finds that discrimination has occurred, the employer will be asked to restore the employee, including lost wages or benefits. If necessary, OSHA can take legal action on behalf of the employee.

OSHA agencies are typically divided into consultation and enforcement units. Consultation personnel are invited by the employer to assist with identification and control of hazards. The consultations are confidential and free of charge. If consultation personnel identify hazards, the employer is provided an opportunity to correct them in a reasonable time. If the employer fails to correct the problem, placing workers at risk, then the consultant must notify the enforcement division. After an inspection or referral, employers who do not comply with OSHA standards may receive citations and penalties (Table 20–1).

After a complaint, employees may request an informal review of any decision not to issue a citation but cannot contest citations, amendments to citations, penalties, or lack of penalties. They may contest the time granted by OSHA to abate a hazardous condition. Employees may request a review of OSHA action by submitting a written objection to OSHA. The OSHA area director then forwards these objections to the Occupational Safety and Health Review Commission, which operates independently of OSHA.

Similarly, an employer may request an informal meeting with OSHA's area director to discuss the case. Employee representatives may be invited to attend the meeting. The area director is authorized to enter into settlement agreements that revise citations and penalties to avoid prolonged legal disputes. Employers may also request review from the Occupational Safety and Health Review Commission.

Federal OSHA standards fall into four major categories: general industry (29 C.F.R. 1910), construction (29 C.F.R. 1926), maritime–shipyards, marine terminals, longshoring (29 C.F.R. 1915–9), and agriculture (29 C.F.R. 1928). Each of these four categories imposes requirements targeted to that industry, although, in some cases, they are identical for each category of employer. Among the standards that impose similar requirements on all industry sectors are those for access to medical and exposure records, personal protective equipment, and hazard communication.

Access to medical and exposure records

The Access to Medical and Exposure Records Standard[15] requires that employers preserve and grant employee access to any exposure monitoring or medical records maintained by the company that relate to a worker's own exposure to hazardous substances or processes. These records must be maintained for 30 years after the worker's period of employment. Employees must also be no-

TABLE 20–1. Occupational Safety and Health Act (OSHAct) Violations and Penalties

VIOLATION	EXPLANATION AND PENALTIES
Other-than-serious violation	A violation that has a direct relation to job safety and health but probably would not cause death or serious physical harm. A proposed penalty of up to $7000 for each violation is discretionary. A penalty for an other-than-serious violation may be adjusted downward by as much as 95%, depending on the employer's good faith (demonstrated efforts to comply with the OSHAct), history of previous violations, and size of business. When the adjusted penalty amounts to less than $50, no penalty is proposed
Serious violation	A violation in which substantial probability exists that death or serious physical harm could result and in which the employer knew, or should have known, of the hazard. A mandatory penalty of up to $7000 for each violation is proposed. A penalty for a serious violation may be adjusted downward, based on the employer's good faith, history of previous violations, gravity of the alleged violation, and size of business
Willful violation	A violation that the employer intentionally and knowingly commits. The employer either knows that what he or she is doing constitutes a violation or is aware that a hazardous condition exists and has made no reasonable effort to eliminate it. The OSHAct provides that an employer who willfully violates the Act may be assessed a civil penalty of not more than $70,000 but not less than $5000 for each violation. A proposed penalty for a willful violation may be adjusted downward, depending on the size of the business and its history of previous violations. Usually no credit is given for good faith. If an employer is convicted of a willful violation of a standard that has resulted in the death of an employee, the offense is punishable by a court-imposed fine or by imprisonment for up to 6 months or both. A fine of up to $250,000 for an individual, or $500,000 for a corporation (authorized under the Comprehensive Crime Control Act of 1984 [1984 CCA], not the OSHAct), may be imposed for a criminal conviction
Repeated violation	A violation of any standard, regulation, rule, or order where, on reinspection, a substantially similar violation is found. Repeated violations can bring a fine of up to $70,000 for each such violation. For a repeat citation, the original citation must be final; a citation under contest may not serve as the basis for a subsequent repeat citation
Failure to correct prior violation	Failure to correct a prior violation may bring a civil penalty of up to $7000 for each day the violation continues beyond the prescribed abatement date

Additional violations for which citations and proposed penalties may be issued are as follows: *(1)* falsifying records, reports, or applications; on conviction can bring a fine of $10,000 or up to 6 months in jail or both; *(2)* violations of posting requirements can bring a civil penalty of up to $7000; and *(3)* assaulting a compliance officer or otherwise resisting, opposing, intimidating, or interfering with a compliance officer in the performance of his or her duties is a criminal offense, subject to a fine of not more than $250,000 for an individual and $500,000 for a corporation (1984 CCA) and imprisonment for not more than 3 years. Citation and penalty procedures may differ somewhat in states with their own occupational safety and health programs.

tified of the existence of these records and their right to access and review
them.

Personal protective equipment

The Personal Protective Equipment Standard,[16] included separately in the standards for each industry segment (except agriculture), requires that employers
provide workers with appropriate personal protective equipment. This may include protective helmets or hard hats, respirators, eye protection, hearing protection, hard-toed shoes, or other specialized equipment (e.g., welding goggles
or face shields). The employer is expected to provide this equipment without
charge to the employee, except for prescription safety glasses and hard-toed
safety shoes.

Hazard communication

The Hazard Communication Standard[17] is designed to provide employees with
a "right to know" the chemical hazards that they encounter in their workplace.
This standard requires that manufacturers and importers of hazardous materials
conduct a hazard evaluation of the products they manufacture or import. If the
product is found to be hazardous under the terms of the standard, containers of
the material must be appropriately labeled, and the first shipment of the material
to a new customer must be accompanied by a Material Safety Data Sheet
(MSDS).

   If employees work with compounds that are divided from the original con-
tainer into smaller containers, these containers also must have appropriate labels
and warnings. Employees must be given access to MSDS on request, and the
sheets must be easily accessible. Employers must train their employees to recognize and avoid the hazards that the materials present.

   The Hazard Communication Standard also gives health-care providers an important right of access to information about the identity and quantity of ingredients that are listed as "trade secrets" on the MSDS. When a medical emergency
exists or immediate first aid is required, manufacturers must immediately disclose the "trade secret" information and can subsequently request a confidentiality agreement and statement of need. In nonemergent situations, the manufacturer can require a written request including a statement of need and the
execution of a confidentiality agreement including assurances that means exist
to protect against further disclosure.

Record keeping

Section 8(c)(1) of the OSHAct states that "Each employer shall make, keep,
and preserve . . . such records regarding his activities relating to this Act . . .
necessary or appropriate for the enforcement of this Act or for developing in-

formation regarding the causes and prevention of occupational accidents and illnesses." [18]

Employers with more than 10 employees must maintain OSHA-specified records of job-related injuries and illnesses, except for certain low-hazard industries such as retail, finance, insurance, real estate, and some service industries.

OSHA Form 200 is an injury/illness log, with a separate line entry for each recordable injury or illness (excluding minor injuries that require only first aid treatment and that do not involve medical treatment, loss of consciousness, restriction of work or motion, or transfer to another job). A summary section of OSHA Form 200, which includes the total of the previous year's injury and illness experience, must be posted in the workplace for the entire month of February each year. OSHA Form 101 is an individual incident report that provides added detail about each individual recordable injury or illness.

Employers with 10 or fewer employees or employers in traditionally low-hazard industries are exempt from maintaining these records unless they are selected to be part of a national survey of workplace injuries and illnesses conducted by the Department of Labor's Bureau of Labor Statistics (BLS) each year. Selected employers are notified to begin keeping records during the survey year, and technical assistance on completing these forms is available.

All employers, regardless of the number of employees or industry category, must report to the nearest OSHA office within 8 hours any accident that results in one or more fatalities or hospitalization of three or more employees. OSHA investigates these "catastrophic" accidents to determine whether violations of standards contributed to the event.

The Federal Mine Safety and Health Act

The Federal Mine Safety and Health Act (MSH Act) of 1977[19] covers all miners and others working on mine property; it is administered by the Labor Department's Mine Safety and Health Administration (MSHA). This law revised and expanded the earlier Federal Coal Mine Health and Safety Act of 1969 and brought metal and nonmetal (noncoal) miners under the same general standards as coal miners.

Each mine in the United States must be registered with the MSHA. Many mine operators are also required to submit plans to the MSHA for approval before beginning operations. Required plans cover most operational aspects such as ventilation, roof control, and miner training. The MSHA must inspect every underground mine at least four times a year and every surface mine at least twice a year. Mine operators are required to report each individual mine accident or injury to the MSHA. In addition, the Act provides authority for closure of mines in cases of imminent danger to workers or failure to correct violations within the time allowed.

Mine safety and health regulations cover numerous hazards, including respiratory exposure to dust and its toxic contaminants; noise; machinery and mobile equipment; roof falls; flammable and toxic gases; electrical equipment; fires; explosives; and access and egress. The MSHA also conducts training and assists the mining industry in reducing deaths, serious injuries, and illnesses.

Other Relevant Authorities

Congress enacted the Toxic Substances Control Act (TSCA) of 1976[20] to test, regulate, and screen all chemicals produced or imported into the United States. The TSCA requires that any chemical that reaches the consumer marketplace be tested for possible toxic effects before commercial manufacture. TSCA also includes extensive record keeping and reporting requirements for toxic chemicals. Section 8(c) requires chemical manufacturers, processors, and distributors to maintain records of "significant adverse reactions" for 30 years. Section 8(e) requires manufacturers, processors, and distributors to report to the U.S. Environmental Protection Agency (EPA) any "information which reasonably supports the conclusion that such substance or mixture presents a substantial risk of injury to health or the environment." Medical providers or public health authorities may find that data collected under these sections provide another source of information regarding the potential health adverse effects of new or poorly characterized substances.

After the public outcry over pollution disasters in Love Canal, New York, and Times Beach, Missouri, Congress passed the Comprehensive Environmental Response, Compensation and Liability Act of 1980 (CERCLA),[21] which provided liability for past polluters, as well as current owners of polluted sites. CERCLA created a federal "Superfund" to clean up uncontrolled or abandoned hazardous-waste sites as well as accidents, spills, and other emergency releases of pollutants and contaminants into the environment. Through the Act, the EPA was given the power to seek out parties responsible for any release and ensure their cooperation in the clean up. CERCLA also created the Agency for Toxic Substances and Disease Registry (ATSDR) and provided a framework for health and safety regulation of workers at hazardous waste sites.

In the wake of the disaster in Bhopal, India, The Superfund Amendments and Reauthorization Act of 1986 reauthorized CERCLA to continue clean-up activities around the country. Title III of SARA included the Emergency Planning and Community Right-to-Know Act (EPCRTKA).[22] This law was designated to help local communities protect public health, safety, and the environment from chemical hazards. In addition to its provisions addressing emergency preparedness and community right-to-know issues, both EPCRTKA and CERCLA contain provisions that grant medical providers access to information regarding the identity and quantity of chemical ingredients considered "trade secrets" similar to the OSHA Hazard Communication standard.

Preparation and use of pesticides are regulated under The Federal Insecticide Rodenticide and Fungicide Act.[23] This Act gives the EPA jurisdiction to protect the health and safety of agricultural workers and commercial pesticide applicators who are exposed to these substances.[24]

Employment Discrimination and Benefits Law

Title VII of the Civil Rights Act and the Pregnancy Discrimination Act

Title VII of the Civil Rights Act prohibits discrimination based on sex, race, religion, or national origin. Discrimination based on pregnancy, childbirth, or related medical conditions constitutes unlawful sex discrimination under Title VII.[25] Women affected by pregnancy or a related condition must be treated in the same manner as other applicants or employees with similar abilities or limitations.

An employer cannot refuse to hire a woman because she is pregnant if she is able to perform the major functions of her job. Nor may an employer single out pregnancy-related conditions for special procedures to determine an employee's ability to work.

If an employee is temporarily unable to perform her job because of pregnancy, the employer must provide the same benefits afforded to any other temporarily disabled employee, such as modified work, temporary reassignment, or disability leave. Pregnant employees must be permitted to work as long as they are able to perform their jobs, and employers may not have a rule that prohibits an employee from returning to work for a predetermined length of time after childbirth.

Employers must hold open jobs for employees with pregnancy-related conditions the same length of time they hold open jobs for employees on sick or disability leave.

Health insurance provided to employees must cover pregnancy-related expenses in the same manner that they cover costs for other medical conditions. Coverage amounts can be limited only to the same extent as costs for other conditions, and employees with pregnancy-related disabilities must be treated the same as other temporarily disabled employees regarding seniority and benefits.

The Age Discrimination in Employment Act of 1967

The Age Discrimination in Employment Act of 1967 (ADEA)[26] protects persons aged 40 years or older from employment discrimination based on age. The

ADEA's protections apply to both current employees and applicants. The ADEA forbids discrimination against a person because of his or her age with respect to any term, condition, or privilege of employment. The ADEA also precludes age preferences, limitations, or specifications in job notices or advertisements.

The Rehabilitation Act and the Americans with Disabilities Act

The Rehabilitation Act of 1973 [27] prohibits disability-based discrimination in federal employment and by federal contractors. The Act served as the forerunner and model for the Americans with Disabilities Act of 1990 (ADA),[28] which greatly expanded and refined the protections for persons with disabilities. The ADA prohibits private employers, state and local governments, employment agencies, and labor unions from discriminating against qualified persons with disabilities in job application procedures, hiring, firing, advancement, compensation, job training, and other terms, conditions, and privileges of employment. According to the Act, an individual with a disability is a person who (1) has a physical or mental impairment that substantially limits one or more major life activities; (2) has a record of such an impairment; or (3) is regarded as having such an impairment.

A qualified employee or applicant with a disability is an individual who can perform the essential functions of the job with or without reasonable accommodation. Reasonable accommodation may include making existing facilities used by employees readily accessible to and usable by persons with disabilities; restructuring the job, modifying work schedules, or reassigning to a vacant position; acquiring or modifying equipment or devices; adjusting or modifying examinations, training materials, or policies; and providing qualified readers or interpreters.

An employer is required to accommodate the known disability of a qualified applicant or employee if it would not impose an "undue hardship" on the operation of the employer's business. Undue hardship is defined as an action requiring significant difficulty or expense when considered in light of factors such as an employer's size, financial resources, and the nature and structure of its operation. An employer is not required to lower quality or production standards to make an accommodation, nor is an employer obligated to provide personal-use items such as glasses or hearing aids.

Employers may not ask job applicants about the existence, nature, or severity of a disability. Applicants may, however, be asked about their ability to perform specific job functions. A job offer may be conditioned on the results of a medical examination only if the examination is required for all entering employees in similar jobs. Medical examinations of employees must be job related and consistent with the employer's business needs.

Employees and applicants currently engaging in the illegal use of drugs are not covered by the ADA when an employer acts on the basis of such use. Tests for illegal drugs are not subject to the ADA's restrictions on medical examinations. Employers may hold illegal drug users and those with alcoholism to the same performance standards as other employees.

Family and Medical Leave Act of 1993

The Department of Labor's Employment Standards Administration, Wage and Hour Division administers and enforces the Family and Medical Leave Act (FMLA)[29] for all private, state, and local government employees and some federal employees. Most federal and certain congressional employees are also covered by the law and are subject to the jurisdiction of the U.S. Office of Personnel Management or the Congress.

The FMLA entitles eligible employees to take up to 12 weeks of unpaid, job-protected leave in a 12 month period for specified family and medical reasons. To be "eligible" for FMLA leave, an employee must work at a worksite within 75 road miles of which that employer employs at least 50 employees; must have worked at least 12 months (which do not have to be consecutive) for the employer; and must have worked at least 1250 hours during the 12 months immediately preceding the date of commencement of FMLA leave. The FMLA provides an entitlement of leave for the following reasons: birth or adoption of the employee's child; to care for an immediate family member (spouse, child, parent) who has a serious health condition; or the employee's own serious health condition.

An employer must maintain group health benefits that an employee was receiving at the time leave begins during periods of FMLA leave, at the same level and in the same manner as if the employee had continued to work. Under most circumstances, an employee may elect or the employer may require use of any accrued paid leave (e.g., vacation, sick, personal) for periods of unpaid FMLA leave. The FMLA leave may be taken in blocks of time less than the full 12 weeks on an intermittent or reduced leave basis. Taking intermittent leave for the birth, placement for adoption, or foster care of a child must be approved by the employer.

When leave is foreseeable, an employee must provide the employer with at least 30 days' notice of the need for leave. If the leave is not foreseeable, then notice must be given as soon as practicable. An employer may require medical certification of a serious health condition from the employee and may require periodic reports during the period of leave of the employee's status and intent to return to work, as well as "fitness-for-duty" certification on return to work in appropriate situations.

When the employee returns from FMLA leave, he or she is entitled to be restored to the same job or to a job equivalent to the job the employee left when leave commenced. An equivalent job is one with equivalent pay, benefits, and responsibilities. The employee is not entitled to accrue benefits during periods of unpaid FMLA leave, but he or she must be returned to employment with the same benefits at the same levels that existed when leave began. Any unused benefits accrued at the time leave began are retained by the employee.

Labor Law

Labor organizations have made an essential and undeniable contribution to the health and safety conditions of American workplaces. Although labor law is a complex system of legal and administrative elements and remedies, the National Labor Relations Act of 1935 (Wagner Act) is the primary rule book of labor–management relations in the United States. Once a union is organized and certified under the Act, much of the relationship between workers and management in a particular company or industry is defined in a collective bargaining agreement. Most importantly, both labor and management have a legal duty to bargain collectively. Failure to do so constitutes an "unfair labor practice." Safety and health rules and practices within the organization are mandatory subjects of collective bargaining.[30] Additionally, many collective bargaining agreements provide for joint labor–management safety committees that review safety practices, investigate accidents, and suggest or implement safety policies.

Unions have been important and influential advocates for worker health and safety. They can be important or even indispensable partners in epidemiologic investigations, education and training activities, or other worksite-based health and wellness interventions.

Relevant State Statutes

In addition to federal statutes and rules, many states have specific provisions that address radiation safety; building safety; hazardous material handling; worker and community right-to-know issues; and other laws or rules addressing specific work exposures, conditions, or duties. Workers' compensation law is largely a state-based system; it plays a varying role, directly and indirectly, on the health and safety of workers within each jurisdiction. Provision of resources for injury and illness prevention, research, and integration with OSHA consultative and enforcement activities also varies among the states.

State public health statutes or administrative rules may include mandatory reporting requirements for some or all occupational diseases. State workers' compensation systems may include programs for occupational injury and illness surveillance as well as prevention activities.

Criminal prosecution for intentional or grossly negligent worker injury or death is also possible under state criminal statutes. Federal preemption arguments have been offered as defenses to criminal charges brought in state court, but at least two state supreme courts have held that the OSHAct does not pre-empt state criminal jurisdiction.[31]

Other Authorities

Other government agencies

Other federal and state departments or agencies may have jurisdiction or re-sponsibility for specific occupations or exposures. For example, the Department of Transportation (DOT) has specific occupational safety and health standards for commercial vehicles (Federal Highway Administration), railroads (Federal Railroad Administration [FRA]), aviation (Federal Aviation Administration [FAA]), public transit (Federal Transit Administration), and maritime (U.S. Coast Guard). The Department of Energy and the Nuclear Regulatory Commission largely regulate worker exposure to ionizing radiation, and the CDC plays a key role in recommending occupational safety and health practices for laboratory and health-care workers and other workers exposed to biologic agents.

Nongovernment organizations

Many national and international organizations develop and disseminate occupational health and safety standards. The American Conference of Government Industrial Hygienists (ACGIH) is particularly influential in the development of exposure limits for chemical and physical hazards. In fact, many of the original OSHA permissible exposure limit (PEL) standards adopted under Section 6(a) of the OSHAct were adopted from the ACGIH Threshold Limit Value standards that were current at the time. The American National Standards Institute has contributed a number of industry- or process-specific standards such as laser safety, respirator selection and use, and radiation protection. Safety testing and standards of the National Safety Council are important guides, as are the national fire and electrical codes of the National Fire Protection Association.

Although these private organization standards or guidelines do not have the force of law, they are often based on extensive research or careful professional consensus. They serve as models or evidence for government legislation or rule making or are voluntarily adopted by individual employers or industry groups. Courts also value the indirect authority of these documents, particularly if they have been widely accepted in an industry or professional community.

Professional organizations

Professional societies such as the American College of Occupational and Environmental Medicine, the American Association of Occupational Health Nurses, American Industrial Hygiene Association, American Society of Safety

Engineers, and the American Thoracic Society play an important role in promoting occupational health and safety, raising public awareness, and issuing position statements and guidelines.

LEGAL ISSUES AND CONTROVERSIES

OSHA Challenges

Soon after its passage, the OSHAct was the subject of lawsuits that challenged several of its basic provisions. The feasibility component of standard setting was considered in *Industrial Union Department, AFL-CIO v. Hodgson*, 499 F.2d 467 (D.C. Cir. 1974). The court found that Congress did not intend OSHA to create standards that would require the use of equipment that was not available with existing technology or would threaten the financial viability or continued existence of an industrial sector or process. The Court also stated, however, that some methods might be economically feasible even if they were financially burdensome, reduced profits, or placed some individual employers out of business.

Similarly, in *The Society of the Plastics Industry, Inc. v. Occupational Safety and Health Administration*, 509 F.2d 1301 (2d Cir. 1975), manufacturers and users of vinyl chloride monomer challenged an OSHA standard that lowered the PEL to 1 part per million, stating that it was infeasible. The Court, however, believed that the industry was capable of attaining this limit and stated, "In the area of safety, we wish to emphasize, the Secretary is not restricted by the status quo. He may raise standards which require improvements in existing technologies or which require the development of new technology, and he is not limited to issuing standards based only on devices already fully developed."

Later, the "technology forcing" provision was scaled back somewhat in *American Iron and Steel Institute v. OSHA*, 577 F.2d 825 (3rd Cir. 1978). Here, the court found that "the Secretary can impose a standard which requires an employer to implement technology "looming on today's horizon," but could not "place an affirmative duty on each employer to research and develop new technology."

In its first review of an OSHA standard, *Industrial Union Department v. American Petroleum Institute*, 448 U.S. 607 (1980), the U.S. Supreme Court considered a challenge to the OSHA Standard for benzene. The petroleum industry contended that the "reasonably necessary" and "feasible" provisions of the OSHAct required a "cost–benefit analysis" before issuing a new or revised OSHA standard. The Supreme Court did not address the "cost–benefit analysis" issue but instead articulated a "significant risk" requirement for standard setting. The Court concluded that because OSHA had determined that no safe level of exposure existed, it had set the PEL at the lowest technologically feasible level.

The Court was concerned, however, that OSHA had failed to demonstrate the practical effect of this lowered PEL and therefore never made a threshold determination that the standard was "reasonably necessary and appropriate to remedy a significant risk of material health impairment" as required by Section 3(8) of the Act.

The Court stated that, before issuing a standard, the Secretary had to determine that a place of employment was "unsafe" and had to determine what level of risk constituted a "significant risk" that required a standard for worker protection. The Court endorsed the use of quantitative risk assessment but left to the agency the determination of what was a significant risk and the methods and assumptions of the risk assessment.

A short time later, the U.S. Supreme Court addressed the issue of cost–benefit analysis directly in *American Textile Manufacturers Institute, Inc. v. Donovan*, 542 US 490 (1981). The Court specifically rejected any contention that the feasibility requirement of the OSHAct required an analysis of costs and benefits. The Court concluded that, after finding that a significant risk was present, the OSHAct required OSHA to place "worker health above all other considerations save those making attainment of this 'benefit' unachievable."

Right of Access to Information

Initially, requests by OSHA and NIOSH for access to employee medical records were challenged on constitutional grounds. The Department of Labor responded by promulgating a rule that provided access to employee exposure and medical records.[32] In a challenge before the Circuit Court of Appeals of the District of Columbia, the standard was upheld as constitutional on the grounds that it satisfied a legitimate government purpose and no immediate harm was shown.[33]

Right of Access to Workplaces

Inspections of private workplaces were sanctioned by the OSHAct, and OSHA inspectors were assumed to have authority to enter workplaces to conduct unannounced and involuntary inspections. In *Marshall v Barlow's*, 436 U.S. 307 (1978), however, the U.S. Supreme Court found that OSHA inspectors could not conduct warrantless inspections of the nonpublic areas of a business without the employer's permission. If an employer refused entry there was no "probable cause" requirement to obtain the warrant as long as OSHA could demonstrate that the request was part of an administrative program designed to meet agency goals or priorities for workplace safety. The Court noted that this was not a difficult threshold to cross but felt that the added requirement for a court-issued warrant provided an appropriate procedural safeguard for an employer's Fourth Amendment rights.

Roles and Responsibilities for Ensuring Health and Safety

The inability of OSHA to routinely inspect all workplaces (approximately 2000 compliance officers and 76.5 million workplaces) has required the agency to develop priorities for inspection and enforcement actions. Priorities are determined on the basis of (*1*) concerns about "imminent danger" to workers, (*2*) catastrophes or fatal accidents, (*3*) need for response to employee complaints, (*4*) targeted inspections of "high hazard" industries or employers with high injury and illness rates, and (*5*) follow-up inspections to determine whether previously identified hazards have been abated.

Public health agencies may develop different priorities or have different strategies to ensure workplace health and safety. For example, in Oregon, the state public health authority receives notification from laboratories of all blood lead levels over 25 µg/dL in adults. The state's health division then notifies and sends educational material regarding the health effects of lead to the worker and the employer. This blood lead level is significantly lower than the OSHA threshold of 40 µg/dL. Using the data collected from this system, the public health agency recently conducted an epidemiologic investigation and offered consultative assistance to an employer whose employees consistently had blood lead levels greater than 25 µg/dL.

Similarly, the public health agency has responsibility for investigating reported cancer clusters and for recording infectious disease cases. Many states have added occupational diseases to their list of reportable illnesses, and many participate in NIOSH-sponsored surveillance programs (e.g., the Sentinel Event Notification System for Occupational Risk).

Genetic Screening in the Workplace

Genetic testing of workers is a particularly thorny issue. It has become even more controversial with scientific advances that have allowed more precise testing (e.g., genome analysis vs. morphologic chromosomal aberrations) and identification of genetic markers of disease susceptibility.

Controversy has been primarily about privacy issues, consequences of disclosure, and the potential for "genetic discrimination" within and outside of the workplace. The Supreme Court's opinion of sex-based exclusion in *Johnson Controls*[34] suggests, by analogy, that selecting or reassigning workers on the basis of genetic susceptibility to specific exposure would probably be looked on with disfavor. Similarly, the U.S. Equal Employment Opportunity Commission (EEOC) has identified such actions as discriminatory under the "regarded as" definition of disability under the ADA. President Clinton issued an Executive Order prohibiting federal departments and agencies from basing employment decisions on genetic information.[35]

Proper application of the burgeoning developments in genomic science is still being debated. This is likely to be an active area of scientific and legal ferment in the future.

ADA-Related Issues

In 1999, the Court simultaneously reviewed three cases that considered the definition of disability under the ADA.[36] The Court held that the question of whether a person was a qualified individual with a disability had to be analyzed in light of any treatments, medications, aids, or prostheses that corrected or mitigated the impact of the underlying medical or psychological condition. The Court stated, for example, that severely myopic individuals were not disabled if their myopia could be corrected with glasses or contact lenses. Similarly, individuals with hypertension were not disabled if their condition could be controlled with medication. The Court also reaffirmed that disability had to be considered from a range of jobs that the individual was qualified for, not a specific job, and that other federal standards (e.g., FAA or DOT medical standards) were not preempted by the ADA.

Another area that is likely to garner Supreme Court review is the issue of when an applicant or employee is not qualified because he or she constitutes a "direct threat" to health or safety in the workplace. The ADA specifies that the direct threat analysis could be extended only to the threat of serious harm or injury to coworkers or the public. The EEOC, however, in promulgating its interpretive rules, adopted the general understanding and practice that direct threat would also include a significant risk to the disabled employee. Recently, the Ninth Circuit Court of Appeals ruled that the statute was plain on its face and that considerations of harm to self were improper.[37]

The ADA continues to generate substantial litigation in the federal courts. Issues regarding the coverage of the ADA, what constitutes a disability, and the relation of the ADA to collective bargaining agreements have been or will be reviewed by the U.S. Supreme Court.

PRACTICE CONSIDERATIONS

Worker Protection

Despite significant improvements in worker safety and health during the past 30 years, OSHA has many critics. Industry has characterized OSHA regulation as petty, burdensome, and unnecessary. Unions and worker advocacy groups believe that OSHA has not gone far enough to protect workers and the environment. In contrast to the central authority and large appropriations of the EPA, responsibility for worker health and safety is fragmented and lacks the same public and political support that protecting the environment enjoys.

Rule-making efforts are almost universally challenged by industry as excessive and by unions as insufficient. These legal challenges have prevented or delayed standard development so that, after 30 years, fewer that 40 substance-specific standards have been promulgated.

Significant reform is unlikely, however. Several attempts at OSHA reform were introduced in previous Congressional sessions by conservative politicians but focused largely on decreasing OSHA jurisdiction and authority. Attempts at reform were unsuccessful, and the OSHAct remains largely unchanged from its original form.

Accessing and Developing Surveillance Data Useful for Targeting Interventions

OSHA logs may provide valuable information to epidemiologists conducting research or investigating outbreaks of disease, but data may be limited, incomplete, or unavailable. The time delay in submitting data and the limited sampling of some occupations gives these data limited utility as a surveillance tool.

Other sources of surveillance data may include mandatory laboratory or physician reporting of specific occupational diseases or injuries; analysis of workers' compensation, group health, disability, or other insurance claim data; sentinel health providers; or surveys of worker populations. Unions or community-based organizations also may be important sources of epidemiologic data. Accessing data sources may require cooperative agreements with other government entities, confidentiality agreements, or other privacy safeguards such as encryption or stripping data of personal identifiers.

Courts have upheld government access or collection of data where a legitimate interest has been demonstrated, the public interest outweighs any potential risk to individuals, and adequate privacy safeguards have been implemented. Access by private or nongovernment organizations is more limited, and informed consent is probably necessary when personally identifiable data are used.[38]

Seeking Technical Assistance

Federal and state OSHA agencies provide free consultation services to employers. This consultation service is provided confidentially and distinct from the enforcement activities of the agency. Employers can request consultation without fear of fine or citation, as long as they agree to remedy any serious hazards identified during the consultation period. OSHA consultants are obligated to refer serious hazards to the enforcement division if the employer does not abate the hazard in a reasonable time.

NIOSH provides extensive consultation and training opportunities for employers. NIOSH investigates hazards associated with specific substances, processes, or industries and offers suggestions to reduce or eliminate those hazards. NIOSH performs research on exposure-control methods and equipment, safety, and health training and prevention methods and recommends new or revised standards to OSHA. NIOSH also provides many of the training opportunities for occupational safety and health professionals directly or through grant programs.

One of the most powerful tools to obtain technical assistance with an occupational health issue is to request a NIOSH Health Hazard Evaluation (HHE). An HHE is a structured investigation of a workplace to identify and characterize potential health hazards. Health Hazard Evaluations can be requested by employees, labor unions, or employers. An individual employee can request an HHE if two other employees co-sign the request. Labor unions can initiate the request for their members.

Health Hazard Evaluations are designed to investigate new or incompletely understood occupational hazards or exposures. Examples include unusual illness clusters, concerns about disease excess among worker populations, new or infrequently encountered substances or exposures, or combinations of exposures. The evaluations are not intended to provide routine assistance where the hazards have been clearly recognized and effective control measures are available. In this situation, referral to OSHA is more appropriate. More information regarding the NIOSH HHE program is available at the NIOSH website, http://www.cdc.gov/niosh/hhepage.html.

EMERGING ISSUES

Genetic Screening

Few employers have instituted genetic testing programs because of the legal and ethical controversies regarding their use among working populations. Burlington Northern Santa Fe Railroad (BNSF) began using a genetic screening test on its employees who had filed workers' compensation claims for carpal tunnel syndrome (CTS). The test was designed to identify a genetic marker for CTS susceptibility and thereby establish that the condition was not work related.

The EEOC viewed this as a discriminatory work practice and filed a suit under the ADA asking for a preliminary injunction in February 2001. The EEOC alleged "genetic bias," noting that testing was performed without worker consent or knowledge and that at least one worker was threatened with dismissal for failing to provide a blood sample. In April 2001, the suit was settled with an Agreed Order that prohibited BNSF from continuing its genetic testing program. The EEOC stated that it would "respond aggressively" to allegations of discrimination based on genetic tests.[39]

The EEOC does not appear to have addressed the issue of BNSF's activity within the context of workers' compensation law, in which evidentiary standards have traditionally allowed employers to collect or discover information that reasonably relates to their defense of the claim. Workers' compensation claimants are sometimes compelled to participate in medical examinations and undergo tests by medical experts selected by the insurer or employer. Similarly, workers may sometimes be placed under "hidden camera" surveillance when fraud or malingering is suspected. How and why these other investigative techniques differ from genetic testing with the workers' compensation arena have yet to be articulated.

Disability Discrimination and Employments Benefit Law

The complex interactions of the ADA, the FMLA, and similar state laws regarding disability discrimination, family leave, and workers' compensation create a confusing legal environment for employers and employees. Unfortunately, the goals and provisions of these laws, administered by different departments and agencies, sometimes conflict, and resolution of the conflicts continues to generate litigation. Several important ADA-related cases regarding reasonable accommodation, seniority and collective bargaining agreements, public accommodation, and remedies will undergo Supreme Court review in the near future, and plaintiffs, employers, governments, and employment lawyers will follow these developments closely.

Confidentiality

The Health Insurance Portability and Accountability Act (HIPAA; i.e., the Kennedy-Kasselbaum Act) was passed in 1999. It sought to address issues regarding the coverage and transferability of employer-sponsored health insurance. The Act also contained provisions to facilitate the use of electronic data transfer for claims processing while improving the protection of confidential medical information. This section of the Act, termed "Administrative Simplification" called on the U.S. Congress to pass a comprehensive medical record privacy law by August 1, 2000. If Congress failed to pass this legislation, then the Act authorized the Secretary of the DHHS to promulgate rules to this effect. Congress missed the deadline, and the DHHS rules[40] were formally adopted on April 14, 2001, after a brief delay following the inauguration of President George W. Bush.

The DHHS Privacy Rule promulgated under HIPAA establishes parameters for electronic data transfer and places restrictions on the collection and use of medical records by covered entities. The Rule permits disclosure of personal health information if required by law, and therefore public health reporting statutes or rules are not preempted. Public health authorities can continue to receive and collect data on injuries, illnesses, births, and deaths and investigate health risks and outcomes. The use of personally identifiable data for research is also regulated by the Rule and requires patient consent except in limited circumstances.[41]

The full impact of HIPAA on the American health-care system is not yet clear, but many health-care and insurance organizations anticipate high costs for compliance and have opposed its implementation.

ACKNOWLEDGMENTS

The author gratefully acknowledges the assistance of Greg Wagner, M.D., M.P.H. (National Institute for Occupational Safety and Health, CDC, Morgantown, West Virginia), and Mark Rothstein, J.D. (University of Louisville, Louisville, Kentucky), who reviewed and offered comments on a draft of the manuscript.

References

1. Page RM, Cole GE, Timmreck TC. *Basic Epidemiological Methods and Biostatistics.* Boston: Jones and Bartlett, 1995: pp. 3–4.
2. Carter T. Diseases of occupations—a short history of their recognition and prevention. In: Baxter PJ, Adams PH, Aw TC, Cockcroft A, Harrington JM, eds. *Hunter's Diseases of Occupations*, 9th ed. London: Arnold, 2000 p. 920.
3. Hamilton A. *Exploring the Dangerous Trades: The Autobiography of Alice Hamilton, M.D.* Boston: Little, Brown, 1943.
4. Ashford N, Caldart C. *Technology, Law and the Working Environment*, rev ed. Washington, DC: Island Press, 1996: pp. 3–9.
5. Rothstein M. *Occupational Safety and Health Law*, 4th ed. St. Paul, MN: West Group, 1998: pp. 1–10.
6. NIOSH. *Worker Health Chartbook, 2000.* DHHS (NIOSH) Publication No. 2000-127, 2000.
7. NIOSH. *Proposed National Strategies for the Prevention of Leading Work-Related Diseases.* DHHS (NIOSH) Publication Nos. 89-128, 89-129, 89-130, 89-131, 89-132, 89-133, 89-134, 89-135, 89-136, 89-137, 1989.
8. NIOSH. *National Occupational Research Agenda.* DHHS (NIOSH) Publication No. 96-115, 1996.
9. NIOSH. *Work Related Lung Disease Surveillance Report 1999.* DHHS (NIOSH) Publication No. 2000-105.
10. U.S. Department of Labor. Census of fatal occupational injuries. Bureau of Labor Statistics News. Available at http://www.bls.gov/news.release/cfoi.toc.htm. Accessed April 3, 2002.
11. United States Constitution, Article I, Section 8.
12. The Occupational Safety and Health Act. 29 U.S.C. § 651 *et seq.*
13. United States Constitution, Article VI.
14. 29 C.F.R. Part 1975.
15. 29 C.F.R. § 1910.20.
16. 29 C.F.R. § 1910.132; see also Parts 1910, 1915, 1917, 1918, 1926.

17. 29 C.F.R. § 1910.1200.
18. 29 C.F.R. § 1904.
19. Federal Mine Safety and Health Act of 1977, Pub. L. 91-173, as amended by Pub. L. 95-164.
20. The Toxic Substances Control Act, Pub. L. 94-469, 15 U.S.C. § 2601 *et seq.*
21. 42 U.S.C. § 9601, *et seq.*
22. 42 U.S.C. § 11001 *et seq.*
23. 7 U.S.C. § 136.
24. 40 C.F.R. § 170.
25. 42 U.S.C. § 2000.
26. 29 U.S.C. §§ 621–34.
27. 29 U.S.C. §§ 701–96.
28. 42 U.S.C. §§ 12101 *et seq.*
29. The Family and Medical Leave Act. 29 U.S.C.§§ 2601 *et seq.*
30. *National Labor Relations Board v. Gulf Power Company*, 384 F.2d 822 (5th Cir. 1967)
31. *People v. Chicago Wire Magnet Corp.*, 126 Ill. 2nd 356 (1989); *People v. Hegedus*, 432 Mich. 598 (1989).
32. Occupational Safety and Health Administration. Access to Medical and Exposure Records, 29 C.F.R. 1910.20.
33. *United Steelworkers v. Marshall*, 647 F.2d 1189 (D.C. Cir. 1980).
34. *Automobile Workers v. Johnson Controls*, 499 U.S. 187 (1991).
35. Executive Order 13145, February 8, 2000.
36. *Sutton v. United Airlines, Inc.*, 119 S.Ct. 2139 (1999); *Murphy v. United Parcel Service, Inc.*, 119 S.Ct. 2133 (1999); *Albertsons, Inc. v. Kirkingburg*, 119 S.Ct. 2162 (1999).
37. *Echazabal v. Chevron USA, Inc.*, 226 F.3d 1063 (9th Cir. 2000).
38. Rischitelli DG. The confidentiality of medical information in the workplace. *J Occup Environ Med* 1995;37:583–93.
39. Available at http://www.eeoc.gov/press/4-18-01.html. Accessed October 15, 2001.
40. Standards for the Privacy of Individually Identifiable Health Information. 65 *Federal Register* 82462 (December 28, 2000).
41. 45 C.F.R. §§ 164.501, 164.508(f), 164.512(i).

Index